Recent Advances in Gerontology

Recent Advances in Gerontology

Editor: Mason Button

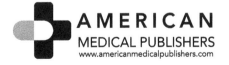

AMERICAN
MEDICAL PUBLISHERS
www.americanmedicalpublishers.com

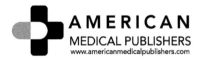
AMERICAN
MEDICAL PUBLISHERS
www.americanmedicalpublishers.com

Cataloging-in-Publication Data

Recent advances in gerontology / edited by Mason Button.
    p. cm.
Includes bibliographical references and index.
ISBN 978-1-63927-009-5
1. Older people--Health and hygiene. 2. Older people--Medical care.
3. Gerontology. 4. Aging--Physiological aspects. I. Button, Mason.
RA564.8 .R43 2022
362.198 97--dc23

American Medical Publishers,
41 Flatbush Avenue,
1st Floor, New York,
NY 11217, USA

ISBN 978-1-63927-009-5 (Hardback)

Contents

Preface

The purpose of the book is to provide a glimpse into the dynamics and to present opinions and studies of some of the scientists engaged in the development of new ideas in the field from very different standpoints. This book will prove useful to students and researchers owing to its high content quality.

The diverse aspects of aging, such as social, psychological, biological, cognitive and cultural aspects, are studied within the discipline of gerontology. It draws concepts and researches from a variety of fields like biology, medicine, nursing, political science, dentistry, physical and occupational therapy, psychiatry, psychology and sociology. Gerontology helps in government planning, evaluating the impact of the elderly people on the society and the operation of nursing homes. Some of the major sub-specialties within this field are biogerontology, environmental gerontology, social gerontology and jurisprudential gerontology. Biogerontology seeks to intervene in the aging process as well as prevent diseases which are related to aging. This book unfolds the innovative aspects of gerontology which will be crucial for the progress of this field in the future. From theories to research to practical applications, case studies related to all contemporary topics of relevance to this field have been included in it. This book will serve as a valuable source of reference for graduate and post graduate students.

At the end, I would like to appreciate all the efforts made by the authors in completing their chapters professionally. I express my deepest gratitude to all of them for contributing to this book by sharing their valuable works. A special thanks to my family and friends for their constant support in this journey.

Editor

Neurocognitive Implications of Tangential Speech in Patients with Focal Brain Damage

Nora Silvana Vigliecca

Abstract

There are no studies on the neurocognitive implications of tangential speech (TS). This research aims to take a step forward in the study of narrative processing, by evaluating TS in a sample that helps to detect this deficit when it is neurogenic and recently manifested. The relationship between TS, secondary to focal brain injury, and neuropsychological and neuroanatomical variables was explored. A comprehensive neuropsychological battery was administered to 175 volunteers: 95 alert inpatients, without aphasia, without psychiatric history and without TS history, and 80 healthy participants, without TS. Results: TS (prevalence 16%) was independent of type or site of injury. An adverse effect of TS on global neuropsychological performance was observed. This effect was significantly related to attentional errors along with prolonged processing times but not to correct responses. Reliability and validity indices for the present TS screening scale were provided. Conclusion: Present results support the hypothesis that this neurogenic inability to spontaneously find, organize and communicate verbal information, beyond single words, depends on extended brain networks involving processes such as sustained attention, complex-syntax comprehension, the (implicit) interpretation and spontaneous recall of a narrative, and emotional and behavioral alterations. Early TS detection is advisable for prevention and treatment at any age.

Keywords: communication disorders, language disorders, disconnected speech, focal cerebral lesions, goal-directed speech, mild cognitive impairment, narrative processing, sustained attention, time of day orientation

1. Introduction

The organization of spoken language involves the selection and maintenance of the topic of the conversation (with logical sense and pertinence) according to the context and the listener. Ferstl et al. [1] affirm that language processing in context requires more than merely comprehending words and sentences: important processes such as inferences for bridging successive utterances, the use of background knowledge, discourse context and pragmatic interpretations need to be considered. Besides, the study of language processing in context also requires the analysis of its behavioral or expressive mechanisms, in particular, the presence of failures in goal-directed speech. Considering the method of analysis on these mechanisms, it is probable that the presence of failures in the quality and consistency of the discourse can be screened with a single (but comprehensive) measure, thus avoiding fragmentation into multiple variables, as previously considered in the field of communication disorders (see, e.g., [2]).

Currently, there is growing interest in the neurobiology of language beyond single words or short phrases [3–5] and, consequently, beyond aphasia. Aside from those basic studies, and going to the clinical practice, health professionals are often faced with patients (without aphasia) who cannot adequately explain a certain topic, for example, the reason for consultation. This may be a non-trivial problem. The impossibility of finding or pondering the proper verbal information to narrate an event (even when the most basic linguistic elements to construct the narrative are preserved) may be related to illness. The identification and causes of such impossibility require suitable evaluations as well as better definitions.

Excessive speech and incoherent or disorganized speech involve two different systems of classification. However, they are commonly linked. The terms logorrhoea; verbosity; tachyphemia; pressured speech; cluttered speech; disorders of speech, fluency, communication or language in general; circumstantial speech; tangential speech (TS); disconnected speech; flight of ideas; formal thought disorder; 'word salad'; loss of goal; loss of topic; etc., are ambiguously defined in the literature. The definitions change notably throughout the different disciplines or authors involved. There are even some methodological problems to differentiate, for example, a lot of speech, which may be just a style of speech, from logorrhoea, which includes failures in the quality and consistency of speech; these problems may become evident when tests of fluency are used as indicators of logorrhoea [6].

In order to increase understanding on the matter, it is necessary to study each of those terms or constructs more systematically, from different perspectives. In particular, the use of comprehensive approaches in which pure language impairments are integrated with the rest of the cognitive functions is a necessary endeavor. Concurrently, and since the newest approaches in neuroimaging, for example, tend to study restricted language tasks and brain regions, the complement among different perspectives is for this reason doubly advisable.

There is a lack of study aimed at systematically analyzing TS in order to delimit and organize its conceptual and methodological basis. In this work, TS is attempted to be studied as pure language impairment because losing the focus or topic of the conversation has been found to be a common factor among several manifestations of irrelevant or incoherent speech. Besides, the concept of TS in itself links two attributes of the narrative: its content and quality (the 'what') with its organization and consistency (the 'how').

This study may represent the first attempt in the scope to generate hypotheses about a feature that usually has been explored as part of the larger attribute of pragmatics, with extremely variable conceptions and approaches.[1] Toward controlling this source of variability, and taking into account that discourse processing has been considered a typical skill associated with pragmatics, some of the measures which have been previously reported as valid indicators of discourse processing (see, e.g., [8–10]), were included in the present study approach.

The evaluation of spontaneous speech is a crucial step in any neuropsychological assessment to detect aphasia, but not to detect TS. Probably this is so because a simple easy-to-administer scale for measuring this comprehensive behavior has not been designed yet, particularly in clinical settings and for screening purposes. To design such a TS scale, the analysis (and eventual integration) of previous concepts on the matter is required.

Harvey and Bowie [11] described two types of disturbances in the production of goal-directed speech as common symptoms in schizophrenia: verbal underproductivity and disconnected speech. The first is characterized by a reduction in the amount of speech or in the breadth of information; the second, by illogical or tangential connections between words or sentences as a result of which the speaker often fails to return to the goal of the discourse.

In the field of brain injury, unlike the above described classification, disconnected or underproductive discourses could in principle suggest either delirium (involving disturbance/ clouding of consciousness) or aphasia (involving lack/impairment of fluency or naming). Discarding delirium and aphasia such types of verbal symptoms may mimic psychiatric ones which, incidentally, have been considered for some authors manifestations of right hemisphere communication dysfunctions ([12–16], also see below).

Some of the neuropsychiatric constructs that have been cited together with TS are quite similar in many respects to TS, in particular when the attributes of coherence, consistency, stability and/or relevance are involved.

Tanner [17] stated that logorrhea is a garrulous and incoherent talking; the speech is rambling and has no point or conclusion; words are not connected semantically. The author also states that TS lacks of continuity and consistency and the train of thought wanders. Tangentiality is defined by Andreasen [2] as replying in an irrelevant manner; it refers only to immediate replies to questions (stimulus-response mode) and not to transitions in spontaneous speech. Tangentiality is theoretically distinguished from several other disorders such as: derailment, in which the errors are similar to tangentiality but they occur in the spontaneous conversational mode; poverty of content of speech, where the speech is adequate in amount but conveys little information; distractible speech, where inappropriate changes of topic only occur in response to external environmental stimuli; circumstantial speech, where the speech is indirect or delayed in reaching the goal, but the goal is eventually reached, etc. [2].

---

[1]A similar methodological heterogeneity has been described for TS, within the perspective of discourse analysis [7].

In the present work, and trying to achieve a unified construct, previous studies on TS as well as on disconnected speech, logorrhoea, circumstantial speech and any other dysfunction which affect the quality and consistency of information in the topic of the discourse were reviewed.

Disconnected speech, logorrhoea and TS have been associated with psychiatric and/or cognitive disorders not neurologically lateralized [17–27], including schizophrenia,[2] dementia, mania, autism, semantic pragmatic disorder, attention-deficit hyperactivity disorder and traumatic brain injury.

Concerning the neuroanatomical bases of disconnected speech, logorrhoea and TS, ambiguous findings have been reported when using the lesion-based approach. As a rule, these reports do not clearly demonstrate the double dissociation between, for example, the left and the right hemispheres, and the frontal lobe and the rest of the lobes [12, 28–34]. Considering just TS, and excluding subcortical structures, Marini [33] supports the hypothesis that there is a major involvement of frontal right hemispheric areas to the process of organization of information in a narrative discourse: the individuals with right hemisphere damage produced descriptions with normal levels of microlinguistic processing but with more tangential errors and conceptually incongruent utterances, that is, with more impairments in macrolinguistic processing. Within this framework, the right hemisphere has been associated with the ability to correctly communicate prosodic, discourse and pragmatic aspects of language, including topic maintenance [29]. On the contrary, the involvement of the left hemisphere on TS has rarely been reported. Ferstl et al. [35] state that damage to frontal areas has been associated with nonaphasic language disturbances in which word and sentence level processes remain largely intact but text level processes are impaired. These authors studied several sites of lesions, including non-frontal ones, and analyzed text comprehension in nonaphasic patients. Ferstl et al. [35] observed that patients with left-frontal or bilateral frontal lesions cannot make use of instructions which require a change of perspective for recalling a story; besides, left-frontal damage leads to an impairment of goal-directed text-processing skills. Despite such specific finding, and under the lesion-based approach, the involvement of the left hemisphere and the non-frontal lobes on TS is scarce or unclear.

The dissociation between the left and the right hemisphere has been more frequently studied, and the results are contradictory, when the so-called pragmatic and/or emotional abilities of the right hemisphere (considered as a whole) were analyzed [10, 14, 36–39]. Taking into account these specific abilities of the right hemisphere, the quality and consistency of information in the topic of the discourse has always been an essential feature

---

[2]In the field of schizophrenia, Holshausen et al. [23] exclude the indicator of poverty of content [2] from the concept of disconnected speech. However, in the present study it is assumed that if a patient speaks fluently but he/she conveys little information, then such information is irrelevant; additionally, if the information conveyed is superficial or indirect, as in the case of circumstantial speech, such information is also irrelevant. Holshausen et al. [23] did include the indicator of circumstantial speech [2] within the concept of disconnected speech. However, the supposed property of circumstantial speech by which the goal of the conversation is 'eventually reached' [2] is not here assumed as a true event; instead, the degree by which that goal is actually reached is analyzed.

to be analyzed. However, the presence of failures in the processing of this feature, along with its neurological, cognitive and behavioral implications has not been elucidated yet. Neuropsychologically speaking, and as stated by Zanini et al. [39], the strong dichotomy of denotative versus connotative language, as processed by the left versus right hemispheres, respectively, has been recently challenged. Interestingly, some of the supposed abilities of the right hemisphere are nowadays separately analyzed in studies of social cognition, emotional connotation, valence, neuropragmatics, mentalizing, communication and narrative processing, among other processes [1, 3–5, 8, 40–48]. Such studies usually describe extended brain networks and bilateral involvement in their communication or language models.

The influence of the left hemisphere and the non-frontal lobes on TS might be indirectly inferred from those studies which, to date, have mainly involved healthy participants (HP) and language comprehension tasks. Nevertheless, when a language expression task (i.e., narrative production) was additionally evaluated in two neurofunctional studies with healthy participants [8, 40], Awad et al. [40] observed a common bilateral functional system, predominantly left lateralized, for both narrative comprehension and production. This functional system was most apparent in the left anterior temporal neocortex and the left temporal-occipital-parietal junction. As well, while the left and right hippocampus and adjacent inferior temporal cortex were active during speech comprehension, activity was reduced during speech production. AbdulSabur et al. [8] observed that the language system was integrated with regions that support other cognitive and sensorimotor domains, that is, they observed that, in addition to traditional language areas (e.g., left inferior frontal and posterior middle temporal gyri), both narrative production and comprehension engaged regions associated with mentalizing and situation model construction, as well as premotor areas. These authors reported strong associations between language areas and the superior and middle temporal gyri during both tasks. However, only during narrative production were the language-related regions connected to cortical and subcortical motor regions. AbdulSabur et al. [8] reported marked bilateral involvement for narrative comprehension alone (including right hemisphere homologs of perisylvian language areas), and predominantly left lateralized (and anterior) involvement for narrative production alone.

Complementary research exploring the relationship between patients with focal brain lesions and language expression tasks, excluding aphasia, is necessary. TS has been poorly studied in patients with focal brain lesions, especially in patients with left hemisphere damage and in patients differentiated by frontal and non-frontal lobe damage. A comprehensive neuropsychological study of goal-directed speech is necessary in the scope, not only to help elucidate the TS neuroanatomical correlates but also the TS cognitive and behavioral nature. This research aims to take a step forward in the study of narrative processing, by evaluating TS in a sample that helps detect this deficit when it is neurogenic and recently manifested. Due to the lack of clear antecedents on the matter, the main objective for the present study was to explore the relationship between TS, secondary to focal brain injury, and neuropsychological and neuroanatomical variables.

The present study is part of a bigger research project which aims at developing efficient tests, that is, brief and/or easy to apply neuropsychological techniques without neglecting the goals of accuracy and validity (see, e.g., [49–51]). Since theory and validity are interlaced, it is expected that the present data are not only useful to hypothesize about the bases of TS, but also to explore the viability, validity and reliability of the present scale to assess TS in a natural situation, by the bedside of the patient.

In summary, the present study aimed to explore, in patients with focal brain injuries, if TS is associated with cognitive, emotional or behavioral impairments and with specific sites of brain injury. Complementarily, the present study aimed to explore if a hypothetical pattern of neuropsychological and/or neuroanatomical impairments can be identified for TS as well as if reliability and validity indices can be obtained for the present TS screening scale.

In view of the reviewed, and in an attempt to delimit the conceptual definition of TS, only communication dysfunctions which affect the quality and consistency of information in the topic of the discourse, without affecting the most basic resources to carry out such discourse, were considered. More specifically, when: (a) the deficit was secondary to brain injury, (b) the patient was alert, without aphasia, without psychiatric history and without TS history and (c) according to the conditions which were expressed in the first paragraph of this work, the topic of the conversation was missing (i.e., the topic was irrelevant to the interview situation, or it was not well preserved or focused during the interaction) the resulting speech was defined as tangential.

In view of the exploratory nature of the study, a comprehensive neuropsychological battery was administered because all the battery tests and subtests were in principle considered potential factors for explaining TS. However, and bearing in mind that the tasks of narrative comprehension, memory and production have been previously recognized as valid measures of discourse processing (DP) [8–10], they were specially evaluated. Considering that tests of fluency have been used as indicators of logorrhoea [6], and that logorrhoea includes failures in the quality and consistency of speech, the performance in tasks of spoken and written verbal fluency were also evaluated.

2. Material and methods

2.1. Material

The battery of Neuropsychological Tests Abbreviated and Adapted for Spanish Speakers, a valid and reliable instrument developed to detect dementia, aging and cognitive impairment, including the probable site of brain impairment, was administered [52–55]. Sixty-seven indicators of 25 basic subtests were analyzed. The present battery assessed the task completion time [i.e., the processing time (T)] in several subtests as well as: (1) spontaneous speech (in its aphasic manifestations); (2) personal orientation; (3) time and place orientation, and errors (E) in time orientation; (4) phonemic discrimination (letter 'A') by auditory cancelation (verbal auditory selective and sustained attention: omission and commission E); (5) figure discrimination (triangle) by visual cancelation [nonverbal visual selective and sustained attention: correct responses (CR) as well as errors and time (E&T)]; (6) direct and reverse serial order (months forward and backwards: E&T); (7) spatial memory (five hidden objects: accuracy (remembered objects and places) as well as four different types of E); (8) copy of alternating or repetitive graph series; (9) copy and naming (written response) of simple figures; (10) constructional praxia (cube and clock drawing in response to commands: CR and T); (11) syntax-complex verbal comprehension; (12) verbal auditory attention span (digits: forward and backwards); (13) writing abilities such as writing one verbal automatism (the name), writing by copying and by dictation and writing-legibility; (14) written verbal fluency [quantity: number of words, quality: syntactic complexity, legibility: overall score and legibility regardless of quantity (average score per word)]; (15) written arithmetic operations; (16) mental calculations (subtracting serial sevens: CR and T); (17) oral verbal fluency (number of words beginning with 'F'); (18) reading (a story): oral expression and abstraction/comprehension; (19) visual memory: face recognition; (20) visual memory: retrieval of a complex figure; (21) graphesthesia; (22) finger recognition; (23) a delayed story recall (spontaneous and cued, using two indicators: the interviewer's global impression during administration, and a standardized and detailed scoring of 25 passages after administration); (24) the paired-associate word learning, which included three trials and a delayed recall of easy and hard pairs and (25) semantic verbal memory/naming by picture confrontation. [Note: In general, accuracy (CR) was assessed unless otherwise indicated by E, T, and/or E&T.] The tasks of the battery related with DP were complex verbal comprehension (i.e., syntax-complex verbal comprehension and story comprehension) in addition to storytelling [i.e., a delayed story recall (spontaneous and cued)]. The tasks of the battery related with fluency were written verbal fluency (quantity: number of words) and oral verbal fluency (number of words beginning with 'F'). Details of test administration and scores are explained elsewhere [49–56].

The emergence of the following disorders as a consequence of brain injury as reported by the caregiver during the initial interview were also registered (scale range: 0–3): sensory deficits; motor deficits; perceptual-cognitive disorders (i.e., difficulty in recognizing known persons, places, moments or objects, independently of sensory acuity); sleeping disorders (i.e., insomnia, somnolence during the day, etc.); language disorders (i.e., paraphasias, anomies, echolalia, intrusions, reduced verbal comprehension or fluency, dysarthria, etc.); behavioral disorders (i.e., abnormal responses, anxiety, irritability, depression, lack of sphincter control, difficulty in organizing action, changes of personality, etc.); and thought disturbances (i.e., hallucinations, delusions, loss of sense of reality, dissociative symptoms, etc.). The presence of seizures was also registered.

Some complementary behavioral observations, which are usually evaluated during the administration of the comprehensive battery were also analyzed: the behavioral observations computed in this study were: degree of cooperation (0–3, i.e., absent: 0, very poor: 1, poor: 2, good: 3); emotional state (−1 to 1, i.e., inhibited: −1, normal: 0, excited: 1); disability awareness (0–3, i.e., null: 0, bad: 1, regular: 2, good: 3); language speed (−1 to 1, i.e., slow: −1, normal: 0, rapid: +1); voice volume (0–4, i.e., whispered: 0, hypophonic: 1, low: 2, normal: 3, hyperphonic: 4) and prosody (0–3, i.e., total or severe dysprosody: 0, moderate prosody: 1, slight prosody: 2, normal expression or prosody: 3). The presence of emotional lability, aggression, hallucinations, delusions and verbal perseverations (including words and/or thoughts) was also registered.

2.2. Subjects and procedures

Data were obtained from a sample of 175 Argentine Spanish-speaking right-handed volunteers. Clinical data were obtained from a sample of 95 patients who were consecutively recruited from the Neurological and Neurosurgery Service of the Cordoba Hospital, a public hospital for adults. Demographically matched healthy participants (HP) were recruited from cultural, recreational and retirement centers in the province of Cordoba. HP were included if they were independent and adapted to daily life demands, without any known neurological or psychiatric disease. HP were excluded if they had: (i) TS or any type of language impairment, (ii) symptoms of neurological or psychiatric disorders, (iii) risk of neurological damage by disease or accident, (iv) any kind of medical condition which could affect neuropsychological performance or (v) sensorial or motor difficulties which could prevent them from carrying out the tests fluently. The recruitment method is better described elsewhere [49–51, 54, 57]. Patients were included if they had focal brain lesions confirmed by MRI and complementary diagnostic studies, and if they were preoperative inpatients. Patients were excluded if they: (i) had multiple or diffuse brain damage, (ii) had any other (previous or simultaneous) associated neurological disease, (iii) had history of psychiatric disorders, (iv) had history of TS, (v) were treated with psychotropic medication, (vi) had aphasia, hemianopia, hemineglect, hemihypesthesia or minimum signs of clouding of consciousness, according to the coincident report among the physician (before administering the battery), the caregiver (during the initial interview), as well as the neuropsychologist (during the administration of the battery). The data collected during the initial interview with the caregivers was taken as evidence of the premorbid condition. The comprehensive neuropsychological battery was administered and scored blindly to neuroanatomical data and the TS scale, which was applied by other member of the research team.

Patients grouped by TS were compared on their demographic variables as well as on type and site/side of lesion, disease duration (reported in months), risk factors (malnutrition, frequent contact with toxic agents, hypertension, heart disease, obesity, diabetes, genetic component of the illness, alcohol or drug consumption, etc.), and the presence of brachial and crural hemiparesis. Regarding the sites of lesion, they were divided into anterior hemisphere (frontal) lesions (A) versus posterior hemisphere (temporal, parietal or occipital) lesions (P). Lesions located in inferior structures (such as thalamus, basal ganglia, internal capsule, etc.) were classified as subcortical (SC) lesions; and lesions located in the frontal lobe and any of the posterior lobes, or in regions located between the frontal lobe and the posterior lobes, were classified as antero-posterior (AP) ones. As well, lesions were divided into left (L), right (R) and bilateral (B), according the injured hemisphere.

The emergence of TS was registered as a feature of spontaneous speech, different from the aphasia symptoms usually assessed by this item. In the item of spontaneous speech, the patients' ability to describe their own disease is explored. The interviewer's question in the TS item was: *'Tell me what happened to you and why you are here. (When did the problem start? How was it...?).'*

If the topic of the conversation was missing at any moment of the interaction, and digressive responses were maintained irreversibly, without spontaneous recovering, throughout the three successive statements, the resulting speech was empirically defined as tangential. TS was coded as present. Subsequently, the interviewer gave a prompt. (In order to corroborate the interviewees' own ability to get back to the point, interviewers did not have to give indications or ask questions which facilitate the recall of the topic of the conversation.) If TS was repeated three times (maximum four prompts), the interview was finished.

The following scale was applied:

0 = Empty talk; pointless speech (the thread of the conversation is missing); inconsistency with the context and with a line of communication; disconnected from the listener; permanent irrelevant comments. The discourse is impaired. Topic recovering is 0%.

1 = Speech disconnected from the goal of the conversation, or difficult to insert into a coherent line of communication, most of the time or in most of the expressions; interviewee may or may not get back to the point by means of an interviewer's prompt such as 'and so?' The discourse is relatively or mostly impaired. Topic recovering is >0% and ≤50%.

2 = Speech that may drift into nonessential details without straying too far from the main topic of conversation. Although it has a fluctuating direction (sometimes it approaches the topic and sometimes it scatters for no apparent reason), the interviewee can usually get back to the point at the request of the interviewer. The discourse is rarely impaired. Topic recovering is >50%.

3 = Correct or normal speech in its logical sense and adequacy to the context. If at times it deviates a bit from the topic, involving marginal comments, the main idea or gestalt returns spontaneously. The discourse is not impaired.

The interviewee's verbatim response was recorded (hand-written format) and the interviewer's prompts or questions were registered with a vertical line. Transcripts were reanalyzed by a second rater to assess inter-rater reliability. In order to carry out this study, transcripts were rated blindly by two trained neuropsychologists, members of the research team. [Note: As the prompts for TS cannot be changed, each TS prompt was binary-coded as 0 (disagreement) or 1 (agreement). The reason for that was to avoid magnifying the correlation by reevaluating only those patients within the range of TS. If all the indications were reassessed with a value of 0 (100% disagreement), the patient's score (initially <3) was increased by one point. If no prompt was provided in the first instance, and in the second evaluation, it was thought that the interviewee should have received at least one prompt, the patient's score (initially = 3) was decreased in one point].

2.3. Ethical statements

This study was performed pursuant to the ethical standards established in the 1964 Declaration of Helsinki. The participants or the patient's caregivers gave their written informed consent and the approval of the Research and Ethics Committee of the Cordoba Hospital was obtained. The neuropsychological evaluation did not pose any risk to the participants who, in all cases, were alert, and willing to perform the complete battery of tests, independently of their relative capacity or willingness to perform some of the subtests in particular. Participants did not receive any payment for their contribution.

2.4. Statistical analysis

Demographic data were analyzed by ANOVA for Age (TS as grouping variable) or by Chi square (χ^2) for education (three levels: 1st level: primary school, 2nd level: high-school and 3rd level: college or superior) and gender (two levels: men and women).

If the obtained number of TS cases was so small that the presence of empty cells and/or lack of variance could be observed, the original scale of TS was planned to be recoded. Under this condition, and unless otherwise indicated, the groups representing TS were patients without TS (non-TSP), patients with TS (TSP), as well as HP.

The effect of TS on neuropsychological performance was analyzed. With this purpose, a representative measure of the performance in the comprehensive battery was searched by multiplying the errors and times by (−1), and by studying the internal consistency of all the individual indicators through the Cronbach alpha coefficient. If the Cronbach alpha coefficient was satisfactory (0.70 or greater), the individual indicators were added thus obtaining a representative measure of the general neuropsychological performance (GNP). This variable was analyzed by ANOVA with TS as grouping variable and the Bonferroni post-hoc test for pairwise comparisons.[3] The possibility of selecting representative measures of both CR and E&T was also analyzed. If that possibility was viable, a bivariate MANOVA with TS as grouping variable and CR and E&T as univariate dependent variables was carried out, using the Bonferroni post-hoc test for pairwise comparisons. The possibility of selecting a representative measure of DP was also analyzed. If that possibility was viable, the individual indicators of the tasks of the battery related with DP were added, and this variable was analyzed by ANOVA with TS as grouping variable and the Bonferroni post-hoc test for pairwise comparisons. If the ANOVA indicates both a significant main effect of TS, and significant pairwise comparisons among the three groups, the association between TS and DP was also analyzed as a way to contribute to the study of the validity of the TS scale (see below). With this purpose, the association by cross tabulation was studied and the percentile partition with the highest χ^2 was reported.

---

[3]ANOVA is a statistical dependency test. Each significant difference implicates a significant correlation between the independent and dependent variables. In this work no causal relationship between TS and the neuropsychological performance was assumed. The relationship between both variables was studied by ANOVA and, whenever a significant effect was reported, a double implication between the two variables was implicit. Such relationship was always emphasized in the text.

The indicators of number of words in the tasks of either spoken or written verbal fluency were analyzed by ANOVA, using the Bonferroni post-hoc test for pairwise comparisons.

The relationship between TS and the report of the caregiver during the initial interview, on the one hand, and the complementary behavioral observations during the administration of the battery, on the other hand, were studied through the Spearman's rank-order coefficient (r) for ordinal scales or by χ^2 for dichotomous ones.

2.4.1. Complementary statistical information

Additional data were searched with the purpose of discovering the nature of the cognitive impairments associated with TS. Explicitly, if TSP impairment was verified for GNP in general, and for CR or E&T in particular, further analyses on the individual indicators of the GNP component that produced a significant difference between TSP and both non-TSP and HP were performed, thus trying to see the qualitative pattern of TS impairments. MANOVA with TS as grouping variable and the individual indicators of the pertinent GNP components as dependent variables was performed, using Bonferroni post-hoc test for pairwise comparisons. Similarly, if the representative measure of DP produced a significant difference between TSP and both non-TSP and HP, further analyses on its individual indicators were also performed with the same purpose. MANOVA with TS as grouping variable and the individual indicators of DP as dependent variables was performed, using Bonferroni post-hoc test for pairwise comparisons.

In order to outline a hypothetical pattern of cognitive impairments associated with TS all the statistical analyses, including the complementary ones, were taken into account. If some of those cognitive impairments were coincident with measures which have been previously reported as valid indicators of DP, that coincidence was taken as evidence of the validity of the present TS scale. Additionally, inter-rater reliability was analyzed by the intra-class correlation coefficient (ICC). The difference between both evaluations was analyzed by the Wilcoxon paired-sample test.

3. Results

3.1. Main outcomes

A total of 15 cases with a value different from 3 in the TS scale were observed. Only one case was observed with a score of 0 and four cases with a score of 2. Due to such small number of cases, and in order to get better inferences, TS was recoded using 0 when the symptom was absent (non-TSP) and 1 (TSP) when the symptom was present (prevalence 16%).

Table 1 shows that TSP, non-TSP and HP did not differ in their demographic data.

Table 2 shows that there were no significant differences on type of lesion between non-TSP and TSP. Malignant tumors represented the most frequent type of lesion. By grouping the cells with fewer cases (i.e., the cells with the rest of the lesions), a non-significant difference

Group	Age (mean ± SD)	Education (three-level frequency)	Gender (men frequency)	N
non-TSP	41.90 ± 14.50	42 32 6	49	80
TSP	42.26 ± 14.23	6 8 1	8	15
HP	44.40 ± 16.85	34 40 6	40	80
Total	43.07 ± 15.56	82 80 13	97	175
	$F(2, 172) = 0.53$	$\chi^2 = 2.11$; df: 4	$\chi^2 = 2.08$; df: 2	
	$p = 0.57$	$p = 0.71$	$p = 0.35$	

Table 1. Demographic data.

between non-TSP and TSP was also observed when malignant tumors were compared with the rest of the lesions ($\chi^2 = 0.02$; df: 1; $p = 0.87$).

Non-significant differences were observed between non-TSP and TSP when A versus P lesions, excluding other lesions, were compared [non-TSP: A = 53% (A lesions/A + P lesions): (31/59), P = 47% (P lesions/A + P lesions): (28/59); TSP: A = 45% (5/11), P = 55% (6/11) ($\chi^2 = 0.19$; df: 1; $p = 0.67$)], or when R versus L lesions, excluding other lesions, were compared [non-TSP: R = 59% (R lesions/R + L lesions): (34/58), L = 41% (L lesions/R + L lesions): (24/58); TSP: R = 56% (5/9), L = 44% (4/9) ($\chi^2 = 0.03$; df: 1; $p = 0.86$)]. Non-significant differences were observed between non-TSP and TSP when specific site lesions [i.e., A, P, AP, SC ($\chi^2 = 2.89$; df: 3; $p = 0.41$); L, R, B ($\chi^2 = 0.97$; df: 2; $p = 0.61$)] were compared, or even when specific lobe lesions were compared ($\chi^2 = 8.48$; df: 9; $p = 0.49$) (percentages not shown, but available upon request).

Lesion	Group	
Type	Non-TSP	TSP
AVM	8	2
BEN TU	18	4
MAL TU	25	5
ISQ STR	6	1
HEM STR	4	1
TBI	6	2
OTHER	13	0
Total	80	15
$\chi^2 = 3.27$; df: 6; $p = 0.77$		

AVM: arteriovenous malformation, BEN TU: benign tumor, MAL TU: malignant tumor, ISQ STR: ischemic stroke, HEM STR: hemorrhagic stroke, TBI: traumatic brain injury, OTHER [name (N)]: subdural hematoma (1), aneurysm (2), mesial temporal sclerosis (4), abscess (2) and cyst (4).

Table 2. Classification of the focal cerebral lesions based on their type.

Both groups of patients did not differ on disease duration [(mean ± SD): non-TSP: 29.04 ± 65.25, TSP: 35.66 ± 79.31 [F (1, 93) = 0.12, p = 0.73], in the number of any additional risk for cognitive impairment [non-TSP: 1.15 ± 1.03, TSP: 1.4 ± 1.06 [F (1, 93) = 0.74, p = 0.39], or in the presence of hemiparesis [brachial: non-TSP: 31% (partial/total count) (25/80), TSP: 27% (4/15): ($\chi 2$ = 0.12, df = 1, p = 0.72); crural: non-TSP: 31% (25/80), TSP: 20% (3/15) ($\chi 2$ = 0.77; df = 1, p = 0.38)].

The Cronbach alpha coefficient for all the indicators of the comprehensive battery considered as a whole (representing GNP) was 0.94. The Cronbach alpha coefficients for CR and E&T were 0.92 and 0.77, respectively. Therefore, GNP, on the one hand, in addition to CR and E&T, on the other hand, were analyzed. The Cronbach alpha coefficient for all the indicators of DP was 0.70; therefore, a representative measure of DP was also analyzed. (Note: In all the significant differences reported from now on, TSP was always more impaired than non-TSP, and both groups of patients were more impaired than HP).

The ANOVA with TS as grouping variable and GNP as dependent variable (see **Figure 1**) indicated a main effect of TS (F (2, 172) = 25.55, p < 0.0001) with significant pairwise comparisons (Bonferroni post-hoc tests: non-TSP vs. TSP: p = 0.0017; HP vs. either non-TSP or TSP: p < 0.0001).

The bivariate MANOVA with TS as grouping variable and CR and E&T as univariate dependent variables (see **Figure 2**) indicated that CR and E&T produced significant effect on GNP (Wilks lambda = 0.73, F (4, 342) = 14.77, p < 0.0001) and that a main effect of TS was produced on the two components of performance (univariate effect of CR: F (2, 172) = 12.32, p < 0.0001, univariate effect of E&T: F (2, 172) = 28.35, p < 0.0001). However, non-TSP and TSP did not differ in CR but they did differ in E&T when pairwise comparisons were analyzed (Bonferroni post-hoc tests: non-TSP vs. TSP in CR: p = 0.2439, non-TSP vs. TSP in E&T: p < 0.0001; HP vs.

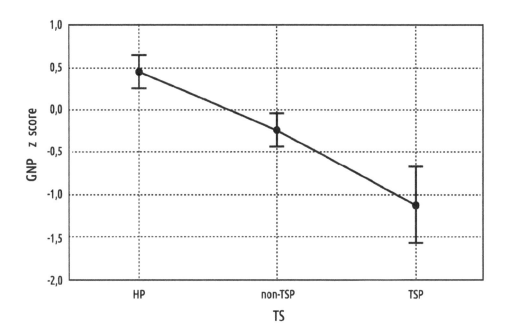

Figure 1. GNP (total score) as a function of TS (HP, non-TSP and TSP). LS means effective hypothesis decomposition. Vertical bars denote 0.95 confidence intervals.

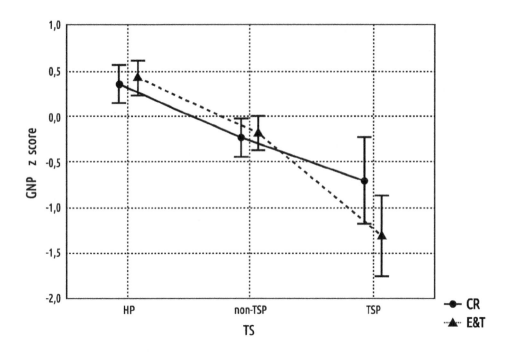

Figure 2. CR and E&T (total score) as a function of TS (HP, non-TSP and TSP). LS means effective hypothesis decomposition. Vertical bars denote 0.95 confidence intervals. E&T were multiplied by (−1).

either non-TSP or TSP: $p < 0.0003$ in any of the univariate measures). (Note: Since CR and E&T have different units of measurement, z-scores were used to show GNP results, which were identical to the results obtained with the raw scores).

The ANOVA with TS as grouping variable and the representative measure of DP as dependent variable indicated a main effect of TS ($F_{(2, 172)} = 34.61$, $p < 0.0001$), with significant pairwise comparisons among the three groups using Bonferroni post-hoc test: that is, difference between non-TSP and TSP: $p = 0.002$, difference between HP and either non-TSP or TSP: $p < 0.0001$. A significant association between TS and DP was demonstrated (see **Table 3**): By taking the 25th percentile (P25) of the whole sample as cutoff point, 95% of the HP and 63% of the non-TSP had a score greater than the P25, while 80% of the TSP had a score equal or less than the P25.

The ANOVA with TS as grouping variable and the number of words in written verbal fluency as dependent variable indicated a main effect of TS ($F_{(2, 172)} = 12.63$, $p < 0.0001$),

Group	≤ Percentile 25	> Percentile 25	Total
HP	4	76	80
Non-TSP	30	50	80
TSP	12	3	15
$\chi^2 = 46.24$; df: 2; $p < 0.0001$ (25th percentile = 36.00)			

Table 3. Distribution of frequencies according to 25th percentile on the representative measure of DP.

with non-significant pairwise comparisons between non-TSP and TSP (Bonferroni post-hoc test: p = 1); significant pairwise comparisons between HP and either non-TSP or TSP were observed (Bonferroni post-hoc tests: p < 0.003). The ANOVA with TS as grouping variable and the number of words in oral verbal fluency as dependent variable indicated a main effect of TS (F (2, 172) = 25.02, p < 0.0001), with non-significant pairwise comparisons between non-TSP and TSP (Bonferroni post-hoc test: p = 0.621); significant pairwise comparisons between HP and either non-TSP or TSP were observed (Bonferroni post-hoc tests: p < 0.0001).

Regarding the report of the caregiver during the initial interview, the r (rank-biserial) between TS and: (a) sensory deficits, (b) motor deficits, (c) sleeping disorders, (d) perceptual disorders, (e) language disorders, (f) behavioral disorders and (g) thought disturbances were: 0.06, −0.14, 0.07, 0.08, 0.00, 0.29 and 0.43, respectively, the last two coefficients being statistically significant. The association between TS and the presence of seizures was non-significant: non-TSP: 51% (41/80), TSP: 33% (5/15) (χ2 = 1.62, df = 1, p = 0.20).

Regarding the complementary behavioral observations registered during the administration of the neuropsychological battery, the r (rank-biserial) between TS and: (a) degree of cooperation, (b) emotional state, (c) language speed, (d) disability awareness, (e) voice volume and (f) prosody were: −0.36, 0.23, 0.32, −0.19, 0.14 and 0.08, respectively. Of these, the first three coefficients were statistically significant. A non-significant association with the presence of emotional lability was observed: non-TSP: 6% (5/80), TSP: 20% (3/15) (χ2 = 3.09, df = 1, p = 0.08). A non-significant association with the presence of verbal perseverations was also observed: non-TSP: 8% (6/80), TSP: 13% (2/15) (χ2 = 0.56, df = 1, p = 0.46). There were no patients who showed aggression, hallucinations or delusions, during the administration of the battery.

3.2. Complementary statistical information

Since the GNP component that produced a significant difference between TSP and both non-TSP and HP in pairwise comparisons was E&T, its individual indicators were analyzed. The MANOVA with TS as grouping variable and the E&T indicators as dependent variables indicated that all the dependent variables produced a significant effect on the multivariate measure of performance (Wilks lambda = 0.38, F (34, 312) = 5.75, p < 0.0001). A main effect of TS was observed in all the components of the model except for E in time orientation to year as well as two types of E in hidden objects (all significant univariate effects: F (2, 172) ≥ 3.11, p < 0.05; all non-significant univariate effects: F (2, 172) ≤ 1.41, p ≥ 0.2466). Significant differences between non-TSP and TSP according to Bonferroni post-hoc test involved E in verbal auditory sustained attention [omission E (p = 0.004) and commission E (p = 0.0002)], T in nonverbal visual sustained attention (p < 0.0001), as well as E in the time of day (p = 0.0003). The two groups of patients did not differ in the rest of the indicators (Bonferroni post-hoc tests: non-TSP vs. TSP all p ≥ 0.0627). [Note: Considering pairwise comparisons, when a significant difference between non-TSP and TSP was observed, a significant difference between TSP and HP was also observed with p < 0.0001; besides, by taking the P25 of the whole sample as cutoff point for these significant indicators, 93% of the HP (74/80) and 68% of the non-TSP (54/80) had a score greater than the P25, while 80% of the TSP (12/15) has a score equal or less than the P25 (results available upon request).] As shown, the presence of TS for the E&T indicators (individually considered) appeared as a rather nonspecific factor in terms of the stimuli involved, that is, TS was not related to a certain modality of cognitive impairment such as the verbal or the nonverbal one.

Additionally, and given that the representative measure of DP also produced a significant difference between TSP and both non-TSP and HP, its individual indicators were analyzed. The MANOVA with TS as grouping variable and the indicators of DP as dependent variables indicated that all the dependent variables produced a significant effect on the multivariate measure of performance (Wilks Lambda = 0.52, $F (12, 334) = 10.71$, $p < 0.0001$). A main effect of TS was produced on all the components of the model except for the interviewer's global impression during administration of the cued story recall (all significant univariate effects: $F (2, 172) \geq 8.78$, $p < 0.0002$; the non-significant univariate effect: $F (2, 172) = 1.48$, $p = 0.2305$). When pairwise comparisons were analyzed, non-TSP and TSP did not differ in the standardized and detailed scoring of the 25 passages after administration of the cued story recall (Bonferroni post-hoc test: $p = 0.3179$) but they did differ in the rest of the components (Bonferroni post-hoc tests: non-TSP vs. TSP all $p \leq 0.0220$). Considering HP, significant differences between HP and TSP were observed in any of the univariate measures, excluding cued recall (Bonferroni post-hoc tests: HP vs. TSP all $p < 0.0001$). Therefore, not all the indicators of DP, individually considered, produced significant differences between non-TSP and TSP as it can be inferred from the cued recall in its both indicators. [Note: all univariate results described in the present study were confirmed with nonparametric tests (results available upon request)].

Regarding inter-rater reliability, the ICC was 0.86 without difference between both raters according to the Wilcoxon paired-sample test ($z = 0.00$, $N = 95$, $p = 1$). [Note: the ICC for the dichotomized TS scale was 0.79 [Wilcoxon paired-sample test ($z = 0.40$, $N = 95$, $p = 0.685$)].

4. Conclusion

Present results support the hypothesis that the emergence of TS (with a prevalence of 16% in this sample) not only may be a consequence of focal brain lesions, of any type or site, but also is associated with cognitive impairment. TSP showed, as a whole, an impaired GNP relative to non-TSP and HP. The implication of TS on cognition was more related to E&T, rather than to CR, that is, although both CR and E&T contributed with the differences observed in GNP, when the two components of performance were differentiated, E&T were significantly associated with TS whereas CR were not. Alternatively, the tasks of the battery related with DP were significantly associated with TS whereas the tasks related with verbal fluency were not. More detailed analyses carried out to discover the cognitive nature of the TS correlates, indicated that the effect of TS on E&T involved tasks of different modality such as verbal and nonverbal sustained attention and attention (orientation) to the time of day. On the contrary, the effect of TS on the tasks related to DP involved, specifically, complex verbal comprehension and the spontaneous, implicit and delayed recall of a story, excluding cued recall. The association between TS and recognized measures of discourse processing (such as narrative comprehension, memory and production [8–10]) provided support for the viability and validity of the present screening scale to assess TS. A satisfactory inter-rater reliability for the TS scale was also observed. Additionally, TS was associated with emotional and behavioral alterations in the clinical sample: significant correlations were observed between TS and the emergence of behavioral and thought disturbances, as reported by the caregiver during the initial interview, as well as between TS and the complementary behavioral observations of emotional excitement, rapid speech and diminished cooperation, as reported by the neuropsychologist during the battery administration. Regarding intervening clinical variables, and aside from the type and site of injury (see above), TS was independent of demographic variables, presence of neurological risks and disease duration.

5. Discussion

In the most recent research on verbal communication, AbdulSabur et al. [8] and Awad et al. [40] analyzed the processes involved in sharing knowledge through narrative processing, and described extended brain networks and bilateral involvement in their neurofunctional studies with healthy participants. Consistent with this view, Jouen et al. [5] observed in a combined fMRI and DTI study with healthy participants that understanding sentences and pictures revealed bilateral involvement and a common fronto-temporo-parietal network for both modalities. This semantic network was not limited to sensorimotor systems but extended to the highest levels of cognition, including autobiographical memory, scene analysis, mental model formation, reasoning and theory of mind. Present results agree with those studies since no focal brain lesions were identified for TS. To be precise, present results agree with the hypothesis that this neurogenic inability to spontaneously find, organize and communicate verbal information for a specific topic, and beyond single words, may be caused by several sites of brain damage or, most probably, by aberrant interactions within extended brain networks.

In trying to understand how TS is integrated with the rest of the cognitive functions, present results indicated that TSP showed an overall impaired cognitive performance relative to non-TSP; however, the contribution of the GNP components of E&T and CR showed distinctive patterns: the relative weight of E&T was superior to that observed in CR, thus finally producing a significant effect only on E&T. More thorough analyses carried out to discover the nature of the cognitive impairments associated with TS provided illustrative results: by considering just those individual indicators of E&T related to sustained attention, which were significantly associated with TS, it can be noticed that one task involved verbal auditory stimuli and the other task involved nonverbal visual stimuli; besides, one task involved number of errors and the other task involved the time for solving the task. Therefore, neither the type of stimulus nor the type of failure seemed to be relevant to this finding. Additionally, and bearing in mind that tests of sustained attention are characterized by being monotonous and simple, some interviewees may be tempted to think that such type of tasks can be carried out with minimal effort, which may increase E&T. Nevertheless, such type of tasks only increased E&T in TSP regarding non-TSP. The errors in the time of day were also significantly associated with TS. Given that these errors not only involve other type of stimulus, but they also may be seen as a failure of sustained attention,[4] the nature of the significant TS impairments in E&T (and sustained attention) as a whole appeared to be independent of the type of the stimulus. In this context, it can be speculated that TS impairments in E&T may have insidiously influenced all type of tasks, although only some of those tasks showed significant impairments. (In passing, and methodologically speaking, present results highlight the need of assessing the presence and magnitude of the E&T; otherwise, valuable information can be lost. Likewise, an increased time to respond correctly, which may sometimes be a subtle difficulty (see, e.g., [58]) could represent relevant data to be assessed, as indicated by the results obtained in the E&T in general, and in the T of nonverbal sustained attention, in particular).

On the other hand, the individual indicators of DP that produced a significant difference between non-TSP and TSP were: (a) syntax-complex verbal comprehension; (b) reading a story: abstraction/comprehension and (c) a delayed (and spontaneous) story recall. So, it can be stated that TS was also associated with high-level and/or complex linguistic tasks involving processes such as verbal comprehension, attention and memory. Regarding this finding, it can be relatively understood that if patients have problems to narrate an event (e.g., the reason for consultation), they can also have problems to narrate other event (e.g., the story involved in DP). The nature of the cognitive demands involved in this particular task of story recall, however, provide additional information in relation to the factors which were combined with the narration itself: specifically, the items (b) and (c) involved implicit attention and memory, that is, those tasks were intentionally designed to be effortlessly or automatically carried out by leaving them unprompted. For example, the comprehension and recall of a story were both included as components to a series of reading tasks, in which the command was just 'read' (neither 'think about what you read' nor 'remember what you read'). Therefore the cognitive demands of interpreting and later recalling a story required that the information be spontaneously registered and organized by the interviewee. By integrating these findings with those described above concerning sustained attention, it can be observed that most of the individual tasks associated with TS required a high degree of spontaneous (unassisted/self-controlled) organization. If failures in cognitive engagement interfere with such organization, then the appearance of irrelevant commentaries or task-unrelated thoughts (mind-wandering) could be favored. In this way, it is probable that E&T increase and the final performance (GNP) decrease. In other words, the process that goes

---

[4]If the time of day is seen as the target stimulus, and the ability to maintain focused awareness on it during continuous period is seen as the attention task condition, then paying attention to the time of day is a form of sustained attention.

from 'knowing the correct response', as inferred from CR, to the final result can be delayed or obstructed with errors.

Franklin et al. [59] assessed lapses of attention (mind-wandering) with experience-sampling thought probes during a standard implicit learning, in a serial reaction time task. Their results revealed an adverse effect of mind-wandering on implicit learning. Such results would be in agreement with the present ones because TSP, who had lower scores on tasks of sustained attention, also showed an impaired implicit learning in story recall with regard to non-TSP.

It is currently accepted that when automatic tasks are carried out, other cognitive and emotional associations are more prone to be spontaneously processed in the form of, for example, mind-wandering (see [59–61]). Since in the present study, TS was associated with automatic and complex linguistic tasks, it can be hypothesized that TS is an exacerbated manifestation of mind-wandering linked to high-level and verbal cognitive impairment. As verbal language interacts with the rest of the cognitive and behavioral functions thus helping to voluntarily organize thoughts and actions of any kind, dysfunctions in this domain can seriously affect many other skills [62]. What is more, the left inferior frontal gyrus involved in inner speech [63], which is an essential part of the executive-control language network, has been related to the monitoring of self-generated thoughts and divergent thinking [60].

In addition, and considering just the two groups of patients, TS was associated with emotional and behavioral alterations. Although there were no patients who showed aggression, hallucinations or delusions during the administration of the battery, there was an association between TS and either the behavioral and thought disturbances as perceived by the caregiver[5] or the presence of diminished cooperation, emotional excitement and rapid speech as registered by the neuropsychologist.

Within this context, it is worth mentioning that, although language speed was found to be higher in TSP than in non-TSP, both groups of patients did not differ in spoken and written verbal fluency tests. This finding suggests that the clinical interpretation of rapid speech in TSP was probably produced by the presence of many irrelevant words during a certain period of observation. Furthermore, the interaction of TS with diminished cooperation, or emotional excitement, may have as well affected the outcome: the process of selecting (finding and pondering) the correct verbal information to be expressed, necessarily involves an inhibitory adjustment, as only some parts of the total thoughts linked to the target topic will be expressed. If the emotional balance between excitatory and inhibitory mechanisms is affected, the cognitive organization which goes from nonspecific/divergent utterances to specific/convergent ones may be obstructed. Alternatively, tests of fluency, unlike spontaneous speech, are required to follow certain constraints, which may have prevented TSP from communicating irrelevant information (compared with the relevant one) during such tasks. So, it seems

---

[5]When the semantics and syntax in a sentence do not represent a problem, as in the case of nonaphasic patients, that is, when the ability to use, understand or connect words is not impaired, then impairments in the semantics and (high-level) 'syntax' in a narrative, can be interpreted as a manifestation of thought (see, e.g., [17]).

that both the type of task constraints and the cognitive engagement to effectively prioritize between competing internal and external demands [64] were implicated in TS.

The interaction among emotional, behavioral and verbal language functions may have also influenced present anatomical results. The ability to deliberately stop intrusive thoughts and pay attention to the context, the relevant goal and the interviewer's signals (verbal and nonverbal) pertains to the more encompassing function of communication and social interaction. Kuhlen et al. [65] affirm that, for successful communication, conversational partners need to estimate each other's current knowledge state. These authors observed that nonverbal facial and bodily cues can reveal relevant information for such knowledge and also proposed that an integrative account of the mirroring and mentalizing networks can explain their results. Accordingly, Prochnow et al. [66] found that both supra- and subliminal emotional facial expressions shared a widespread network of brain areas, many of which have been implicated in empathy and social encounters. Since emotional and behavioral disturbances were observed in TSP, including nonverbal social processes, a disruption of distributed brain networks concerning such processes is conceivable for these patients.

The psychiatric and/or cognitive disorders that have been linked to TS also involve complex brain functions and networks. For example, and considering the implications for understanding the functional neuroanatomy of bipolar disorder, Satzer and Bond [67] observed in their review about mania and focal brain lesions that mania occurs most commonly with lesions affecting frontal, temporal and limbic-brain areas: bilateral prefrontal emotion-modulating regions and a probable imbalance between left-sided excitatory and right-sided limbic-brain inhibitory lesions have been proposed to understand the pathophysiology of mania. Considering the functional relationship between language and mood disorders, Cuesta and Peralta [68] observed that disorganization was the main language dimension accounting for the broader construct of formal thought disorder [2], which is usually studied in patients with psychiatric disorders.[6] Taken together, these studies underline a relationship among disorganization of language, emotional disturbances and a disruption of distributed brain networks, agreeing with the present anatomical results.

Another psychiatric disorder that has been linked to TS is schizophrenia. Under this background, and also related to the concepts of disorganization of language and formal thought disorder, Holshausen et al. [23] hypothesize that executive functioning may play a role in maintaining the topic of conversation, planning upcoming speech and inhibiting inappropriate or unrelated discourse. (The authors also suggest employing a neurocognitive battery to elucidate this question in further studies.) Given that, in the present study, TSP and non-TSP showed differences in global cognition, and that global cognition and executive functioning are closely related [49, 56], it cannot be discarded that TSP showed impairment

---

[6]A radical difference between the psychiatric approach and the present one is that the construct of formal thought disorder and, particularly, its subcomponent of disconnected or disorganized speech include incoherence below the level of the sentence. These two different levels of analysis may lead to discover different levels of linguistic impairment.

in executive function compared with non-TSP. In line with this notion, Barbey et al. [9] suggest that core elements of discourse processing emerge from a distributed network of brain regions that support specific competencies for executive, social and emotional processes (see also [69–73]).

On the other hand, sustained attention [69], discourse abilities [8] and internally oriented mental processes such as: autobiographical memory; theory of mind; self-referential processing; future thinking and scene construction [60, 74], that is, the retrieval and integration of elements of previous experiences into a coherent event [74], have been related to the default mode network. Since all these cognitive processes are comprised in the spontaneous (self-referential) speech by which patients describe their own disease, the link between TS and the default mode network cannot be discarded either.

In summary, this work highlights the importance of studying a single and comprehensive item, that is, spontaneous speech, thus emphasizing the registration of one of its pathological expressions. As demonstrated here, TS was related to illness, to a neurogenic cognitive and behavioral disorder which, apparently, comprised a distributed brain network. Understanding the psychobiological correlates of TS may result in better strategies for interpreting such a disorder, in particular, to avoid errors in clinical practice. Since TS may be a non-trivial feature, its early detection is advisable for prevention and treatment: in the same way as finding and organizing words are essential points to be analyzed in the aphasic component of spontaneous speech, finding and organizing topics are essential points to be analyzed in the discourse component of spontaneous speech. People who show the failures associated with TS, even if those failures are subtle or insidious (like an increase in the frequency of apparently harmless lapses, interruptions of sustained attention, increased time to respond correctly, difficulty understanding or expressing complex texts, inability to (implicitly) attend and recall recent conversations, along with emotional and behavioral changes), may be suffering of a neurogenic disorder, with implications in global cognition and high-level language processing. If those failures are not early detected and treated, they may evolve to a more serious condition.

The combination of failures in selective and sustained attention along with the special characteristics of the language impairments observed in this study, allowed to outline a hypothetical pattern of cognitive symptoms associated with TS to be verified in further research. The association between TS and recognized measures of discourse processing, namely, complex verbal comprehension and story recall/storytelling, provided support for the viability and validity of the present TS screening scale, which was also reliable between raters.

By using efficient scales, aphasia and TS could be simultaneously screened during the first step of the doctor-patient interview. In this work, one complex function was assessed with a simple but carefully designed scale, which facilitates both saving time and controlling intervening variables during the interview interaction. The property of saving time during neuropsychological language evaluations is valuable, particularly in public hospitals. Additionally, the structure of evaluation proposed here for TS might serve as a model to be totally or partially applied to other conversational items, or even to other scientific disciplines interested in discourse processing and cognition. Since aging is a factor associated with cognitive impairment and cognitive impairment is a factor associated with TS, the presence of TS in the elderly must not be ignored.

Acknowledgements

This study was supported by funds from the National Council of Scientific and Technological Research in Argentina (CONICET), from which Vigliecca is an employee. I am grateful to Silvia Molina and Marisa Peñalva for their participation in the study and to the doctors of the Neurosurgery Service of the Cordoba Hospital.

Conflict of interest

The author declares no conflicts of interest in this paper.

Author details

Nora Silvana Vigliecca

Address all correspondence to: nsvigliecca@gmail.com

National Scientific and Technical Research Council (CONICET), Institute of Humanities (IDH-CONICET), Service of Neurology and Neurosurgery of Cordoba Hospital, National University of Cordoba (UNC), Cordoba, Argentina

References

[1] Ferstl EC, Neumann J, Bogler C, et al. The extended language network: A meta-analysis of neuroimaging studies on text comprehension. Human Brain Mapping. 2008;**29**:581-593. DOI: 10.1002/hbm.20422

[2] Andreasen NC. Thought, language, and communication disorders. I. Clinical assessment, definition of terms, and evaluation of their reliability. Archives of General Psychiatry. 1979;**36**:1315-1321. http://www.ncbi.nlm.nih.gov/pubmed/496551

[3] Bašnáková J, Weber K, Petersson KM, et al. Beyond the language given: The neural correlates of inferring speaker meaning. Cerebral Cortex. 2014;**24**:2572-2578. DOI: 10.1093/cercor/bht112

[4]   Hagoort P, Indefrey P. The neurobiology of language beyond single words. Annual Review of Neuroscience. 2014;**37**:347-362. DOI: 10.1146/annurev-neuro-071013-013847

[5]   Jouen AL, Ellmore TM, Madden CJ, et al. Beyond the word and image: Characteristics of a common meaning system for language and vision revealed by functional and structural imaging. NeuroImage. 2015;**106**:72-85. DOI: 10.1016/j.neuroimage.2014.11.024

[6]   Robles-Bayón A, Santos-García D, Rodríguez-Osorio X, et al. A clinico-anatomical correlation study of logorrhoea. Revista de Neurologia. 2009;**49**:633-638. https://www.ncbi.nlm.nih.gov/pubmed/20013715

[7]   Ellis C, Henderson A, Wright HH, et al. Global coherence during discourse production in adults: A review of the literature. International Journal of Language & Communication Disorders. 2016;**51**:359-367. DOI: 10.1111/1460-6984.12213

[8]   AbdulSabur NY, Xu Y, Liu S, et al. Neural correlates and network connectivity underlying narrative production and comprehension: A combined fMRI and PET study. Cortex. 2014;**57**:107-127. DOI: 10.1016/j.cortex.2014.01.017

[9]   Barbey AK, Colom R, Grafman J. Neural mechanisms of discourse comprehension: A human lesion study. Brain. 2014;**137**(Pt 1):277-287. DOI: 10.1093/brain/awt312

[10] Zaidel E, Kasher A, Soroker N, et al. Effects of right and left hemisphere damage on performance of the "right hemisphere communication battery". Brain and Language. 2002;**80**:510-535. DOI: 10.1006/brln.2001.2612

[11] Harvey PD, Bowie CR. Schizophrenia spectrum conditions. In: Weiner IB, Stricker G, Widiger TA, editors. Handbook of Psychology: Clinical Psychology. Vol. 8, 2nd ed. Hoboken, NJ: John Wiley & Sons; 2013. pp. 240-261. Available from: https://leseprobe.buch.de/images-adb/da/cf/dacfa0c9-7354-40aa-bcc9-08ab2b87043a.pdf [Accessed: Nov 23, 2016]

[12] Brookshire RH. Introduction to Neurogenic Communication Disorders. 5th ed. St. Louis, MO: Mosby; 1997. Available from: http://www.alibris.com/search/books/isbn/9780815110149?qwork=3315678 [Accessed: Nov 23, 2016]

[13] Gardner H, Brownell H, Wapner W, et al. Missing the point: The role of the right hemisphere in the processing of complex linguistic materials. In: Perecman E, editor. Cognitive Processes in the Right Hemisphere. New York, NY: Academic Press; 1983. p. 169-191. Available from: https://scholar.google.com/scholar?hl=en&as_sdt=0,5&cluster=7916825634030584809 [Accessed: Nov 23, 2016]

[14] Mitchell RL, Crow TJ. Right hemisphere language functions and schizophrenia: The forgotten hemisphere? Brain. 2005;**128**(Pt 5):963-978. DOI: 10.1093/brain/awh466

[15] Searleman A. A review of right hemisphere linguistic capabilities. Psychological Bulletin 1977;**84**: 503-528. DOI: http://dx.doi.org/10.1037/0033-2909.84.3.503

[16] Weintraub S, Mesulam MM. Developmental learning disabilities of the right hemisphere. Emotional, interpersonal, and cognitive components. Archives of Neurology. 1983;**40**:463-468. DOI: 10.1001/archneur.1983.04210070003003

[17] Tanner DC. Communication and dementia. In Tanner DC, editor. Forensic Aspects of Communication Sciences and Disorders. Tucson, AZ: Lawyers & Judges Publishing Company; 2003. p. 275-308. Available from: https://books.google.com.ar/books?id=O7f1j-VPPce4C&dq [Accessed: Nov 23, 2016]

[18] Astell AJ, Harley TA. Accessing semantic knowledge in dementia: Evidence from a word definition task. Brain and Language. 2002;**82**:312-326. DOI: 10.1016/S0093-934X(02)00021-4

[19] Bowie CR, Gupta M, Holshausen K. Disconnected and underproductive speech in schizophrenia: Unique relationships across multiple indicators of social functioning. Schizophrenia Research. 2011;**13**:152-156. DOI: 10.1016/j.schres.2011.04.014

[20] Costello E, Blenner S, Augustyn M. "Different is nice, but it sure isn't easy": Differentiating the spectrum of autism from the spectrum of normalcy. Journal of Developmental and Behavioral Pediatrics. 2010;**31**:720-722. DOI: 10.1097/DBP.0b013e3181fa6b17

[21] Coulter L. Semantic pragmatic disorder with application of selected pragmatic concepts. International Journal of Language & Communication Disorders. 1998;**33**(Suppl.):434-438. DOI: 10.3109/13682829809179464

[22] Glosser G, Deser T. Patterns of discourse production among neurological patients with fluent language disorders. Brain and Language. 1991;**40**:67-88. Available from: http://www.ncbi.nlm.nih.gov/pubmed/2009448

[23] Holshausen K, Harvey PD, Elvevåg B, et al. Latent semantic variables are associated with formal thought disorder and adaptive behavior in older inpatients with schizophrenia. Cortex. 2014;**55**:88-96. DOI: 10.1016/j.cortex.2013.02.006

[24] Mota NB, Vasconcelos NA, Lemos N, et al. Speech graphs provide a quantitative measure of thought disorder in psychosis. PLoS One. 2012;**7**:e34928. DOI: 10.1371/journal.pone.0034928

[25] Robinson G, Ceslis A. An unusual presentation of probable dementia: Rhyming, associations, and verbal disinhibition. Journal of Neuropsychology. 2014;**8**:289-294. DOI: 10.1111/jnp.12041

[26] Ungvari GS, White E, Pang AH. Psychopathology of catatonic speech disorders and the dilemma of catatonia: A selective review. The Australian and New Zealand Journal of Psychiatry. 1995;**29**:653-660. DOI: 10.3109/00048679509064981

[27] Youse KM, Gathof M, Fields RD, et al. Conversational discourse analysis procedures: A comparison of two paradigms. Aphasiology. 2011;**25**:106-118. DOI: 10.1080/02687031003714467

[28] Arseni C, Dănăilă L. Logorrhea syndrome with hyperkinesia. European Neurology. 1977;**15**:183-187. DOI: 10.1159/000114831

[29] Blake ML. Perspectives on treatment for communication deficits associated with right hemisphere brain damage. American Journal of Speech-Language Pathology. 2007;**16**:331-342. DOI: 10.1044/1058-0360(2007/037)

[30] Bogousslavsky J, Ferrazzini M, Regli F, et al. Manic delirium and frontal-like syndrome with paramedian infarction of the right thalamus. Journal of Neurology, Neurosurgery, and Psychiatry. 1988;**51**:116-119. DOI: 10.1136/jnnp.51.1.116

[31] Chatterjee A, Yapundich R, Mennemeier M, et al. Thalamic thought disorder: On being "a bit addled". Cortex. 1997;**33**:419-440. DOI: 10.1016/S0010-9452(08)70228-4

[32] Lehman Blake M. Clinical relevance of discourse characteristics after right hemisphere brain damage. American Journal of Speech-Language Pathology. 2006;**15**:255-267. DOI: 10.1044/1058-0360(2006/024)

[33] Marini A. Characteristics of narrative discourse processing after damage to the right hemisphere. Seminars in Speech and Language. 2012;**33**:68-78. DOI: 10.1055/s-0031-1301164

[34] Trillet M, Vighetto A, Croisile B, et al. Hemiballismus with logorrhea and thymoaffective disinhibition caused by hematoma of the left subthalamic nucleus. Revista de Neurologia. 1995;**151**:416-419. http://www.ncbi.nlm.nih.gov/pubmed/7481408

[35] Ferstl EC, Guthke T, von Cramon DY. Change of perspective in discourse comprehension: Encoding and retrieval processes after brain injury. Brain and Language 1999;**70**:385-420. doi: 10.1006/brln.1999.2151

[36] Borod JC, Rorie KD, Pick LH, et al. Verbal pragmatics following unilateral stroke: Emotional content and valence. Neuropsychology. 2000;**14**:112-124. http://www.ncbi.nlm.nih.gov/pubmed/10674803

[37] Soroker N, Kasher A, Giora R, et al. Processing of basic speech acts following localized brain damage: A new light on the neuroanatomy of language. Brain and Cognition. 2005;**57**:214-217. DOI: 10.1016/j.bandc.2004.08.047

[38] Thomson AM, Taylor R, Fraser D, et al. The utility of the right hemisphere language battery in patients with brain tumours. European Journal of Disorders of Communication. 1997;**32**(3 Spec No):325-332. Available from: http://www.ncbi.nlm.nih.gov/pubmed/9474297

[39] Zanini S, Bryan K, De Luca G, et al. The effects of age and education on pragmatic features of verbal communication: Evidence from the Italian version of the right hemisphere language battery (I-RHLB). Aphasiology. 2005;**19**:1107-1133. DOI: 10.1080/02687030500268977

[40] Awad M, Warren JE, Scott SK, et al. A common system for the comprehension and pro-duction of narrative speech. The Journal of Neuroscience. 2007;**27**:11455-11464. DOI: 10.1523/JNEUROSCI.5257-06.2007

[41] Bögels S, Barr DJ, Garrod S, et al. Conversational interaction in the scanner: Mentalizing during language processing as revealed by MEG. Cerebral Cortex. 2015;**25**:3219-3234. DOI: 10.1093/cercor/bhu116

[42] Catani M, Bambini V. A model for social communication and language evolution and development (SCALED). Current Opinion in Neurobiology. 2014;**28**:165-171. DOI: 10.1016/j.conb.2014.07.018

[43] Engels AS, Heller W, Mohanty A, et al. Specificity of regional brain activity in anxi-ety types during emotion processing. Psychophysiology. 2007;**44**:352-363. DOI: 10.1111/j.1469-8986.2007.00518.x

[44] Hsu CT, Jacobs AM, Citron FM, et al. The emotion potential of words and passages in read-ing Harry Potter – An fMRI study. Brain and Language. 2015;**142**:96-114. DOI: 10.1016/j.bandl.2015.01.011

[45] Mason RA, Just MA. The role of the theory-of-mind cortical network in the compre-hension of narratives. Language and Linguistics Compass. 2009;**3**:157-174. DOI: 10.1111/j.1749-818X.2008.00122.x

[46] Sabb FW, van Erp TG, Hardt ME, et al. Language network dysfunction as a predic-tor of outcome in youth at clinical high risk for psychosis. Schizophrenia Research. 2010;**116**:173-183. DOI: 10.1016/j.schres.2009.09.042

[47] Spielberg JM, Stewart JL, Levin RL, et al. Prefrontal cortex, emotion, and approach/with-drawal motivation. Social and Personality Psychology Compass. 2008;**2**:135-153. DOI: 10.1111/j.1751-9004.2007.00064.x

[48] Varga E, Simon M, Tényi T, et al. Irony comprehension and context processing in schizo-phrenia during remission – A functional MRI study. Brain and Language. 2013;**126**:231-242. DOI: 10.1016/j.bandl.2013.05.017

[49] Vigliecca NS, Baez S. Screening executive function and global cognition with the nine-card sorting test: Healthy participant studies and ageing implications. Psychogeriatrics. 2015;**15**:163-170. DOI: 10.1111/psyg.12104

[50] Vigliecca NS, Baez S. Verbal neuropsychological functions in aphasia: An integrative model. Journal of Psycholinguistic Research. 2015;**44**:715-732. DOI: 10.1007/s10936-014-9316-4

[51] Vigliecca NS, Peñalva MC, Castillo JA, et al. Brief aphasia evaluation (minimum ver-bal performance): Psychometric data in healthy participants from Argentina. Journal of Neuroscience and Behavioral Health. 2011;**3**:16-26. Available from: http://www.aca-demicjournals.org/journal/JNBH/article-abstract/9892DE34603

[52] Vigliecca NS. Neuropsychological tests abbreviated and adapted to Spanish speakers: Review of previous findings and validity studies for the discrimination of patients with anterior vs. posterior lesions. Revista de Neurologia. 2004;**39**:205-212. Available from: http://www.ncbi.nlm.nih.gov/pubmed/15284958

[53] Vigliecca NS, Aleman G. Neuropsychological tests abbreviated and adapted for Spanish speakers: Factor analysis and age correlation. Revista latina de pensamiento y lenguaje y Neuropsychologia latina. 2000;**8**:65-85. Available from: https://www.researchgate. net/publication/305209598_Neuropsychological_tests_abbreviated_and_adapted_for_ Spanish_speakers_factor_analysis_and_age_correlation [Accessed Nov 23, 2016]

[54] Vigliecca NS, Aleman GP. A novel neuropsychological assessment to discriminate between ischemic and nonischemic dementia. Journal of Pharmacological and Toxicological Methods. 2010;**61**:38-43. DOI: 10.1016/j.vascn.2009.10.003

[55] Vigliecca NS, Martini MA, Aleman GP, et al. Neuropsychological tests abbreviated and adapted for Spanish speakers: reliability and validity studies for the discrimination of patients with unilateral brain lesions. Revista latina de pensamiento y lenguaje y Neuropsychologia latina. 2001;**9**:223-244. Available from: https://www.researchgate. net/publication/305179065_Neuropsychological_tests_abbreviated_and_adapted_ for_Spanish_speakers_reliability_and_validity_studies_for_the_discrimination_of_ patients_with_unilateral_brain_lesions

[56] Vigliecca NS, Castillo JA. Construct and concurrent validity of a screening executive test: The nine-card sorting test. In: Goldfarb PM, editor. Psychological Tests and Testing Research Trends. New York: Nova Science Publishers; 2007. pp. 55-81. Available from: https://www.novapublishers.com/catalog/product_info.php?products_id=5497 [Accessed: Nov 23, 2016]

[57] Vigliecca NS, Peñalva MC, Molina SC, et al. Brief aphasia evaluation (minimum verbal performance): Concurrent and conceptual validity study in patients with unilateral cerebral lesions. Brain Injury. 2011;**25**:394-400. DOI: 10.3109/02699052.2011.556106

[58] Condret-Santi V, Barragan-Jason G, Valton L, et al. Object and proper name retrieval in temporal lobe epilepsy: A study of difficulties and latencies. Epilepsy Research. 2014;**108**:1825-1838. DOI: 10.1016/j.eplepsyres.2014.09.001

[59] Franklin MS, Smallwood J, Zedelius CM, et al. Unaware yet reliant on attention: Experience sampling reveals that mind-wandering impedes implicit learning. Psychonomic Bulletin & Review. 2016;**23**:223-229. DOI: 10.3758/s13423-015-0885-5

[60] Beaty RE, Benedek M, Silvia PJ, et al. Creative cognition and brain network dynamics. Trends in Cognitive Sciences. 2016;**20**:87-95. DOI: 10.1016/j.tics.2015.10.004

[61] Fox KC, Spreng RN, Ellamil M, et al. The wandering brain: Meta-analysis of functional neuroimaging studies of mind-wandering and related spontaneous thought processes. NeuroImage. 2015;**111**:611-621. DOI: 10.1016/j.neuroimage.2015.02.039

[62] Vigliecca NS, Peñalva MC, Molina SC, et al. Is the Folstein's mini-mental test an aphasia test? Applied Neuropsychology: Adult. 2012;**19**:221-228. DOI: 10.1080/09084282.2011. 643962

[63] Kühn S, Fernyhough C, Alderson-Day B, et al. Inner experience in the scanner: Can high fidelity apprehensions of inner experience be integrated with fMRI? Frontiers in Psychology. 2014;**5**:1393. DOI: 10.3389/fpsyg.2014.01393

[64] Berger A, Buchman C, Green-Bleier T. Development of error detection. In Posner MI, editor. Cognitive Neuroscience of Attention. 2nd ed. New York: Guilford Press; 2012. p. 312-321. Available from: https://books.google.com.ar/books?isbn=160918985X [Accessed: Nov 23, 2016]

[65] Kuhlen AK, Bogler C, Swerts M, et al. Neural coding of assessing another person's knowledge based on nonverbal cues. Social Cognitive and Affective Neuroscience. 2015;**10**:729-734. DOI: 10.1093/scan/nsu111

[66] Prochnow D, Kossack H, Brunheim S, et al. Processing of subliminal facial expressions of emotion: A behavioral and fMRI study. Social Neuroscience. 2013;**8**:448-461. DOI: 10.1080/17470919.2013.812536

[67] Satzer D, Bond DJ. Mania secondary to focal brain lesions: Implications for understanding the functional neuroanatomy of bipolar disorder. Bipolar Disorders. 2016;**18**:205-220. DOI: 10.1111/bdi.12387

[68] Cuesta MJ, Peralta V. Testing the hypothesis that formal thought disorders are severe mood disorders. Schizophrenia Bulletin. 2011;**37**:1136-1146. DOI: 10.1093/schbul/ sbr092

[69] Bonnelle V, Leech R, Kinnunen KM, et al. Default mode network connectivity predicts sustained attention deficits after traumatic brain injury. The Journal of Neuroscience. 2011;**31**:13442-13451. DOI: 10.1523/JNEUROSCI.1163-11.2011

[70] Cortese S, Castellanos FX, Eickhoff CR, et al. Functional decoding and meta-analytic connectivity modeling in adult attention-deficit/hyperactivity disorder. Biological Psychiatry. 2016;**80**:896-904. DOI: 10.1016/j.biopsych.2016.06.014

[71] Gola KA, Thorne A, Veldhuisen LD, et al. Neural substrates of spontaneous narrative production in focal neurodegenerative disease. Neuropsychologia. 2015;**79**(Pt A):158-171. DOI: 10.1016/j.neuropsychologia.2015.10.022

[72] McDonald S, Code C, Togher L. Communication Disorders Following Traumatic Brain Injury, London: Psychology Press; 2016. Available from: https://books.google.com.ar/ books?id=ewEfDAAAQBAJ&dq=bibliogroup:%22Brain,+Behaviour+and+Cognition%2 2&source=gbs_navlinks_s [Accessed: Nov 23, 2016]

[73] Pina-Camacho L, Villero S, Fraguas D, et al. Autism spectrum disorder: Does neuroimaging support the DSM-5 proposal for a symptom dyad? A systematic review of functional magnetic resonance imaging and diffusion tensor imaging studies. Journal of Autism and Developmental Disorders. 2012;**42**:1326-1341. DOI: 10.1007/s10803-011-1360-4

[74] Xu X, Yuan H, Lei X. Activation and connectivity within the default mode network contribute independently to future-oriented thought. Scientific Reports. 2016;**6**:21001. DOI: 10.1038/srep21001

2

Differentiating Normal Cognitive Aging from Cognitive Impairment No Dementia: A Focus on Constructive and Visuospatial Abilities

Radka Ivanova Massaldjieva

Abstract

Constructive and visuospatial abilities in normal and in pathological aging (cognitive impairment, no dementia, CIND) are investigated. The sample includes 188 participants over 60 years of age, divided in 2 groups: healthy subjects (MMSE ≥28), without cognitive complaints, and individuals with CIND (MMSE between 24 and 27 and subjective cognitive complains). Drawing of cube and drawing of house, Benton Visual Retention Test (BVRT), and Block design are used to test the hypothesis that short visuoconstructive and visuospatial tests can distinguish normal from pathological cognitive aging in its very early stages. Results proved the discriminative sensitivity of BVRT general assessment criteria and of omissions and distortions in CIND. The diagnostic sensitivity of a modification of Moore and Wike [1984] scoring system for house and cube drawing tasks was confirmed as well. Drawing of cube and house could be used for quick screening of CIND in subjects over 60. Principal component analysis with oblimin rotation was performed to explore the different dimensions in the visuospatial and visuoconstructive abilities in old age. A four-factor structure was established, all four factors explaining 71% of the variance.

Keywords: constructive ability, visuospatial ability, cognitive impairment, no dementia (CIND), old age, house and cube drawing, BVRT

1. Introduction

1.1. Mild cognitive impairment and cognitive impairment, no dementia

Age-related cognitive changes are widely discussed by the researchers, and rich evidences about them are reported in the literature [1]. The decline in cognitive functioning has long been traditionally considered a consequence of normal aging [2], and since dementia caused by neurodegenerative diseases has a long preclinical stage [3–7], it may not be recognized for months or even years [8, 9]. Early differentiation of normal aging from neurodegenerative pathology is of great importance in terms of timely adequate treatment helping to postpone further cognitive decline [9–14]. A better understanding of normal aging itself is also extremely important because of the increase in life expectancy and, respectively, of elderly people. This necessitates the implementation of effective measures for successful and active aging, and they require more clarity about the cognitive aging dimensions.

Research related to the early diagnosis of dementia in Alzheimer's disease (AD) and vascular dementia brought about the differentiation of many terms indicating boundary or intermediate conditions of cognitive changes without dementia [3, 5–7, 11, 15–20]. The variety of such terms created over the years and their content are widely discussed in the literature and will not be analyzed here.

The most frequently used term—mild cognitive impairment (MCI)—is defined as an early stage of neurodegenerative pathology, a transient phase between normal aging and dementia. It is a syndrome characterized by a cognitive decline, sufficiently serious to be considered a result of normal aging, but not reaching the criteria for dementia syndrome [6] and associated with an increased risk of developing dementia, most commonly Alzheimer's disease [5, 13, 18]. Criteria for diagnosis of preclinical forms of vascular dementia—mild cognitive impairment of vascular type (MCI-V) and vascular cognitive impairment, no dementia—have been also developed [21, 22].

The definition of MCI syndrome, made by Petersen et al. [23], comprises subjective complaints of memory impairment, normal daily activity, normal cognitive functioning, memory impairment (1–2 standard deviations below the norms), and absence of dementia. This definition is later amplified with impairments of other areas of cognition [24] like naming, abstract thinking, spatial localization, and ability to communicate. The relations between the states of memory decline and conditions of cognitive impairments without significant memory changes are still unclear [11].

Another widely used term for milder impairment of cognition, situated between normal aging and dementia, is "cognitive impairment, no dementia, CIND," characterized by impairment in any objectively tested cognitive area. CIND does not require the determination of the degree or the specific cause of the cognitive decline [24]. It is a condition with similar criteria such as for mild cognitive impairment that could be applied when there is impaired performance of cognitive tests or cognitive complains [25, 26].

As a result of the Third Canadian Consensus conference on the diagnosis and treatment of dementia, Chertkow et al. [4] discuss important recommendations for family physicians in the efforts at providing "practical guidance on definition, diagnosis and treatment of mild cognitive impairment and cognitive impairment, no dementia." They consider it necessary for the general practitioner to know CIND as a condition with an increased risk of dementia and to monitor the patients with this condition.

1.2. Normative (non-pathological) and pathological cognitive aging

It is difficult to establish to what extent the cognitive changes, accompanying aging, are due to the increase in chronological age and to what extent they are associated with illness or life-style [27]. Intensive studies of the impact of age and different diseases on biological, mental, and cognitive changes have not validated sufficiently reliable markers that allow the differentiation of the normal (physiological aging) from pathological aging. The very term "normal" in relation to different characteristics of people in the old age has not enough clear boundaries [21, 28].

For the cognitive changes in elderly, a continuum is used at one end of which is cognitive functioning allowing active and independent life (normal aging) and at the other end significant cognitive impairments typical of dementia. Cognitive aging in late adulthood is one of the most important issues in aging processes research, because of its wide influence on all other aspects of older population life. Taking into account that cognitive aging is too complex to be described briefly, the Committee on the Public Health Dimensions of Cognitive Aging defines it as a lifelong process of change in cognitive functioning. At the same time, the necessity of operational definition is emphasized [29]. Approaching a fuller description and understanding of cognitive changes in later life require responses to different questions of great significance and among them: Are these changes in the elderly global or partial, affecting certain functions earlier? Which components of the cognitive system are the most vulnerable to impairments as a result of aging? How do these components change? How do the changes affect the performance of cognitive tasks, the everyday and social functioning? Are they significantly different patterns of cognitive change allowing accurate and reliable differentiation of normal (normative) from pathological cognitive aging, etc.?

The complexity of the topic has led to a wide variety of approaches and hypotheses. One of the most commonly used ways of thinking is based on Cattell subdivision of cognitive capacities of fluid and crystallized intelligence [30]. The first concept comprises the independent of social experience abilities involved in the processing of new information and problem solving. The second signifies the acquired (learned) cumulative knowledge, e.g., the vocabulary [1, 30, 31]. Results from multiple studies of age-related cognitive changes lead to the development of the so-called classic model of cognitive aging: the crystallized abilities show little or no decline up to 60 years of age or later, whereas fluid abilities decline steadily from age 20 to 80 [31–34]. A recent study exploring cognitive functioning in a representative sample of about 40,000 subjects from the UK, aged 16 to 100, confirmed that the processing effectiveness decreases earlier than the knowledge-based abilities that begin to decline from age 60 [35].

Fluid intelligence is considered connected with Spearman's g (general intelligence—a broad mental capacity underlying specific mental abilities) [see [36]]. Duncan et al. [37] have found that "g" reflects the brain frontal area functions. These findings relate the classic model of cognitive aging with another model, based on the brain localization of cognitive functions and postulating that executive functions, highly related to the frontal lobe, decline earlier than these dependent on the temporal cortex, hippocampus, and limbic system (e.g., memory) [36].

The decline of fluid abilities during the life span find different explanations in two groups of theories: The first group seeks a common factor that influences the worsening of the performance of various cognitive tasks. The age-related slowing of speed of cognitive performance or processing speed is frequently used to explain elders' worse results in neuropsychological testing, compared with younger individuals [1, 34]. The second group relies on diversity—the change of different processes at different speed during adult life [38].

The multifactor intelligence theories differentiate specific capabilities that are equally important for cognitive functioning. According to these theories, there is no common factor of the intelligence. Authors list different numbers of individual abilities from seven to 120 or more. Thurstone [38] distinguishes seven primary mental abilities: numerical, perceptual, verbal comprehension, word fluency, memory, spatial ability, and reasoning abilities [39, 40]. His conceptualization related to primary mental capabilities serves as a basis for H. Gardner's theory about the existence of multiple, relatively independent "intelligences" [41, 42]. Gardner [40] noticed that most intelligence tests measure mainly linguistic (verbal) and logical mathematical abilities, but not spatial, musical, bodily kinetic, and personal intelligence.

The doubts of some cognitive ability researchers, concerning the relevance of factor analysis to the effort to understand human intelligence, lead to the creation of the hierarchical theory of cognitive abilities, describing several general cognitive functions involved in the realization of a large part of the cognitive abilities and more specialized capacities placed higher in the hierarchy of the cognitive system [40]. It is not difficult to see the connection between this hierarchical model and the two-factor theory, according to which the results from each intelligence test depend on the Spearman's common intelligence and on the specific abilities necessary for the performance of each separate test task.

1.3. Constructive and visuospatial abilities and their later life changes

In Mapou's [43] hierarchical model of cognitive abilities, higher level skills depend on the capabilities of the lower levels. The visuospatial functions are modal specific and depend on global functioning (the intelligence) and on basic abilities like attention, sensory and motor functions, executive functions, and problem solving. R. Mapou divides the visual-spatial functions into perceptual abilities, constructive abilities, and spatial awareness. Perceptual abilities are related to the initial processing of the spatial information, which takes place after the sensory basic level and regardless of the motor response. These abilities are responsible for the acquisition of visual information. Constructive abilities include organizational and planning faculties realized through basic visual and motor functions. Spatial awareness involves the ability to orientate in the outer space as well as the awareness of the interior space.

The visuospatial abilities are very important for human everyday functioning, because they are an essential part of the save movement in the environment, that is not possible without a correct estimation of direction, distance, and spatial relationships between objects and places [29, 44]. Different authors depict a different structure of these abilities and propose specific tasks for their assessment [45]. De Bruin et al. [44] present them as composed by spatial visualization, spatial perception, and mental rotation. The definition of Blazer et al. [[29], p. 40], "maintenance and manipulation of visual images," includes producing figures and matching objects and pictures, creating relationships between locations and recognizing faces.

Constructive ability (visual constructive praxis) is also a broad term used for very different types of activities, a common feature of which is assembling, joining individual parts into a single structure—a whole unit. This term refers to combining or organizing behavior in which the relationships between the component parts of the whole object must be understood in order to obtain the desired synthesis between them [46]. The term "constructive apraxia" was introduced by Kleist [see [47]], who defined it in 1914–1918, as an impairment of capacity for spatial organization in assembly, construction, or drawing of a given model, while the motor function is not affected [48]. According to Kleist, constructive apraxia is an executive function deficit that affects also the spatial part of the performance. Bradshaw et al. [49] consider the impairment of the constructive strategy in copying complex figures as part of the so-called dorsolateral prefrontal syndrome that is manifested by executive deficiency. For Kleist, constructive apraxia is independent of both the visual-spatial deficit and the motor disorders. He describes it as impaired integration of these two abilities. Later investigators found that constructive disturbance was almost always associated with a wider visual perceptive or visuospatial impairment [47].

Studies of age influence on cognitive functioning found that the elderly examined showed a decline not only in short-term memory and psychomotor speed but also in constructional and visual-spatial praxis and visual perceptual functions [31, 45, 50]. Constructive impairments can be detected in the early stages of dementia and Alzheimer's disease (AD) [8, 51, 52], but they are better studied in focal brain lesions than in normal aging and dementia. Visuospatial ability's progressive decline is found in patients with dementia in Alzheimer's disease and vascular dementia [8, 47, 53, 54].

A fundamental question, according to A. Benton, is whether patients with general intellectual disabilities have constructive apraxia as well. The author found in a study of 1967 that intellectually impaired patients showed a high incidence of failures in performing constructive tasks, but at the same time, a large number of patients with intellectual disabilities did not have significant difficulties in the performance of such tasks. Therefore, the author concludes that the general intellectual decline is not necessarily related to constructive apraxia [55]. These findings correspond to the subgroup models of cognitive impairments in Alzheimer's disease, expecting decline in particular cognitive domains rather than simultaneous advancing global impairments in the early stages of the disease [see [56]]. Using Factor Analysis of the Severe Impairment Battery results, Pelissier et al. [57] establish relative independence of constructive praxis and visual perceptive function from other cognitive functions. All this is in favor of the need for a separate and specific study of constructional and spatial impairments in normal and pathological aging to allow their better understanding.

1.4. Early recognition of pathological cognitive decline by visuoconstructive and spatial tasks

Assessment of cognitive impairments in the elderly is an important task of modern cognitive neuropsychology. Neuropsychological evaluation can respond to the expectations of valid and reliable differentiation of pathological from normal aging if it is accomplished by sufficiently sensitive, specific, and standardized psychometric tools [14]. The use of such tools is a requirement of the diagnostic algorithm for early discrimination of dementia from normal aging [9, 58]. The widely applied strategy to administer global clinical scales for screening and quantifying the level of individual cognitive deficit has low specificity, particularly in subjects with high or very low level of premorbid cognitive functioning and in the early stages of impairments in elderly [5, 14]. Short tests, assessing specific cognitive dysfunctions, are more accurate than the global cognitive scales [14, 59].

In order to detect age-related visual-spatial and constructive decline early enough, specific neuropsychological techniques are required. Such measures could be efficient and helpful if they take into account the age-related and pathological cognitive changes and assure accuracy of the assessment. Many different neuropsychological instruments are used to test the spatial functions [45]. The visuoconstructive ability is traditionally assessed by drawing of two- or three-dimensional figures [51, 52, 54] and block-building tasks [55] of varying complexity. Drawing neuropsychological tasks can detect the deficits in reproducing shapes, following their relationships in space, but it is difficult to standardize them [51], and in most cases, subject drawings are assessed "intuitively" and very rarely through an objective assessment system [52].

Drawing as a cognitive ability is not well studied in late-life adults. It is a complex multicomponent ability that engages perception, representation, memory, attention, spatial thinking, planning, and motor functions. Better knowledge of the structure of drawing process in old adults as well as of its age-related impairments can contribute to a more successful study of visual constructive and visual-spatial functions and their disturbances in old age.

Our study tests the hypothesis that short and easy-to-use visuoconstructive and visuospatial tests can be used to distinguish normal from pathological cognitive aging in its very early stages if appropriate, accurate, and valid criteria are applied. We use drawing of cube and drawing of house, together with other traditionally used and well-proven neuropsychological instruments—Benton Visual Retention Test (BVRT) and Block design—assessing visual memory, perception, constructional, and spatial abilities.

1.5. Aims of the chapter

The aims of this chapter are to explore the visuoconstructive and visuospatial abilities in normal and in pathological aging (CIND) above 60 years of age and to analyze:

1. The discriminative capacities of a set of visuoconstructive and visuospatial neuropsychological tasks in the differentiation of pathological (CIND) from normal cognitive aging over 60 years of age.

2. The influence of age on the visuoconstructive and visuospatial abilities in healthy elderly and individuals with CIND.

3. The patterns of Benton Visual Retention Test (BVRT) performance in normal aging and in CIND.

2. Method and procedure

2.1. Subjects and recruitment

The participants in this study were individuals over 60 years of age with normal daily functioning and without self-reported history of psychiatric and neurological disorders, residents of Plovdiv region, living independently in the community. The sample was divided in two groups: healthy subjects (MMSE ≥28), without cognitive complaints, and individuals with CIND (MMSE between 24 and 27 and subjective cognitive complains). The decision to accept the diagnostic category CIND was substantiated by the design of the study, which did not include the possibility of conducting detailed clinical, laboratory, and neuroimaging studies. After testing, all the participants from CIND group were advised to seek consultation from a general practitioner or neurologist to accurately identify the cause of the condition and the need for treatment. A total of 216 subjects were recruited for this study with the help of clubs for the elderly; 28 of them dropped out due to age below 60 years, impairments in every day functioning, visual disturbances that hindered neuropsychological testing, data from the interview about mild mental retardation, and test data for severe cognitive deficits. Only participants defining themselves as right handers were included in the study. Basic demographic characteristics of the study groups are shown in **Table 1**.

Groups: Partial testing	Age (years)			Gender		Education		
	Mean	SD	max	Male	Female	1	2	3
				n %		n %		
Healthy	68.11	6.89	88	34	69	20	48	35
				33%	67%	19.4%	46.6%	34.0%
CIND	71.11	7.58	89	37	48	33	33	19
				43.5%	56.5%	38.8%	38.8%	22.3%
Complete testing								
Healthy	67.00	5.19	78	11	29	3	24	13
				27.5%	72.5%	7.5%	60.0%	32.5%
CIND	70.36	6.86	83	8	14	5	10	7
				36.4%	63.6%	22.7%	45.5%	31.8%

Note: 1, primary and secondary school; 2, high school; and 3, college/university.

Table 1. Subject basic demographics.

2.2. Instruments

Assessment of correspondence to the inclusion criteria (administered to all subjects):

1. Mini-Mental State Examination (MMSE) [60], Bulgarian translation [61]—a short global scale for cognitive functioning, with subtests for spatial and temporal orientation, concentration, memory, aphasia, agnosia, and apraxia [8, 62]. The scale is the most widely used screening tool for cognitive impairments in late life in Bulgaria.

2. Semi-structured interview, collecting basic demographic information, and data on neuropsychiatric history and cognitive complains.

3. The Social and Occupational Functioning Assessment Scale—SOFAS (DSM-IV) [3, 63].

Neuropsychological assessment:

1. Benton Visual Retention Test (BVRT), form C, administration "A"—a well-known test of short-term visual memory, visual perception, and constructive ability. The "C" form is considered the easiest BVRT task that makes it appropriate for old adults [64].

2. Raven's Standard Progressive Matrices (RSPM)—a language and culture-free measure of fluid intelligence. The task comprises five sets of 12 black and white matrices, presenting pattern matching tasks with increasing difficulty, used as a test of general intelligence and nonverbal reasoning [65, 66]. The raw score is used in the analyses because of the lack of studies in Bulgaria on late-life RSPM performance.

3. Free drawing of a house and of a cube.

4. Block design—a subtest from Hamburg-Wechsler Intelligence Test, Bulgarian adaptation [67]; the task requires construction of observed patterns—two, four, nine, and 16 elemental figures—from the same multicolored cubes, with standard instruction. The time for task completion is not assessed. The score used in this study is the number of correctly reproduced patterns (accuracy of performance).

2.3. Procedures

The demographic and neuropsychiatric interviewing and the testing were conducted by a licensed clinical psychologist with experience in psychiatric disorder assessment (the chapter author). All the tests were administered individually on 2 separate days. To those who agreed to participate in the full 2-day testing (N = 62), all the study instruments were applied. The other participants (126) were tested with BVRT and RSPM. Subjects were assessed at the elderly club premises in prearranged days and hours.

BVRT cards were reproduced after a 10-s exposition (immediate recall trial) with the standard instruction and assessment: The subject was given 10 white sheets for the reproduction of the 10 test cards and pencil with rubber. Assessment took into account: (1) number of correct reproductions—each card reproduction is judged correct or wrong, and every correct card reproduction received one point— and (2) specific types of errors (quality assessment). Types of errors for which points were awarded were as follows: (a) omissions, (b) distortions, (c) perseverations, (d) rotations, (e) misplacements, and (e) size errors.

Subjects received two white sheets of paper (15 × 21 cm) for the free drawings of cube and house and black pencil with rubber. The drawings were assessed following a modification of the scoring system of Moore and Wyke [52] developed by the author: One point was given for each line drawn from the front, top, and side walls of the cube (maximum nine points). Orientation of the cube was not evaluated. For the additional qualitative criteria of Moore and Wake, quantitative assessment (maximum of four points) was used. One point was given for three-dimensional representation, for the presence of additional elements (interior walls), for the cohesion of the figure, and for lack of spatial distortion (parallelism of the sides and accuracy of the corners).

Written informed consent was obtained from all participants. The study design and procedure were approved by the ethics committee of Medical University in Plovdiv, Bulgaria.

2.4. Data analysis

In order to achieve the study objectives, it was necessary to analyze the differences in test performance between (1) "normal" subjects and subjects with CIND and (2) participants up to and above 70 years of age. Descriptive statistic (frequencies, percents, means, standard deviations) was used to describe the sample as well as for the analysis of results regarding general scoring criteria and error types in study groups; comparison of test performance in different subgroups was made by t-test and Mann-Whitney test; RSPM performance was additionally described using Z-scores and chi-square test. The relationships between study variables were studied with Pearson and Spearman correlations and multiple regression analysis. We performed a principal component analysis to explore the structure of visuoconstructive and visuospatial abilities, involved in the study tests.

3. Results and interpretation

3.1. Performance in the diagnostic groups

Significant differences in BVRT total scores—mean total number of correct reproductions and mean total number of errors—were found when the normal subjects, and the subjects with CIND were compared (p < .001) (**Table 2**). (We use the term "normal" and "healthy" subjects to distinguish between normal and pathological aging, taking into account the conditionality of its use.) There were significantly more omissions and distortions (BVRT) in CIND group than in the normal group (p < .001). These differences can also be seen in the BVRT frequency distribution data—50% of the healthy participants had between three and six correct reproductions and made between seven and 12 errors; 50% of participants with CIND reproduced correctly between two and four cards and made between 10 and 14 errors. As for the different types of

Criteria	Diagnostic group	Mean score	SD	t	p
Total correct	Healthy	4.62	1.805	6.16	< .001
	CIND	3.21	1.328		
Total errors	Healthy	8.91	3.697	-6.23	< .001
	CIND	12.08	3.178		
Omissions	Healthy	1.74	1.925	−3.95	< .001
	CIND	3.14	2.765		
Distortions	Healthy	2.78	1.715	−5.22	< .001
	CIND	4.28	2.153		
Perseverations	Healthy	1.02	1.093	0.93	0.35
	CIND	0.87	1.100		
Rotations	Healthy	1.18	1.135	−2.41	0.17
	CIND	1.58	1.073		
Misplacements	Healthy	1.74	1.335	0.59	0.55
	CIND	1.62	1.291		
Size errors	Healthy	0.46	0.764	−0.98	0.33
	CIND	0.58	0.918		

Note: results from partial testing group.

Table 2. BVRT mean score comparison in the diagnostic groups (t-test).

errors that showed significant differences, 50% of normal subjects made zero to two omissions (one to five in CIND subjects) and, respectively, two to four distortions (2.50 to six in CIND).

Table 3 shows RSPM performance of the participants from both diagnostic groups (percentiles, means, and z-scores). Healthy subjects gave more correct answers than subjects with CIND (p<.001).

Performance of the house and cube drawing, as well as of the Block design tasks, was also significantly worse in the CIND group (Mann-Whitney test, p < .01) (**Table 4**). **Figures 1** and **2** present cube and house drawings in the diagnostic groups.

3.2. Performance in the age groups

When the healthy and CIND study participants were subdivided in age groups, healthy elders up to 70 years of age (N = 70) showed more BVRT correct reproductions and RSPM correct answers (p<.001); they made significantly fewer errors (total errors), as well as fewer omissions and distortions, than the oldest subjects from the same diagnostic group. Younger subjects with CIND (N = 48) made significantly fewer number of errors, as well as fewer omissions (BVRT). They also showed significantly better result in RSPM performance than the subjects over 70 years of age (**Table 5**).

Healthy	RSPM total correct	Mean (SD)	Z score
Minimum	12		−1.505
Maximum	53		2.003
Percentiles			
25	19.00	29.58	
50	28.00	(11.69)	
75	40.00		
CIND			
Minimum	5		−1.716
Maximum	55		4.430
Percentiles			
25	14.00	17.87	
50	16.00	(7.08)	
75	20.00		
		t = 8.462	Chi-square = 1.880
		P < .001	P < .001

Table 3. RSPM results in the diagnostic groups.

No significant differences were found between the age groups with respect to house and cube drawing tasks, as well as to Block design subtest both for healthy and CIND participants (Mann-Whitney test, p >.05).

In the healthy group with partial testing (N = 103), age correlated positively and significantly with BVRT total errors, as well as with omissions, distortion, and rotation scores

Test variables Diagnostic group	Mean rank	Mann-Whitney U	Sig. (Two-tailed)
Total house score	37.04	218.5	P = .001
Healthy	21.43		
CIND			
Total cube score	35.86	265.5	P = .009
Healthy	23.57		
CIND			
Block design score	37.16	213.5	P = .001
Healthy	21.20		
CIND			

Table 4. Mean comparison for cube and house drawing and block design.

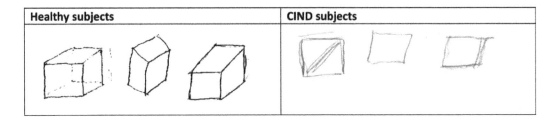

Figure 1. Examples of cube drawings in the diagnostic groups.

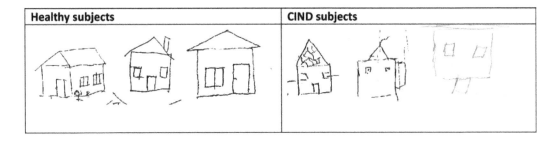

Figure 2. Examples of house drawings in the diagnostic groups.

(r between .213 and .520, p < .05). As expected the relation between age and BVRT total correct score was negative (r = −.397, p < .001).

In the CIND group, age correlated positively and significantly only with BVRT omissions (r = .359, p = .001). The relation between age and size errors score did not reach acceptable significance (r = − .202, p = .064). Negative moderate significant correlation existed between MMSE (r CIND = −.257 and r healthy = −.385) and RSPM total score (r CIND = −.340 and r healthy = −.535) on the one hand and the age, on the other, in both diagnostic groups.

In the group with complete testing, age correlated only with RSPM score, both in the whole group (Pearson correlation), N = 62, and in the diagnostic groups (Spearman correlation)— moderate significant negative correlation (p < .001 and p < .05, respectively).

3.3. Relationships between test measures

3.3.1. Correlation

Most of the measures assessing the performance of the drawing tasks correlate moderately and significantly (Pearson correlation), except for cube total score and BVRT correct and error scores (**Table 6**). As expected Block design and RSPM measures are in a significant relation with all other variables (r between .326 and .591) as well as between them (p < .001). Further analyses (Spearman correlations) were accomplished for the same variables in each diagnostic group separately. In the group of healthy participants, the cube total score cor-relates only with the house total score (r = .345, p = .029). BVRT total correct and total errors correlate highly between them (r = −.886, p < .001) and moderately with RSPM (p < .001). There is a significant correlation between BVRT total errors and Block design score (r = −.318, p = .046).

Healthy	BVRT total correct	BVRT total errors	BVRT O	BVRT D	BVRT P	BVRT R	BVRT M	BVRT SE	RSPM total correct
60-70 years									
N=70									
Mean	5.01	8.04	1.40	2.34	1.04	1.06	1.74	0.46	32.97
SD	1.77	3.56	1.61	1.63	1.03	1.13	1.29	0.77	11.53
>70 years									
N=33									
Mean	3.79	10.76	2.45	3.70	0.97	1.45	1.73	0.45	22.39
SD	1.60	3.37	2.33	1.53	1.24	1.12	1.44	0.75	8.37
T-test	**3.378**	**−3.686**	**−2.347**	**−4.007**	.315	−1.672	.055	.016	**5.273**
	P=.001	**P<.001**	**P=.023**	**P<.001**	P=.753	P=.098	P=.956	P=.987	**P<.001**
CIND									
60-70 years									
N=48									
Mean	3.40	11.44	2.33	4.21	0.98	1.54	1.67	0.69	20.04
SD	1.45	3.32	2.36	2.15	1.10	1.09	1.21	1.05	8.06
>70 years									
N=37									
Mean	2.97	12.92	4.19	4.38	0.73	1.62	1.57	0.43	15.05
SD	1.12	2.81	2.92	2.18	1.10	1.06	1.40	0.69	4.21
T-test	1.515	**−2.178**	**−3.236**	−.359	1.037	−.339	.349	1.275	**3.684**
	P=.133	**P=.032**	**P=.002**	P=.720	P=.303	P=.736	P=.728	P=.206	**P<.001**

Note: O. omissions; D. distortions; P. perseverations; R. rotations; M. misplacements; SE. size errors.

Table 5. Mean comparison for BVRT and RSPM results in the age groups for healthy subjects and CIND.

In the CIND group, results showed a different picture, probably affected by the heterogeneity of cognitive impairments, which is characteristic of this early stage of pathological decline [56, 68]. BVRT total correct and total errors correlate moderately between them ($r = -.447$, $p = .037$), and there is no significant correlation between them and RSPM. The cube total score correlates only with the Block design score ($r = .470$, $p = .027$). The house total score also correlates with Block design score and with Benton total errors($r = -.644$, $p = .001$). Benton total errors correlate with Block design score as well ($r = -.607$, $p = .003$).

Moderate significant correlation was found between BVRT omissions and the cube drawing score ($r = -.378$, $p = .016$) and between BVRT distortions and the Block design score ($r = -.485$, $p = .002$), as well as the RSPM score ($r = -.480$, $p = .002$), in healthy participants. In CIND group the scores for the different types of errors did not correlate with the outcome measures from other tests.

Variables	Age	Block design	Cube score	House score	RSPM	BVRT correct	BVRT errors
Age							
Coefficient r	1	−.071	−.124	−.035	**−.437**	−.113	.130
Sig.		−.071	.335	.788	.000	.382	.315
Block design							
Coefficient r	−.071	1	**.400**	**.448**	**.505**	**.352**	**−.529**
Sig.	.586		.001	.000	.000	.005	.000
Cube score							
Coefficient r	−.124	**.400**	1	**.437**	**.326**	.213	−.204
Sig.	.335	.001		.000	.010	.097	.112
House score							
Coefficient r	−.035	**.448**	**.437**	1	.332	**.400**	**.420**
Sig.	.788	.000	.000		.008	.001	.001
RSPM							
Coefficient r	**−.437**	**.505**	**.326**	.332	1	.573	**−.591**
Sig.	.000	.000	.010	.008		.000	.000
BVRT correct							
Coefficient r	−.113	**.352**	.213	**.400**	**.573**	1	**−.864**
Sig.	.382	.005	.097	.001	.000		.000
BVRT errors							
Coefficient r	.130	**−.529**	−.204	**−.420**	**−.591**	**−.864**	1
Sig.	.315	.000	.112	.001	.000	.000	

Table 6. Intercorrelations between age and visuospatial/visuoconstructive test scores.

In the group with partial testing, we found high significant negative correlation between BVRT total correct and total errors both for healthy and for CIND participants. As for the types of errors, (1) in the group of healthy subjects, the total number correct and total errors correlated moderately and significantly with all types of errors. (2) In CIND group BVRT total correct score correlated moderately and significantly only with the number of omissions and distortions (p=.001) and BVRT total errors—with omissions and distortions (p<.001) as well as with misplacement (p = .016).

3.3.2. Multiple regression analysis

Multiple regression analyses were performed to determine if age continued to predict BVRT score, when education and RSPM (fluid intelligence) score were taken into account. Gender was added as a possible predictor only for BVRT distortions (in healthy group) and for BVRT omissions in CIND group. These were the only variables that correlated with the gender of participants (low negative correlation for distortions, which means more errors in male subjects, and low positive correlation for omissions—more errors, made by females). Dependent variables were the outcome measures that correlated with age in both diagnostic groups. As it could be seen from **Table 7**, age predicted significantly the variance in BVRT omissions, together with fluid intelligence for healthy participants and together with education and fluid intelligence for the participants with CIND. For the other BVRT outcome measures, age is no more significant performance predictor when other demographic variables and fluid intelligence are included in the analyses.

Fluid intelligence contributed to the variance in all the variables analyzed, except for BVRT rotation in the healthy group. Education was a significant predictor only for the total errors, made by healthy participants and for the number of omissions in CIND subjects.

Diagnostic group	Dependent	Predictor	F	B	Beta	t	R²
Healthy	Total correct	Age	11.848***	−.025	−.097	−.967	.264
		Education		.110	.163	1.738	
		RSPM		.057	.372	**3.479****	
	Total errors	Age	24.401***	.087	.162	1.839	.425
		Education		−.250	−.180	**−2.170***	
		RSPM		−.146	−.463	**−4.896****	
	Omissions	Age	11.954***	.092	.329	**3.302****	.266
		Education		.020	.028	.297	
		RSPM		−.045	−.274	**−2.564***	
	Distortions	Age	10.529***	.025	.102	1.036	.301
		Education		−.109	−.170	−1.848	
		RSPM		−.052	−.354	**−3.379****	
		Gender		−.790	−.218	**−2.556***	
	Rotations	Age	3.973*	.003	.020	.183	.107
		Education		−.080	−.189	−1.826	
		RSPM		−.019	−.193	−1.640	
CIND	Omissions	Age	9.353***	.075	.206	**2.001***	.319
		Education		−.337	−.330	**−3.059****	
		RSPM		−.082	−.211	**−2.077***	
		Gender		−.007	−.014	−.138	

Note:
*p<.05;
**p<.01;
***p < .001.

Table 7. Multiple regression analyses of demographic factors and fluid intelligence contributing to BVRT results.

Variables	Factor 1	Factor 2	Factor 3	Factor 4
Block design	.324	.439	.435	.070
House score	.170	.405	.463	−.229
Cube score	.097	.787	.059	−.033
BVRT correct	.840	−.082	.182	−.107
BVRT errors	−.896	.097	−.241	.058
BVRT omissions	−.482	−.404	.572	.305
BVRT distortions	−.050	.021	−.915	.000
BVRT perseverations	−.386	−.079	−.086	−.830
BVRT rotations	−.788	.037	.206	−.208
BVRT misplacements	−.371	.838	−.127	.119
BVRT size errors	−.208	.012	−.035	.664
RSPM total correct	.535	.237	.188	−.186

Table 8. Principal component pattern matrix for the sample with complete testing.

3.4. Principal component analysis

To explore the different dimensions in the visuospatial and visuoconstructive abilities in old age, a principal component analysis was performed with oblimin rotation, because of the comparatively small data set (N = 62) and the postulated interrelations between variables used. A four-factor structure, with eigenvalues bigger than 1, was established, all four factors explaining around 71% of the variance. Item loading above 0.3 on each factor is taken into consideration (**Table 8**). Most of the variables load high on the first factor, which could mean that the same kind of abilities is included in the tasks measured by many of our variables. That is why my suggestion for the name of this factor is "general cognitive ability." I would name the second factor extracted "executive functioning" (planning and executing visuo-constructive and visuospatial tasks). This factor is strongly associated with cube and house drawing, Block design performance, and planning and organization of the BVRT figures on the sheet of paper. It is the second factor on which RSPM score loads (coefficient = .237), and RSPM is proven as an executive test. Factor 3 includes BVRT omissions and distortions, together with house drawing and Block design scores and could be named "visuospatial memory." The characteristics of item loading on factor 4 give reason to label it "visuospatial analysis and visual perception."

4. Discussion

Constructive and visuospatial abilities are complex fluid functions that decline with advancing age [31, 45, 50, 54]. Their impairments are proven characteristics of the pathological aging related to different types of dementia [8, 47, 53], and they are not enough studied in the boundary states, posing a risk for the development of dementia. According to Guerin [69] and

Grossi [51], specific studies are needed to reveal the relations between visuospatial disorders and constructional apraxia.

We found that the global BVRT outcome measures (numbers of correct reproductions and number of errors) can significantly differentiate normal from pathological aging. Our work regarding the qualitative characteristics of BVRT performance is consistent with the view that it is necessary to study the specific patterns of this test results in different diagnostic groups [70, 71]. Most existing studies with BVRT analyze only the number of correct reproductions [71, 72] or the total number of errors [73]. The data about the profiles of errors in different groups, including geriatric, are scarce [74], and as far as they exist, they do not refer to CIND. We can assume that the types of errors that differ significantly in the two studied diagnostic groups—omissions and distortions—reflect the cognitive decline profile in CIND.

House and cube drawing tasks, as well as Block design subtest, also showed good discriminant capacity for differentiation of normal elders from persons with CIND. We compare the results reported here with studies of healthy individuals and dementia, as we were unable to find data on the use of these tests in subjects with cognitive impairment, no dementia. The house drawing test results are consistent with those obtained in Moore and Wyke [52] study, which found a statistically significant difference between the score from house drawing of patients with dementia and control group of healthy subjects. Similar results are reported by Gragnaniello et al. [53], who found mainly omissions of elements and simplification of the drawings of a house by persons with Alzheimer's dementia. Assessment criteria used in our study take into consideration omissions of elements, three-dimensionality, distortion, and cohesion of the figures.

Our results confirm the classic model of cognitive aging, showing a significant decline in fluid intelligence, measured by RSPM, with age, in both diagnostic groups. Concerning the other tests used in this study:

1. Healthy participants up to 70 years of age showed more accurate BVRT reproductions than these over 70 (number correct, number errors, omissions, and distortions). When the education, fluid intelligence, and gender (where correlated with our variables) were included in the model, age was a significant predictor only for BVRT omissions. In age groups over 70, Coman et al. [70] found the greatest decline in mean total number corrects. The error profile was not analyzed in their study. In another study of normal non-demented subjects from 20 to 102 years of age, significant age-related changes in omissions, distortions, and rotations for both genders were found. This made the authors suppose different brain regions involved in the different types of BVRT errors. When longitudinal analyses were performed, authors found more rapid increase of omissions and distortions for the oldest age groups [74].

2. Number of omissions was the only variable upon which age showed a significant effect in subjects with CIND before and after taking into account the other demographic features and RSPM scores. In normals with memory concerns, a negative correlation between age and BVTR total correct was reported [70].

We can conclude that age is a significant predictor of visuospatial memory decline. Accordingly Rabbit et al. [36] reported that age predicted the results from Spatial Working Memory test.

The two age groups did not differ significantly in the performance of house and cube drawing and of Block design task. Data exist about worse perception and presentation of three-dimensionality in cube drawing task by elders [29], but we could not find studies of house and cube drawing in different late-life groups. It could be supposed that the interindividual variability, characteristic of old age in this comparatively small sample, influenced our results. The size of the sample has also prevented the use of a more detailed statistical analysis of the performance of these three tests.

A possible explanation of the results concerning the cube drawing task score and BVTR total outcome measures could be the complexity of the tasks and in particular the three-dimensionality, as a mandatory feature of the cube drawing. These results could be partially explained as well by the structure of the BVRT task, which involves reproduction of geometric shapes by memory. The task of drawing a cube and a house also requires reproduction, but long-term memory is involved here, while Benton test assesses short-term memory. Another difference between Benton test and the drawing of cube and house is related to BVRT patterns themselves—part of them are new, unknown spatial models, and the other part are well-known figures (triangle, square, circle, trapezoid) engaging long-term representations. A comprehensive cognitive model of adults' drawing ability has not yet been developed. What is well known is its "multicomponential nature" [[51], p. 117] confirmed in this study by a principal component analysis of the results from testing healthy adults and individuals with CIND over 60 years of age (four factors extracted).

The global functioning or the intelligence together with attention, sensory, motor, and executive functions is fundamental for the visuospatial and visuoconstructive abilities, following R. Mapou's [43] hierarchical model. The correlations found reflect the relationship between these basic functions and the capabilities required for specific (constructional and spatial) cognitive functions. This explanation is supported by the principal component analysis, according to the results of which global and executive functioning are required for the performance, assessed by a large number of study variables. Interpretation of principal component analysis reveals at the same time the specificity of constructive and spatial functions, based on visuospatial analysis and perception.

As elements of the multiple regression model, education of participants predicted the total number of errors in the group of healthy subjects and the number of omissions in CIND group. In another study without consideration of type of errors, the level of performance of normal older adults aged 61–97 showed dependence on education. In the same paper, in the group of normals with memory concerns from 64 to 74, less educated had worse performance, the difference found not reaching significance over 75. As for the gender effects on BVRT performance, there are no evidences about significant differences between men and women, from most research results available [70]. Resnick et al. [74] reported sex differences for omissions and rotations in subjects from 20 to 102, but they account for very low percentage of the variance (1%). Our multiple regression results gave a gender effect only on distortions, made by healthy subjects.

5. Conclusions

The basic objective of this paper was to analyze the performance of constructive and visuospatial tasks in healthy and in CIND subjects.

The results confirm our hypothesis about significant differences in the level of performance in drawing and construction between persons with CIND and normally aging individuals over 60 years.

We found a prevalence of omissions and distortions in the error profile of CIND and significant difference between CIND and normal aging regarding these two types of errors.

In both diagnostic groups, age of participants showed a significant effect on BVRT omissions, when fluid intelligence, education, and gender were also considered.

Results proved discriminative sensitivity of BVRT general scoring criteria and the separate error types (omissions and distortions) in the preclinical stages of dementia.

We tested a modification of Moore and Wike [52] scoring system for house and cube drawing task in elders, and this study confirmed its diagnostic sensitivity. Drawing of cube and house could be used for quick screening of CIND in subjects over 60.

Results from the principal component analysis (oblimin rotation) reaffirmed the multicomponent structure of the visuospatial and constructive abilities in old age.

The main limitation of this study is the small number of participants with complete neuropsychological testing and the lack of detailed clinical and neuroimaging examination. For the future, it might be interesting to carry out a similar analysis using more detailed description of subjects, including neuroimaging with functional MRT that could give the possibility to conclude about brain structures involved in different task performance.

Author details

Radka Ivanova Massaldjieva

Address all correspondence to: rapsy_99@yahoo.com

Health Care Management Department, Centre for Translational Neuroscience, Medical University, Plovdiv, Bulgaria

References

[1] Harada CN, Natelson Love MC, Triebel K. Normal cognitive aging. Clinics in Geriatric Medicine. 2013;**29**(4):737-752. DOI: 10.1016/j.cger.2013.07.002

[2] Berg L. Does Alzheimer's disease represent an exaggeration of normal aging? Archives of Neurology. 1985;**42**(8):737-739

[3] American Psychiatric Association. Diagnostic and Statistical Manual of Mental Disorders. 4th ed. (DSM-IV) Washington (DC): American Psychiatric Association; 1994. 675 p

[4] American Psychiatric Association. Diagnostic and Statistical Manual of Mental Disorders. 4th ed. Text Revision (DSM-IV-TR) Washington, DC: American Psychiatric Association; 2000

[5] Bischkopf J, Busse A, Angermeyer M. Mild cognitive impairment – A review of prevalence, incidence and outcome according to current approaches. Acta Psychiatrica Scandinavica. 2002;**106**:403-414

[6] Gottfries C, Lehmann W, Regland B. Early diagnosis of cognitive impairment in the elderly with the focus on AD. Journal of Neural Transmission. 1988;**105**(8-9):773-786

[7] World Health Organization The ICD-10 classification of mental and behavioural disorders: Clinical descriptions and diagnostic guidelines. Geneva: World health Organization; 1992

[8] Costa PT, Williams T F, Albert MS, Butters NM, Folstein MF, Gilman S, Gurland BJ, Gwyther LP, Heyman a, Kasrzniak AW, Katz IR, Levy LL, Lombardo NE, Orr-Rainey NK, Phillips LR, Storandt M, Tangalos EG, Wykle ML. Recognition and initial assessment of alzheimer's disease and related dementias: Alzheimer's disease and related dementias guideline panel. Rockvill: Department of Health and Human Services; 1996. 143 p

[9] Golomb J, Kluger A, Ferris S, Garrard P. Clinician's Manual on Mild Cognitive Impairment. London: Science Press; 2001. 277p

[10] Darby D, Maruff P, Collie A, McStephen M. Mild cognitive impairment can be detected by multiple assessments in a single day. Neurology. 2002;**59**:1042-1046

[11] DeCarli Ch. MCI: Prevalence, prognosis, aetiology and treatment. Lancet: Neurology. 2003;**2**:15-21

[12] Henderson S. Early detection. In: Copeland J, Abou-Saleh M, Blazer D, editors. Principle and Practice of Geriatric Psychiatry. Chichester: Wiley; 2002. pp. 191-194

[13] Larrieu S, Letenneur L,Orgogozo J, Fabrigoule C, Amieva, H, Le Carret N, Barberger-Gateau P, Dartigues J. Incidence and Outcome of mild cognitive impairment in a population-based prospective cohort. Neurology. 2002;**59**:1594-1599

[14] Rivas-Vazquez R, Mendez C, Rey G. MCI: New neuropsychological and pharmacological target. Archives of Clinical Neuropsychology. 2002;**596**:1-17

[15] Ritchie K, Touchon J. Mild cognitive impairment: Conceptual basis and current nosological status. The Lancet. 2000;**355**:225-228

[16] Busse A, Bischkopf J, Riedel-Heller S, Argermeyer M. MCI: Prevalence and predictive validity according to current approaches. Acta Neurologica Scandinavica. 2003;**108**: 71-86

[17] Henderson, A. Dementia. Geneva: World Health Organization; 1994. 65 p

[18] Lopez O, Jagust W, DeKosky S. Prevalence and classification of MCI in the Cardiovascular health Study: Cognition Study, Part 1. Archives of Neurology. 2003;**60**:1385-1389

[19] Spinnler H, Della Solo S. The role of clinical neuropsychology in the neurological diagnosis of Alzheimer disease. Journal of Neurology. 1988;**235**:255-271

[20] Welsh-Bolmer K, Madden D. Benign senescent forgetfulness, age-associated memory impairment and age related cognitive decline. In: Copeland J, Abou-Saleh M, Blazer D, editors. Principle and Practice of Geriatric Psychiatry. Chichester: Wiley; 2011. pp. 303-305

[21] Blossom CM S, Matthews F, Khaw KT, Dufouil C, Brayne C. Beyond mild cognitive impairment: vascular cognitive impairment, no dementia (VCIND). Alzheimer's Research & Therapy. 2009;**1**(1):4. DOI: 10.1186/alzrt4

[22] Frisoni G, Galluzzi S, Bresciani L, Zanetti O, Geroldi C. MCI with subcortical vascular features. Journal of Neurology. 2002;**249**:1423-1432

[23] Petersen RC, Smith GE, Waring SC, Ivnik R, Tangalos E, Kokmen E. Mild cognitive impairment: Clinical characterization and outcome. Archives of Neurology. 1999;**56**:303-308. [PubMed]

[24] Chertkow H, Massoud F, Nasreddine Z, Belleville S, Joanette Y, Bocti C, Drolet V, Kirk J, Freedman M, Bergman H. Mild cognitive impairment and cognitive impairment, no dementia: Part A, concept and diagnosis. Canadian Medical Association Journal. 2008;**178**(10):1273-1285. DOI:10.1503/cmaj.070797

[25] Plassman BL, Langa KM, Fisher GG, et al. Prevalence of cognitive impairment without dementia in the United States. Annals of Internal Medicine. 2008;**148**:427-434. PMC 2670458

[26] Plassman BL, Langa KM, McCammon RJ, Fisher GG, Potter GG, Burke JR, Steffens DC, Foster NL, Giordani B, Unverzagt FW, Welsh-Bohmer KA, Heeringa SG, Weir DR, Wallace RB. Incidence of dementia and cognitive impairment not dementia in the United States. Annals of Neurology. 2011;**70**(3):418-426. DOI:10.1002/ana.22362

[27] Metcalfe J. Psychological aspects of ageing. In: Metcalfe J, editor. The Brain: Degeneration, Damage and Disorder. Berlin: Springer; 1998. p. 37-67

[28] Chertkow H, Nasreddine Z, Joanette Y, Drolet V, Kirk J, Massoud F, Belleville S, Bergman H. Diagnosis and treatment of dementia: 3. Mild cognitive impairment and cognitive impairment without dementia: Part A, concept and diagnosis. Alzheimer's and Dementia. 2007;**3**:266-282. DOI:10.1016/j.jalz.2007.07.013

[29] Blazer DG, Yaffe K, Liverman CT, editors. Cognitive Aging: Progress in Understanding and Opportunities for Action/Committee on the Public Health Dimensions of Cognitive Aging, Board on Health Sciences Policy, Institute of Medicine of the National Academies. Washington, DC: The National Academies Press; 2015. 330 p. [PubMed]

[30] Cattell RB. Theory of fluid and crystallized intelligence: A critical experiment. Journal of Educational Psychology. 1963;**54**:1-22. DOI:10.1037/h0046743

[31] Murman DL. The impact of age on cognition. Seminars in Hearing. 2015;**36**(3):111-121. DOI: 10.1055/s-0035-1555115

[32] Hartshorne J, Germine L. When does cognitive functioning peak? The asynchronous rise and fall of different cognitive abilities across the lifespan. Psychological Science. 2015;**26**(4):433-443. DOI:10.1177/0956797614567339

[33] Salthouse T. When does age-related cognitive decline begin? Neurobiology of Aging. 2009;**30**(4):507-514. DOI: 10.1016/j.neurobiolaging.2008.09.023

[34] Salthouse TA. Selective review of cognitive aging. Journal of the International Neuropsychological Society. 2010;**16**:754-760. DOI: 10.1017/S1355617710000706

[35] Whitley E, Deary IJ, Ritchie, SJ, Batty GD, Kumari M, Benzeval M. Variations in cognitive abilities across the life course: Cross-sectional evidence from understanding society: The UK household longitudinal study. Intelligence. 2016;**59**:39-50. DOI: 10.1016/j.intell.2016.07.001

[36] Rabbitt P, Lowe C. Patterns of cognitive ageing. Psychological Research. 2000;**63**(3-4): 308-316

[37] Duncan J, Burgess P, Emslie H. Fluid intelligence after frontal lobe lesions. Neuro-psychologia. 1995;**33**(3):261-268

[38] Kramer AF, Fabiani M, Colcombe SJ. Contributions of cognitive neuroscience to the understanding of behavior and aging. In: Birren JE, Schaie KW, editors. Handbook of the Psychology of Aging. 6th ed. Amsterdam: Elsevier; 2006. p. 57-83

[39] Thurstone LL. Theories of intelligence. The Scientific Monthly. 1946;**62**(2):101-112

[40] Lloyd P, Mayes A. Introduction to Psychology: An Integrated Approach. London: Diamond; 1999. 815 p

[41] Gardner H. Intelligence Reframed: Multiple Intelligences for the 21st Century. New York: Basic Books; 1999. 304p

[42] Rust J, Golombok S. Modern Psychometrics. London: Routledge; 1995. 247p

[43] Mapou RL. A cognitive framework for neuropsychological assessment. In: Mapou R, Spector J, editors. Clinical Neuropsychological Assessment: A Cognitive Approach. New York: Plenum; 1995. p. 295-338

[44] De Bruin N, Devon CB, Jessica NM, Claudia LRG. Assessing visuospatial abilities in healthy aging: A novel visuomotor task frontiers in aging neuroscience. 2016;**8**:7. DOI: 10.3389/fnagi.2016.00007

[45] Techentin C, Voyer D, Voyer SD. Spatial abilities and aging: A meta-analysis. Experimental Aging Research. 2014;**40**(4):395-425

[46] Benton AL, Fogel ML. Three-dimensional constructional praxis: A clinical test. Archives of Neurology.1962;**7**:109-116

[47] Capruso DX, Hamsher K, Benton AL. Assessment of visuocognitive processes. In: Mapou R, Spector J, editors. Clinical Neuropsychological Assessment: A Cognitive Approach. New York: Plenum; 1995. p. 137-183

[48] Forsti H, Burns A, Levy R, Cairns N. Neuropathological basis for drawing disability (constructional apraxia) in Alzheimer's disease. Psychological Medicine. 1993;**23**: 623-629

[49] Bradshaw JL, Mattingley JB. Clinical Neuropsychology. San Diego: Academic Press; 1995. 569 p

[50] Flicker Ch, Ferris S, Reisberg B. A two-year longitudinal study of cognitive function in normal aging and Alzheimer's disease. Journal of Geriatric Psychiatry. 1993;**6**:84-96

[51] Grossi D, Trojano L. Constructional and visuospatial disorders. In: Behrmann M, editor. Disorders of visual behavior. Amsterdam: Elsevier; 2001. p. 99-120

[52] Moore V, Wyke M. Drawing disability in patients with senile dementia. Psychological Medicine. 1984;**14**:97-105

[53] Gragnaniello D, Kessler J, Bley M, Mielke R. Copying and drawing in Alzheimer patients with different stages of dementia. Der Nervenarzt. 1998;**69**:991-998

[54] Lezak MD. Neuropsychological assessment. 3rd ed. New York: Oxford University Press; 1995. 843 p

[55] Benton AL. Constructional apraxia: Some unanswered questions. In: Benton AL, editor. Contributions to clinical neuropsychology. Chicago: The Aldine; 1969. p.129-142

[56] Kirk A, Kertesz A. On drawing impairment in Alzheimer's disease. Archives of Neurology. 1991;**1**:73-77

[57] Pelissier C, Roudier M, Boller F. Factorial validation of the severe impairment battery for patients with Alzheimer's disease. Dementia and Geriatric Cognitive Disorders, 2002;**13**: 95-100

[58] Rascovsky K, Salmon D, Ho G, Galasco D, Peavy G, Hansen L, Thal L. Cognitive profiles differ in autopsy-confirmed frontotemporal dementia and AD. Neurology. 2002;**58** (12):1801-1808

[59] Fillenbaum G, Heyman A, Williams K, Prosnitz B, Burchett B. Sensitivity and specificity of standardized screens of cognitive impairment and dementia among elderly black and white community residents. Journal of Clinical Epidemiology. 1990;**43**(7):651-660

[60] Folstein MF, Folstein SE, McHugh PR. "Mini-mental state": A practical method for grading the cognitive state of patients for the clinician. Journal of Psychiatric Research. 1975;**12**(3):189-198. [PubMed]

[61] Folstein M, Folstein S, McHugh P. MMSE (Bulgarian version). In: Jablenski A, editor. SKAN. 2nd ed. Sofia: FNP; 1996. p. 183-186

[62] Morris RG, Worsley C, Matthews D. Neuropsychological assessment in older people: Old principles and new directions. Advances in Psychiatric Treatment. 2006;6:362-372. DOI: 10.1192/apt.6.5.362

[63] Goldman HH, Skodol AE, Lave TR. Revising axis V for DSM-IV: A review of measures of social functioning. American Journal of Psychiatry. 1992;149:1148-1156

[64] Benton AL. Der Benton-Test: Handbuch. Bern et al.: Hans Huber; 1972. 136 p

[65] Raven J, Raven JC, Court JH. Manual for Raven's progressive matrices and vocabulary scales. Section 3, Standard progressive matrices (including the Parallel and Plus versions) Oxford: OPP Ltd; 2000

[66] Raven JC. Guide to the Standard Progressive Matrices. London: H. K. Lewis; 1960

[67] Kokoshkarova A. Hamburg-Wechsler-Intelligenztest fur Erwachsene (HAWIE). Bern: Hans Huber; 1955. Bulgarian adaptation (1979)

[68] Deary IJ, Corley J, Gow AJ, Harris SE Houlihan LM, Marioni RE, Penke L, Rafnsson SB, Starr JM Age-associated cognitive decline. British Medical Bulletin. 2009;92(1):135-152. DOI: https://doi.org/10.1093/bmb/ldp033

[69] Guerin F, Ska B, Belleville S. Cognitive processing of drawing abilities. Brain and Cognition. 1999;40:464-478

[70] Coman E, Moses JA, Jr, Kraemer HC, Friedman L, Benton AL, Yesavage J. Interactive influences on BVRT performance level: Geriatric considerations. Archives of Clinical Neuropsychology. 2002;17:595-610

[71] Jacqmin-Gadda H, Fabrigoule C, Commenges D, Letenneur L, Dartigues JF. A cognitive screening battery for dementia in the elderly. Journal of Clinical Epidemiology. 2000;53:980-987

[72] Shichita K, Hatano S, Ohashi Y, Shibata H, Matuzaki T. Memory changes in the BVRT between ages 70 and 75. Journal of Gerontology. 1986;41(3):385-386

[73] Arenberg D. Differences and changes with age in the BVRT. Journal of Gerontology. 1978;33(4):534-540

[74] Resnik SM, Trotman K, Kawas C, Zonderman AB. Age associated changes in specific errors on the Benton visual retention test. Journal of Gerontology: Psychological Sciences. 1995;50B(3):171-178

3

Adherence to Medication in Older Adults as a Way to Improve Health Outcomes and Reduce Healthcare System Spending

Luís Midão, Anna Giardini, Enrica Menditto,
Przemyslaw Kardas and Elísio Costa

Abstract

Medications are used as the primary approach to prevent and effectively manage the chronic conditions. Non-adherence to medication is recognized as a worldwide public health problem with important implications for the management of chronic diseases, which affects every level of the population, particularly older adults due to the high number of coexisting diseases and consequent polypharmacy. Estimated rates of adherence to long-term medication regimen are of about 50%, and there is no evidence for significant changes in the past 50 years. The consequences of non-adherence include poor clinical outcomes, increased morbidity and mortality and unnecessary healthcare costs. Factors contributing to non-adherence are multifaceted and embrace those that are related to patients, to physicians and to healthcare systems. Cognitive, sensorial and functional decline, poor social support, anxiety, depression symptomatology and reduced health literacy have been linked to medication non-adherence in the elderly patients. Many interventions to improve medication adherence have been described in the study for different clinical conditions; however, most interventions seem to fail in their aims. In this chapter, a revision of the implications of poor adherence as well as its predictors and available tools to improve adherence is performed.

Keywords: adherence, compliance, persistence, concordance, health literacy, healthcare, elderly

1. Introduction

One of the greatest achievements of mankind in the last century was the increase in average life expectancy, mainly due to advances in public health, technology and medicine. While the twentieth century was the century of population growth, the twenty-first century will be known as the century of aging [1, 2].

Every second, two people celebrate their 60th anniversary [3]. Globally, in 2015, there were 901 million people who were 60 or older, most of whom are the elderly people living in developing countries. This number is expected to be more than double by 2050, reaching 2.1 billion (20% of total population). Interestingly, the number of people aged 80 or older is growing even faster than the elderly in general. By 2015, about 14% of the elderly population (125 million) were 80 or older, and that number is expected to triple by 2050, reaching 434 million (approximately 20% of the senior population) [4].

The speed at which the population is aging is dramatically increasing. For example, France needed 150 years to adapt from a change from 10 to 20% of the population over 60 years. However, developing countries such as India and Brazil have little more than 20 years to adapt to this reality [5]. In these countries, in 2010–2015, the average life expectancy was 68 years, but 78 years in the developed countries [3].

The increase in average life expectancy turns out to be an opportunity for older people and their families. With these extra years, the elderly can devote themselves to school again, can pursue a new career or can chase a lost passion [6]. But all of this depends on one key factor: health. WHO defined health as "a state of complete physical, mental and social well-being and not merely the absence of disease or infirmity" [7].

From the biological point of view, aging occurs due to accumulation of damages, at both cellular and molecular levels. Telomeres are shortened as we age. Aging is characterized by changes in physical appearance such as gradual reduction in height and weight, due to loss of muscle and bone mass, higher reaction times, decline in memory, decreased sexual activity, reduced metabolic rate and a decline in auditory, olfactory and vision functions, as well as diminished lung, immune and renal functions. The speed at which aging occurs is determined by genetic and environmental factors [8]. Physical and social environments, as well as personal characteristics such as gender, ethnicity and socioeconomic status, are factors that affect the aging process from an early age. The environment has a huge influence on both the development and the maintenance of healthy habits. Lifelong healthy behaviors, in terms of diet, exercise and habits, contribute to the prevention of certain diseases [9].

Although this increase in average life expectancy is worthy of celebration, it must be borne in mind that increasing longevity has long-term consequences not only for health but for the health system and for economy too. There are health conditions that are associated with the increase in the elderly population. Cardiovascular diseases, cancer, chronic respiratory diseases and diabetes, the so-called non-communicable diseases are responsible for nearly 60% of the deaths, and they all share an unmodifiable risk factor such as age [10].

The major cause of death among the elderly in developed countries is cardiovascular diseases, accounting for 35% of all deaths [11]. Along with these diseases, cancer is the other major cause of mortality, being responsible for 22% of deaths [12].

The development of these chronic diseases occurs in several ways. There are malignancies such as lung or prostate cancer that are more common in the elderly population. An example of this condition is arthritis that may be present early but only with age it worsens and it manifests due to the senescence of the body in general. There are diseases that turn out to be a combination of the two factors, as with chronic respiratory disease, doubling its prevalence for each decade of life after the 40 years [2].

Usually, older adults have multiple medical problems. Almost 50% of the elderly population has at least three chronic diseases, and of this, approximately 10% has five or more. These diseases can coexist for several reasons such as by random chance, because they are part of the same continuum, because they have risk factors in common or because one triggered the other [2]. Aging and comorbidities together increase the risk of hospitalization and mortality.

This "demographic time bomb" has direct consequences for the economy. With the increase of lifetime expectancy, more people are claiming for pensions, and less number of people are working and paying taxes, which will have an impact on national budgets. The economic growth will also be affected since higher savings for pensions may lead to the reducing of capital investments. At the same time, age-related diseases, comorbidities and geriatric syndromes are gaining attention in society, increasing the demand for health services. The elderly people require more health services, suffer more hospitalizations and occupy the bed longer than any other age group, thus increasing the money spent on healthcare [13].

The main way to treat chronic illnesses is by using medicines. Although they are a powerful tool, its potential is not fully used, since half of the patients do not take them as prescribed, meaning they either do not take them or they do, but in the wrong dosage or in the wrong timing, failing to realize full benefits of treatments [14, 15]. Non-adherence is a huge problem that is directly linked with an increase in morbidity and mortality, costing between $100 and 300 billion per year, in the United States (**Figure 1**) [16].

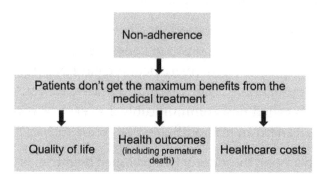

Figure 1. Non-adherence consequences.

2. Medical adherence taxonomy

"Drugs don't work in patients who don't take them" is the often-cited statement of Surgeon General of the United States C. Everett Koop (1985). Non-adherence is the major problem for pharmacotherapy in ambulatory patients. It is more prevalent than would be expected. It is highly associated with increased morbidity and mortality, and is an aspect that until recently was neglected. Despite its importance and all the efforts that have been made to understand it, non-adherence is still misunderstood. This behavior, in addition to the direct effects on the patient, since it compromises the preservation and the quality of her/his life, also has economic consequences. Therefore, in recent years, therapeutic adherence has been extensively studied from pharmacological, behavioral, economical perspectives [17]. Despite all the studies, the lack of uniformity in the methods of analysis and the absence of a universal taxonomy/terminology are a major obstacle when making/analyzing systematic reviews, as it makes it difficult to draw conclusions.

Compliance, adherence, concordance and *persistence* are the four widely used terms that have been used interchangeably. *Adherence* and *compliance*, the mostly used terms have different connotations in the patient's attitude regarding medication. *Compliance* comes from the Latin word *complire*, meaning to fulfil a promise/to complete an action, implying that the patient has a passive role on the process. *Adherence* derives from the Latin word *adhaerere*, which means remain constant, keep close, having the patient agreed with the prescription [15, 18, 19]. Of the other two terms, *Concordance* implies that the patient and the professional healthcare came to an agreement about the treatment that the patient should follow, acknowledging that they may have different points of view, while *persistence* relates to the time interval between the first and the last dose of medicine [19–21].

Given this heterogeneity, it was necessary to obtain a consensus on the terminology and taxonomy in the field of non-adherence. The ABC project (Ascertaining Barriers to Compliance) was created under the seventh Framework Program, and the main objective was to provide consensus taxonomy and terminology in non-adherence medication and to provide concise and adequate definitions that could serve the needs of both clinical research and medical practice [22].

Medication adherence is defined as an active, cooperative and voluntary participation of the patient in following recommendations from a healthcare provider. This is a multifactorial behavior that involves three critical steps (**Figure 2**).

Management of adherence has a main purpose to increase the benefit to the patient, and minimize the risk of harm, caused by the medication. It encompasses healthcare systems, providers, patients and their family/friend's networks, and serves to monitor and support patient's adherence to medication [22].

Adherence-related sciences include all the disciplines that study the causes and consequences of non-adherence, including medicine, nursing, sociology, biostatistics, pharmacy, behavioral science, pharmacometrics and health economics [19].

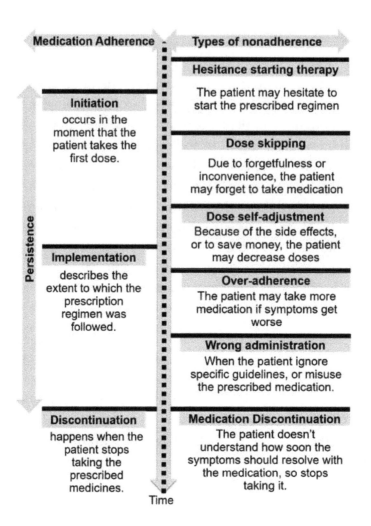

Figure 2. The ABC taxonomy of medication adherence describing its three key elements and demonstrating how patients can deviate.

The ABC taxonomy relies on these three elements, making a clear distinction between procedures that describe actions through routines that have been established (*medication adherence* and *management of adherence*) and the sciences that study those procedures (*adherence-related sciences*) [22].

Of note, currently, the use of compliance has diminished, as this very term, for historical reasons, mostly, was perceived as the one that implies paternalistic relation between the doctor and patients. Therefore, this term is not advised by the ABC taxonomy.

3. Determinants of non-adherence

Non-adherence to therapy is a public health problem in general, with a special focus on the elderly population. Non-adherence causes the patient outcome to be compromised, resulting in decreased effective disease control, increased risk of hospitalization and increased morbidity and mortality [23].

To improve the adherence, we must first understand the causes, predictors and determinants responsible for non-adherence. Many of them have been described so far [24]. According to WHO, there are five large sets of factors by which people are non-adherent (**Figure 3**) [25]:

- socioeconomic factors;

- health system related;

- therapy related;

- patient related; and

- condition related.

The socioeconomic status is correlated with adherence to therapy. Of these factors, the professional situation, social support, housing conditions, distance to treatment, transportation and medication prices as well as social inequalities are the utmost importance. The existence of support provided either by the family or by friends has a very positive influence on adherence. The lack of involvement of family and friends leads to a state of social isolation, which is one of the determinants of non-adherence [26]. The professional situation is also important, since people with economic difficulties must set priorities in budget management, with food and housing being the first, often leaving the medication to second option [22].

The relationship between health professionals and patients is extremely important in adherence, since they play a critical role of technical and psychosocial support, giving the individual the basic skills to adhere to medication, developing beliefs about his/her ability to deliver on medications and on the benefits of therapy. However, the lack of knowledge and availability of health professionals, the overloading of health services, which translates into difficulties in access to consultations and the short duration of these, the lack of capacity of the system to promote psychoeducational programs, and the inexistence of follow-up mechanisms are some of the causes responsible for non-adherence [23]. Perhaps, there is a need to adapt the arrangements of the healthcare services to the needs of the growing number of old and very old persons.

The duration of, and the complexity of drug regimens may have consequences for adherence to therapy, since the longer and more difficult the treatment is, the greater the likelihood of discontinuation. Thus, it is necessary to develop simpler schemes, which require small changes in living habits, facilitating adherence. However, these are not the only characteristics on medication that lead to non-adherence. Side effects of some medications, including nausea, vomiting, fatigue and other metabolic changes as well as drug-drug interactions or adverse reactions to medications may also lead to treatment withdrawal [15, 23].

The cognitive and intellectual characteristics of the patients, as well as their personality and behaviour, and their knowledge of the disease and treatment and their motivation are the determinants related to the patient, which lead to non-adherence. To adhere, the patient must understand what is transmitted to him/her and understand the reason for the prescription.

Thus, it is important to focus on health literacy, understood as the ability of individuals to make healthy decisions based on the information provided. Since, adherence is a decision made by the individual based on their beliefs about the consequences of adherence to therapy, when the patients recognize that they have a responsibility to their health and that their behaviour may bring benefits, which improves adherence [15].

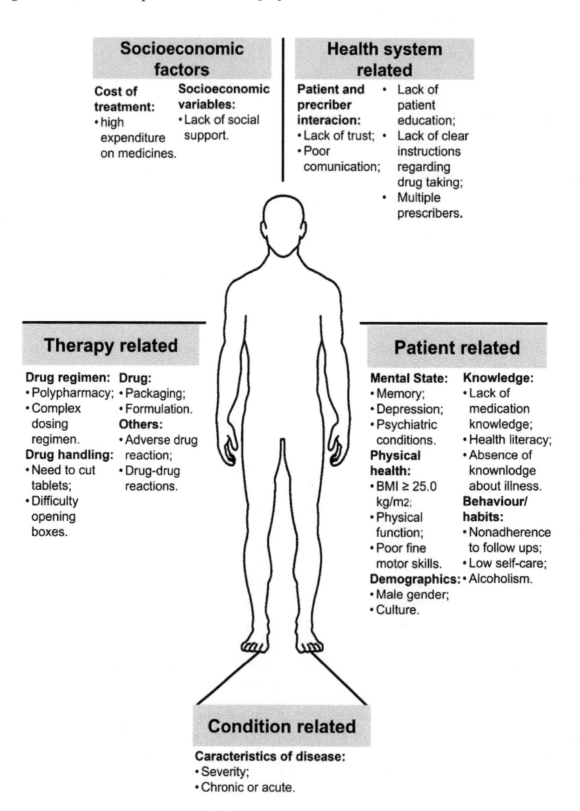

Figure 3. Predictors of non-adherence to medication, modified from WHO [25].

The characteristics of the disease such as severity and the symptomatic/asymptomatic nature are factors related to the condition that affects adherence. It is considered that the severity of the disease and the disability that symptoms cause at physical, psychological and social levels are most frequently associated with non-adherence. Individuals with chronic asymptomatic diseases do not adhere to treatment frequently, since the absence of symptoms lower their motivation to take their drugs continuously. In addition, the existence of other concomitant diseases that are treated with various medications (i.e., polypharmacy) is also one of the major factors that contribute to non-adherence [17, 25, 27].

4. Costs associated with non-adherence

With the increase of life expectancy, the greater the spending on health. Accord-ing to an OECD study, people over 65 accounts for 40–50% of health spending in Europe and their per capita costs are 3–5 times higher than those under 65. And, this tends to increase over time [28].

There are not many researches that investigate the impact of non-adherence on the economy, since it is difficult to assess. In addition to the direct impact on both patient health and non-adherence healthcare costs such as avoidable hospitalizations, emergencies, drugs, and so on, non-adherence leads to an indirect impact on the economy. In fact, per year, non-adherence leads to an average of 2.62 days that the employee missed work, leading to a decrease in the productivity [29]. Moreover, few articles focus on the costs of non-adherence among the elderly. The following paragraphs review the costs of non-adherence in several diseases that often affect the elderly such as chronic cardiovascular diseases, chronic obstructive pulmonary disease, diabetes, arthritis, and osteoporosis.

Will et al., in 2016, found that hospitalizations were eight times more frequent in non-adherent hypertension patients. Expenditures with these patients were four times higher compared to adherent patients. According to the author's estimates, in the United States of America, the outcome of non-adherence was $ 41 million, over 3 million for non-adherent hypertensive patients, over a period of 8 years. These costs were related to the cost of outpatient medication and preventable hospitalizations [30].

Bansilal et al., in 2016, studied the association between the levels of adherence and long-term major adverse cardiovascular events and resource utilization in coronary artery disease patients. The authors found that non-adherent patients have higher associated medical costs, with $ 719 associated with hospitalizations per patient and $ 821 associated with revascular-ization surgeries, being these patients also related to higher emergency visits. Thus, it is pos-sible to deduce that non-adherence to treatments, in addition to the risk to the patient, leads to increases in expenses associated with secondary cardiac events [31].

In congestive heart failure, Esposito et al., in 2009, assessed the impact that adherence to therapy would have on the related costs in patients with congestive heart failure. Non-adherent patients (17,496 compared to 19,122 adherent patients) had higher costs for the health system (US$ 25,312 compared to US$ 19,402 for adherent patients), mainly explained by the increase in hospital admissions (42% of the total value), in terms of higher frequency/duration compared to adherent patients [32].

Simoni-Watilla et al., in 2012, demonstrated that adherent patients with chronic obstructive pulmonary disease had higher costs related to prescription medications than non-adherent patients. However, these were cost-effective since the adherent patients have much lower costs than the non-adherent patients, in terms of hospitalizations and outpatient [33]. Halpern et al., in 2011, drew the same conclusions. Although pharmacy costs were higher in adherent patients, non-adherent patients incurred higher total expenditures [34].

Ho et al., in 2006, evaluated the impact of non-adherence in Type 2 Diabetes. Higher HbA$_1$c, blood pressure and LDL cholesterol levels were recorded in non-adherent patients, leading to the increased risk of mortality and morbidity. The economic impact of non-adherence is continually increasing, resulting in long-term complications [35]. Dall et al., in 2010, estimated that $ 218 billion per year (indirect costs spent for treating diabetes) spent in the USA. Although the cost of treating diabetes is high, representing approximately 7% of health spending, the return on this investment is enormous. Per year, non-insulin and non-antihyperglycemic drugs, insulin and oral hyperglycemic agents cost $ 776, while avoidable hospitalizations cost $ 886 per patient [36].

Tang et al., in 2008, found that arthritis adherent patients have higher costs in the pharmacy than non-adherent patients. However, costs related to outpatient, inpatient and laboratory services, related to non-adherence, exceed the amount spent in the pharmacy [37]. Pasma et al., in 2017, demonstrated that decreased adherence leads to an increase in healthcare costs (in anti-TNF therapies, synthetic DMARDs and rheumatology outpatients) [38].

In osteoporosis, poor adherence reduces the potential effectiveness of the drug, resulting in decreased health outcomes and incurring heavy costs. Hiligsmann et al., in 2009 evaluated the economic outcome of non-adherence in osteoporosis patients. Non-adherent patients suffer from more fractures than adherent patients, leading to higher healthcare spending, in comparison to the costs associated with medication adherence [39].

In general, all adherent patients have higher drug costs for obvious reasons. However, in the long run, they incur lower expenses than the non-adherent patients, since visits to the emergency rooms, inpatient and outpatient are decreased [40]. One of the reasons that lead the elderly to non-adherence is the high price of medicines. For pensioners with poor retirement, they must manage the budget to pay for basic needs, being in the medicines no longer a priority [41]. One of the ways to overcome this problem is to increase support for the elderly in the purchase of medicines or to reduce their taxes. Although this will mean higher expenses initially, it will pay off in the long-term [42].

5. Interventions to promote adherence

To improve adherence to therapy in the elderly, there are many questions that need to be addressed and deserve all the attention, once they are the basis for deciding what course to take (**Figure 4**) [43].

Socioeconomic factors:

• Is the patient able to care for himself? Does he have some family/friends support?

Health care system factors:

• Is the patient on polypharmacy? Is the shared patient record available to allow all the healthcare professionals in need to check which medicines is the patient taking?
• Has the patient enough health literacy?

Health care providers factors:

• Is the healthcare team aware of problems that the patient is facing at home with drug taking?
• Has the patient approached the health care team demonstrating the trust that he has on them?

Medication factors:

• Does the medication need to be cut?
• Has the patient any adverse reaction to the drug?
• Are there any chances to simplify the regimen?

Patient factors:

• How is the patient's knowledge about his medicines and disease?
• Is the patient able to handle his own medication?
• Is the patient willing to take his medicines?

Figure 4. Questions to be addressed to the patient to choose how adherence can be improved.

Just as there are many reasons for a patient to not adhere to the therapy, there is no single solution to this problem. Interventions should be planned and appropriate to each patient, since each patient is unique, with her/his particularities and specificities. Therefore, health professionals should develop strategies that focus not only on the problem of adherence to therapy but also on all aspects that have directly or indirectly influenced it. The intervention of health professionals, to promote behavioural changes, should be based on the creation of a link with the patient and the informal care provider, through the establishment of an empathic relationship, always considering the sociocultural characteristics and the need for social support [12, 14].

To improve adherence, educational and behavioural interventions are needed. Educational interventions are simple measures that promote knowledge regarding both illness and medication and allow the provision of individual and/or group information, whether through oral, written, audiovisual and/or computerized transmission. To avoid barriers between the health professional and the patient, the language should be clear and objective, in line with the patient's level of knowledge and easy to memorize. Educational interventions that involve the patient, relatives or caregivers, are promoters of changes in adherence to the therapeutic regimen. Moreover, communication between health professionals and patients is an extremely important step toward promoting adherence to treatment. The preparation of the patient for adherence must include health literacy, once patients with basic or below basic health literacy may be unable to understand what information the box and the medicine data sheet has. Also, the patient should be provided with all specific information about the treatment such as the objectives of the therapy, the risks and benefits and expected results as well as the consequences of adherence or non-adherence. Behavioural interventions aim to:

- Involve patients in treatment;
- Simplify therapeutic regimens;
- Facilitate compliance with proposed treatments;
- Incorporate adaptation mechanisms into daily practice; and
- Provide supporting documentation and reward for improved adherence [14].

Patients should be actively involved in their treatment using strategies to prevent non-adherence. For that, the medicinal regimen should be changed as little as possible, since it interferes with the memorization, leading to forgetfulness and, consequently, non-adherence. Medical or nursing appointments are used to communicate or advise the patient and his/her family, keeping them informed of progress and results [15].

Counselling includes information about the drugs, their indications, side effects and how to overcome them. To encourage adherence to therapy, health professionals can use the following strategies [25]:

- listen to the patient;
- ask the patient to repeat the actions he/she should take;
- provide clear instructions as to drug taking, preferably in writing;
- propose a simpler therapeutic regimen that considers patient routines;
- use methods of counting medicines taken;
- contact the patient if he or she misses an appointment;
- adapt the frequency of consultations according to the needs of the patients, always referring to the importance of adherence to the therapeutic regimen; and
- reinforce positive behaviours and involve the family in the process of adherence.

According to Osterberg and Blaschke [17], the methods to increase adherence to the therapeutic regimen can be grouped into four categories:

1. patient education;
2. communication between health professionals and the patient;

3. the posology and type of medicine; and

4. the availability of health services.

According to the WHO proposal, increased adherence is based on three measures:

1. adequate and continuous information;

2. training of health teams in motivational strategies; and

3. adoption and continued application of these strategies [25].

Regardless of the classification used, the improvement in therapeutic adherence passes through the link between information and motivation. Knowing the concepts about diseases and treatments may result in the adoption of long-lasting behaviours and attitudes that favour adherence to treatment by patients.

6. Concluding remarks

As the population is aging, people are more prone to chronic diseases. Pharmacotherapy is the best treatment to follow. Approximately, half of the elderly have at least three chronic diseases, which result in polypharmacy. Complicated drug delivery regimens cause the elderly to eventually give up treatment. Another reason for treatment discontinuation is the high prices of medicines. Failure to adhere to treatment has a negative impact not only on the patient's health, increasing the risk of morbidity and mortality, yet also on the sustainability of entire healthcare care systems, due to higher number of avoidable hospitalizations and emergency visits, and finally, on the economy.

Thus, it becomes mandatory to find a way to overcome this problem, and it is necessary to implement techniques that increase adherence. These changes start with patient education. Providing the patients with all the necessary information about their illness, treatment, prognosis, and the consequences of non-adherence is the prerequisite of the right decisions. However, this should be followed with the use of other adherence-targeting interventions, tailored to the individual needs.

Finally, more studies are needed in this area, as the impact of non-adherence to therapeutics by the elderly on the economy has not yet been fully unveiled.

Acknowledgments

This work received financial support from the European Union (FEDER funds POCI/01/0145/ FEDER/007728) and National Funds (FCT/MEC, Fundação para a Ciência e Tecnologia and Ministério da Educação e Ciência) under the Partnership Agreement PT2020 UID/MULTI/ 04378/2013.

Author details

Luís Midão[1], Anna Giardini[2], Enrica Menditto[3], Przemyslaw Kardas[4] and Elísio Costa[1*]

*Address all correspondence to: emcosta@ff.up.pt

1 UCIBIO, REQUIMTE and Faculty of Pharmacy, University of Porto, Porto, Portugal

2 Psychology Unit, Instituti Clinici Scientifici Maugeri Spa – Società Benefit, Care and Research Institute, IRCCS Montescano, Italy

3 School of Pharmacy, CIRFF/Center of Pharmacoeconomics, University of Naples Federico II, Naples, Italy

4 Department of Family Medicine, Medical University of Lodz, Lodz, Poland

References

[1] Lunenfeld B, Stratton P. The clinical consequences of an ageing world and preventive strategies. Best Practice & Research Clinical Obstetrics & Gynaecology. 2013;27(5):643-659. DOI: 10.1016/j.bpobgyn.2013.02.005

[2] Divo MJ, Martinez CH, Mannino DM. Ageing and the epidemiology of multimorbidity. European Respiratory Journal. 2014;44(4):1055-1068. DOI: 10.1183/09031936.00059814

[3] HelpAge International. Global Ageing Statistics [Internet]. Sep 22, 2017. Available from: http://www.helpage.org/resources/ageing-data/global-ageing-statistics/

[4] World Health Organization. World Population Ageing. 2015. DOI: ST/ESA/SER.A/390. http://www.un.org/en/development/desa/population/publications/pdf/ageing/WPA2015_Report.pdf

[5] World Health Organization. Global Health and Aging 2011. DOI: 11-7737. http://www.who.int/ageing/publications/global_health.pdf

[6] Breyer F, Costa-Font J, Felder S. Ageing, health, and healthcare. Oxford Review of Economic Policy. 2010;26(4):674-690. DOI: 10.1093/oxrep/grq032

[7] World Health Organization. Constitution of the world health organization. Basic Documents. 1946. DOI: 12571729. http://www.who.int/governance/eb/who_constitution_en.pdf

[8] Partridge L. The new biology of ageing. Philosophical Transactions of the Royal Society B. 2010;365:147-154. DOI: 10.1098/rstb.2009.0222

[9] Hernandez LM, Blazer DG. The Impact of Social and Cultural Environment on Health [Internet]. USA: National Academies Press; 2006. Available from: https://www.ncbi.nlm.nih.gov/books/NBK19924/ [Accessed: Oct 3, 2017]

[10] World Health Organization. Noncommunicable Diseases [Internet]. WHO. World Health Organization; 2017. Available from: http://www.who.int/mediacentre/factsheets/fs355/en/ [Accessed: Oct 3, 2017]

[11] Lionakis N. Hypertension in the elderly. World Journal of Cardiology. 2012;**4**(5):135. DOI: 10.4330/wjc.v4.i5.135

[12] Marengoni A, Monaco A, Costa E, Cherubini A, Prados-Torres A, Muth C, et al. Strategies to improve medication adherence in older persons: Consensus statement from the senior Italia Federanziani advisory board. Drugs and Aging. 2016;**33**(9):629-637. DOI: 10.1007/s40266-016-0387-9

[13] Marešová P, Mohelská H, Kuča K. Economics aspects of ageing population. Procedia Economics and Finance. 2015;**23**:534-538. DOI: 10.1016/S2212-5671(15)00492-X

[14] Costa E, Giardini A, Savin M, Menditto E, Lehane E, Laosa O, et al. Interventional tools to improve medication adherence: Review of literature. Patient Preference and Adherence. 2015;**9**:1303-1314. DOI: 10.2147/PPA.S87551

[15] Brown MT, Bussell JK. Medication adherence: WHO cares? Mayo Clinic Proceedings. 2011;**86**(4):304-314. DOI: 10.4065/mcp.2010.0575

[16] Bosworth HB, Granger BB, Mendys P, Brindis R, Burkholder R, Czajkowski SM, et al. Medication adherence: A call for action. American Heart Journal. 2011;**162**(3):412-424. DOI: 10.1016/j.ahj.2011.06.007

[17] Osterberg L, Blaschke T. Adherence to medication. The New England Journal of Medicine. 2005;**353**:487-497. DOI: 10.1056/NEJMra050100

[18] Aronson JK. Compliance, concordance, adherence. British Journal of Clinical Pharmacology. 2007;**63**(4):383-384. DOI: 10.1111/j.1365-2125.2007.02893.x

[19] Vrijens B, De Geest S, Hughes DA, Przemyslaw K, Demonceau J, Ruppar T, et al. A new taxonomy for describing and defining adherence to medications. British Journal of Clinical Pharmacology. 2012;**73**(5):691-705. DOI: 10.1111/j.1365-2125.2012.04167.x

[20] Cramer JA, Roy A, Burrell A, Fairchild CJ, Fuldeore MJ, Ollendorf DA, et al. Medication compliance and persistence: Terminology and definitions. Value in Health. 2008;**11**(1):44-47. DOI: 10.1111/j.1524-4733.2007.00213.x

[21] Hugtenburg JG, Timmers L, Elders PJM, Vervloet M, van Dijk L. Definitions, variants, and causes of nonadherence with medication: A challenge for tailored interventions. Patient Preference and Adherence. 2013;**7**:675-682. DOI: 10.2147/PPA.S29549

[22] Ascertaining Barriers for Compliance: Policies for safe, effective and cost-effective use of medicines in Europe. ABC Project Final Report. 2012. http://abcproject.eu/img/abc%20final.pdf

[23] Martin LR, Williams SL, Haskard KB, Dimatteo MR. The challenge of patient adherence. Therapeutics and clinical risk management. 2005 Sep;**1**(3):189-199

[24] Kardas P, Lewek P, Matyjaszczyk M. Determinants of patient adherence: A review of systematic reviews. Frontiers in Pharmacology. 2013;**4**:1-16. DOI: 10.3389/fphar.2013.00091

[25] WHO. Adherence To long-TermTherapies: Evidence for action. World Health Organization; 2003. DOI: 10.1016/S1474-5151(03)00091-4

[26] Miller TA, Dimatteo MR. Importance of family/social support and impact on adherence to diabetic therapy. Diabetes, Metabolic Syndrome, and Obesity: Targets and Therapy. 2013; **6**:421-426. DOI: 10.2147/DMSO.S36368

[27] Stewart D, Mair A, Wilson M, Kardas P, Lewek P, Alonso A, et al. Guidance to manage inappropriate polypharmacy in older people: Systematic review and future developments. Expert Opinion on Drug Safety. 2017 Nov 25;**16**(2):203-213. DOI: 10.1080/147403 38.2017.1265503

[28] La Maisonneuve CD, Martins JO. Public spending on health and long-term care: A new set of projections. Vol. 6. OECD Economic Policy Papers. 2013. https://www.oecd.org/ eco/growth/Health%20FINAL.pdf

[29] Rizzo JA, Simons WR. Variations in compliance among hypertensive patients by drug class: Implications for healthcare costs. Clinical Therapeutics. 1997;**19**(6):1446-1457. DOI: 10.1016/ S0149-2918(97)80018-5

[30] Will JC, Zhang Z, Ritchey MD, Loustalot F. Medication adherence and incident preventable hospitalizations for hypertension. American Journal of Preventive Medicine. 2016; **50**(4):489-499. DOI: 10.1016/j.amepre.2015.08.021

[31] Bansilal S, Castellano JM, Garrido E, Wei HG, Freeman A, Spettell C, et al. Assessing the impact of medication adherence on long-term cardiovascular outcomes. Journal of the American College of Cardiology. 2016;**68**(8):789-801. DOI: 10.1016/j.jacc.2016.06.005

[32] Esposito D, Bagchi AD, Verdier JM, Bencio DS, Kim MS. Medicaid beneficiaries with congestive heart failure: Association of medication adherence with healthcare use and costs. American Journal of Managed Care. 2009;**15**(7):437-445

[33] Simoni-Wastila L, Wei YJ, Qian J, Zuckerman IH, Stuart B, Shaffer T, et al. Association of chronic obstructive pulmonary disease maintenance medication adherence with all-cause hospitalization and spending in a medicare population. American Journal of Geriatric Pharmacotherapy. 2012;**10**(3):201-210. DOI: 10.1016/j.amjopharm.2012.04.002

[34] Halpern R, Baker CL, Su J, Woodruff KB, Paulose-Ram R, Porter V, et al. Outcomes associated with initiation of tiotropium or fluticasone/salmeterol in patients with chronic obstructive pulmonary disease. Patient Preference and Adherence. 2011;**5**:375-388. DOI: 10.2147/PPA.S19991

[35] Ho P, Rumsfeld J, Masoudi F, McClure D, Plomondon M, Steiner J, et al. Effect of medication nonadherence on hospitalization and mortality among patients with diabetes mellitus. Archives of Internal Medicine. 2006;**166**(17):1836-1841. DOI: 10.1001/archinte. 166.17.1836

[36] Dall TM, Zhang Y, Chen YJ, Quick WW, Yang WG, Fogli J. The economic burden of diabetes. Health Affairs. 2010;**29**(2):297-303. DOI: 10.1377/hlthaff.2009.0155

[37] Tang B, Rahman M, Waters HC, Callegari P. Treatment persistence with adalimumab, etanercept, or infliximab in combination with methotrexate and the effects on healthcare costs in patients with rheumatoid arthritis. Clinical Therapeutics. 2008;**30**(7):1375-1384. DOI: 10.1016/S0149-2918(08)80063-X

[38] Pasma A, Schenk C, Timman R, Van't Spijker A, Appels C, Van Der Laan WH, et al. Does non-adherence to DMARDs influence hospital-related healthcare costs for early arthritis in the first year of treatment? PLoS One 2017;**12**(2):1-14. DOI: 10.1371/journal.pone.0171070

[39] Hiligsmann M, Ethgen O, Bruyère O, Richy F, Gathon HJ, Reginster JY. Development and validation of a markov microsimulation model for the economic evaluation of treatments in osteoporosis. Value in Health. 2009;**12**(5):687-696. DOI: 10.1111/j.1524-4733.2008.00497.x

[40] Roebuck MC, Liberman JN, Gemmill-Toyama M, Brennan TA. Medication adherence leads to lower healthcare use and costs despite increased drug spending. Health affairs (Project Hope). Jan 1, 2011;**30**(1):91-99. DOI: 10.1377/hlthaff.2009.1087

[41] Luz TCB, Loyola Filho AI de, Lima-Costa MF. Perceptions of social capital and cost-related non-adherence to medication among the elderly. Cadernos de Saude Publica. 2011;**27**(2):269-276. DOI: S0102-311X2011000200008 [pii]

[42] Rosenbaum S. The patient protection and affordable care act: Implications for public health policy and practice. Public Health Reports. 2011;**126**(1):130-135. DOI: 10.1177/00 3335491112600118

[43] Yap AF, Thirumoorthy T, Kwan YH. Medication adherence in the elderly. Journal of Clinical Gerontology and Geriatrics. Jun 1, 2016;**7**(2):64-67. DOI: 10.1016/j.jcgg.2015.05.001

4

Decision-Making Experiences and Patterns in Residential Care Homes for Older Residents, Family Members and Care Providers

Lisa Pau Le Low

Abstract

Aim: To explore the decision-making experiences and processes taking place in residential care homes from older residents, their families and staff members, particularly how residents' needs were met and their degree of involvement in making decisions.

Methods: A constructivist grounded theory study was used to interview 28 residents, 22 family members and 31 staff. Results: Three processes illuminated the residents' approaches to decision-making over time. These processes demonstrated how residents settled into the homes and began to develop their decision-making approaches in conjunction with their family and staff members. The degree of negotiation and compromises in decision-making that was possible for older people could be captured in the data.

Conclusions: The influence of family members and staff in supporting or hindering residents from decision-making highlighted the subtle discussions, delicate negotiations and compromises that occurred. Findings presented will be discussed with the wider literature on caring for older people in these homes.

Keywords: decision-making, family, qualitative, residential care homes, residents, staff

1. Introduction

As residential care homes play a progressively more important role in the lives of Chinese older people it is important to ensure that the care provided 'in their new home' is of a high standard and that their multiple needs are recognized and met. Like other countries around the world, Hong Kong (HK) is faced with an aging population. However changing family structures and the socio-economic context have made it particularly challenging for families to keep older people at home, even with supportive services. This has seen a growing number of residential care homes emerging. As these homes are becoming important for older people, it is pivotal to understand how they make decisions and how their family members and care providers support them, or not, to meet their wishes and preferences. Indeed, few studies have examined the roles of these key stakeholder groups (i.e., residents, families and care providers), their level of involvement in decision-making, and influences they have on decisions that determine older people's lives. By examining these various perspectives the aim is to understand the 'what' and 'how' of decisions; that is, the processes that drive decision-making and their subsequent outcomes. Currently, little is known about the respective roles adopted by key stakeholders, their level of involvement in decision-making and the influence they have on decisions that determine the residents' lives. If older people in these homes are to enjoy the same rights as those living in the community then a better understanding of how decisions are made in these homes is necessary.

A literature search conducted revealed a scarcity of work (both internationally and locally) that examined decision-making processes and experiences among residents, families and staff in residential care homes. Despite a general lack of literature about 'decision-making in residential care homes', there appears to be an abundant literature on clinical and treatment decision-making, and making decisions to enter residential care homes. Indeed, only two studies were found that specifically examined decision-making and family's experiences in residential care. There were studies on making transitions into residential care homes [1–3], yet in relation to decision-making per se, Edwards et al. [4] concluded in a literature review of 20 papers that there is a paucity of literature that documents the actual decision-making processes. It is known that once admitted into the homes, daily activities become an integral part of the residents' lives, and often involve waiting, daily routines and activities [5]. However, literature exploring how decisions about such matters are made is scant, but closer inspection of that which exists reveal that it is still possible to draw insights of aspects of life in these homes and how resident wish to live and how their lives can be improved.

1.1. Decision-making perspectives: relevance for long-term care residents

In the general literature, the main focus of decision-making highlights the use of a range of strategies such as rational thought, intuition or prior experience in order to choose among the alternatives. Here decision-making is seen to involve a sequence of events or a course of action taken in order to decide what action to take [6–7]. Several authors support a view that decision-making involves using discriminative thinking to choose a particular course of action [6–7]. In this way, decision-making is seen as a complex process involving a series of stages that include observing a situation, evaluating the observed data, and taking actions to achieve the desired outcome [8]. It therefore involves the act of choice following consideration, deliberation and judgment of alternatives [9] through a process of information gathering. This locates decision-making as an active cognitive thought process of making up one's mind about something, and reaching a judgment or decision among a range of alternatives. This of course presumes that alternatives exist, and this may not be the case for many residents in residential care homes.

In the wider health care literature, the type of decision-making described above is usually clinically-oriented and professionally-driven [7, 10]. The main focus has been on making decisions about treatment preferences, monitoring treatment effects, and ethical decision-making [11]. Such studies have contributed to the development of clinical decision-making models to aid healthcare professionals. However, these models have less relevance in residential care homes where decisions may not be primarily clinical, the range of options may be limited as may be the information available to inform decision-making. Another facet of decision-making involves using intuition and prior experience to take action based on the intuitive feeling of the decision-maker [12–15]. This perspective has some potential relevance in residential care homes particularly from the existing literature on the role of intuition in gaining expertise [16]. However, the value of such understanding on how residents make decisions is far from clear.

Of more use is the work of Circielli [17], who examined decision-making of family caregiving for older people. In this decision-making was defined as:

> 'a process where individuals do not always make decisions alone, but make them with others in dyads or groups' (p. 33). It is therefore assumed to be an ongoing process between persons and involves 'shifting from the micro level of the (individual) person to a macro level between persons' (p. 49) in creating perspectives to minimize conflicts in the environment.

This definition appreciates that decision-making is a process that occurs over a period of time, and that potentially involves a number of people. This is likely to be more consistent with the reality of life in a home and will inform the approach to be adopted here.

1.2. Levels and types of decisions in residential care homes

Residential care homes are known to be places where many levels and types of decisions can take place. Although the review by Davies and Brown-Wilson [18] found limited information on the decision-making processes, they mentioned that the types of decisions made in the homes can directly impinge on the lives of residents, families or staff, even though residents may not be directly involved in them. In exploring the range of decisions made in the homes, Rowles & High [19] identified a typology of decision-making approaches based on an ethnographic study of family involvement in several homes. These were 'authoritative decisions', 'given decisions, 'negotiated decisions', and 'reflexive decisions'. While most decisions made in residential care homes will impinge on the daily experiences of residents, authoritative and given decisions are largely made with little input from older residents and their significant others. By definition they should have relatively more involvement in negotiated and reflexive decisions, and these should be the processes involved when decisions concerned with daily matters are made [19]. With reference to Rowles and High's [19] typology of decisions, the last set of reflexive decisions seemed to define residents' levels of control and ability to exercise choice, which may vary within each home. This is consistent with the definition of decisions as defined by Tversky & Kahneman [20], cited in Johnson et al. ([21] p. 359) as:

> 'choices or actions from which a person choose what to or not do, and are based on beliefs about what must happen to achieve goals'.

It would seem that an understanding of decision-making can be retrieved by exploring aspects of daily life that concern older people from previous studies on perceived choice and control, and level of participation/involvement of residents, families and staff.

1.3. Defining the issues at play

In HK, the maintenance of family harmony and filial piety is still very much the core value of the Confucius Chinese traditional practice, despite evidence suggesting that the practice of filial duties has weakened [22–23]. Policy reforms have continued to affirm the view of the 'warm, supportive and stable families are what counts in nurturing the healthy development of individuals' ([24] p. 28). Potentially, there is an expectation that Chinese families still have an important role to play as providers of care, even after older people are admitted into the homes. However, there is very scant information available to understand the respective roles of families and their influences on the care of older people following entry into residential care homes in HK. Despite efforts to involve older people and their significant others in making decisions that affect their care, participation and involvement remain generally minimal and decisions are mainly made by staff based on what they consider to be in the older persons best interests [25]. This is further supported by work undertaken in HK which found that residents became dependent much earlier than needed [26]. It was found that staff acted on behalf of all residents, even for those who did not need their assistance, and perceived the tasks to be within their capabilities. Indeed, there is a need to develop mutual understanding about how to provide care which can truly reflect the competence of older people and minimize unnecessary dependence [27].

Growing old and living in residential care homes need not mean that making decisions becomes a thing of the past. Rather, being able to make informed decisions about personal choices and preferences continues to be important and should be promoted regardless of mental and physical frailty. If the ethos of caring is about understanding what is wanted from older people, merely getting things done for them will not enhance their satisfaction or quality of life. Identifying older people's preferences and values on how care needs ought to be met and their capacity and capability to continue to make decisions about daily living will help to inform appropriate care decisions. Such information will enable staff to re-prioritize and re-organize their work patterns by responding to the older person's expectations of care, and thereby involve those older people who wish to participate in decisions that directly concern their welfare. It is with this intention that this study was undertaken to explore the decision-making experiences and processes taking place in residential care homes from older residents, their families and staff, particularly how residents' needs were met, and their degree of involvement in making decisions.

2. Methodological approach

2.1. Research design

Constructivist grounded theory (conGT) was adopted in this project. This approach was inspired by Rodwell's [28] constructivism approach to research and Charmaz's [29] work on 'Constructing grounded theory: A practical guide through qualitative analysis'. Their writing provided a methodological map in clarifying the strategies and perspectives for understanding the phenomenon on decision-making in residential care homes for older people. In the research process, knowledge was co-created through the reciprocal relationship that was formed between the researcher and participants as they worked towards exploring an interpretative understanding of the participants' experiences and acknowledging they created multiple meanings of their worlds in which they live in [30].

2.2. Sampling and setting

Table 1 depicts the participants and study settings. Purposive sampling was used to recruit the initial sample and to identify participants who were most likely to provide rich information about the experiences or phenomena of interest [31]. As data collection progressed I recruited people with diverse backgrounds to achieve maximum variation and ensure multiple perspectives [28]. Theoretical sampling followed to sample people, activities and events as guided by the emerging codes and categories. The selection criteria were:

- *Resident* refers to newly-admitted persons who were cognitively-intact, spoke Cantonese or Hakkanese and willing to participate. Those refusing to participate in the study and suffering from cognitive impairment were excluded.

- *Family* refers to immediate members such as daughters, sons, spouses or grandchildren who had been identified by the resident as a person of importance in their lives, and were involved in their care to deal with issues at the home.

- *Staff* refers to both professional (social and health care personnel) and non-professional care staff who provided or influenced the physical and/or psychosocial care of residents; at least one staff representative from each rank; and, a willingness to engage in an individual interview with the researcher.

Data collection used a 3 × 3 design with three datasets from residents, families and staff in the three distinct homes. Data collection in home one was completed before commencing concurrent data collection in the second and third homes. In home one, data were collected to provide an orientation and overview of the research problem from the three participant groups. These data informed the selection of another two homes and participants. Homes two and three moved from general discovery of issues to more targeted probing among the participants [28]. The emerging categories were refined to focus on the (co-) constructions that emerged in the data. Data collection terminated when in-depth information, with maximum

Home	Time period	Participants			Interviews		
		Elder	Family	Staff	Elder	Family	Staff
1	10 months	8	6	10	16	6	10
2	11.5 months	12	10	11	22	10	11
3		8	6	10	14	6	10
	Sub-total	28	22	31	52	22	31
	Total		81		105		

Table 1. Overview of participants in the three study homes.

variation in participants' views, and a high degree of consensus about the categories and constructions was achieved.

2.3. Interview procedure

Interviews were the main data collection method used. The main emphasis of interviewing pointed to what, why and how questions were asked, and being able to listen to the participants answering the questions in order to understand the experiences, and deriving interpretations from it [32]. Interviews therefore provided a tentative impetus to make decisions about 'where to go', 'what to look for', 'from whom', and 'how to ask questions' ([28], p. 21). The intention was not to impose a rigid order to the interviews by following each question in a particular sequence, but to allow the interview content to unfold by following the lead of the participants who were telling the story [33]. In fact, the researcher and participants were allowed to go 'beneath the surface of ordinary conversation and examine earlier events, views and feelings' ([29] p. 26–27). The participants were asked to reflect deeply on their experiences and encouraged to talk more. Clarifying and encouraging more information helped to articulate intentions and meanings. Therefore, only a few broad, open-ended semi-structured questions were needed to focus the interviews. A guiding principle in framing the questions was to 'direct questions to collective practices first and then attend to the individual's participation in and views of those practices' ([34] p. 679).

Family and staff members were interviewed once, and residents were interviewed twice (at 2 weeks and between 2 and 3 months after admission). As the study examined how residents made decisions with the support from staff, residents' first interviews and staff interviews were conducted almost simultaneously. Families were interviewed after the residents' second interview. This allowed me to hear the residents' experiences and how staff responded to them before comparing the accounts of residents and staff with the families' to gain fuller perspectives of those experiences.

2.4. Analysis strategy

Simultaneous data analysis and data collection occurred as far as possible. Constant comparative analysis was the method of data analysis used to generate concepts and to develop the theory through an inductive process of defining, categorizing, comparing data and, explaining and seeking relationships in the data [29]. Each interview was transcribed verbatim as soon as possible after each interview. Once the transcripts were checked for accuracy, the data were subjected to initial and focused coding. Initial coding enabled me to examine the fragments of data (words, lines, segments and incidents) and to give them a label that best summarized and described the data [29], using the participants' words to help me stay close to the data. A table of codes was compiled for each participant group, to which constant comparison of data was undertaken to check whether participants from each care home had identified similar concepts. The idea was to keep or reword existing codes, and only add new codes when new information was forthcoming [33]. The table was updated after changes were made to the coding scheme. The table at a glance helped to identify convergent and divergent opinions, and find gaps in the coded data to direct subsequent data collection [29]. Focused coding synthesized larger segments in the data by examining which significant initial codes could be collapsed into broader categories [29]. Similar coded data were compared against the existing extensive data, and the incoming data from other transcripts. The identified sub-categories were compared with the verbatim data and codes to ensure that the 'emergent set of categories and their properties fit the data, work, and were relevant for integrating into a theory' ([35] p. 56). The researcher moved from specific incidents to abstraction, by comparing incidents to incidents and incidents to concepts to determine similarities and differences in an iterative process [33]. Once the codes were all collapsed to form categories, possible relationships among and between the categories were examined to establish a conceptual link between them [29] to theoretically explain decision-making experiences among the stakeholder groups.

2.5. Ethical considerations

Ethical approval was obtained from the Survey and Behavioral Research Ethics Committee of the University to conduct this study. The superintendents of the homes gave me permission to conduct the study. In upholding the ethical principle to respect autonomy, participants were well-informed about the inquiry, and were given time to ask questions before agreeing to consent to participate. The provision of informed information safeguarded the rights and respects the participant's choice to participate. All participants signed the consent form before being interviewed. They were informed of their rights to stop the interviews, refuse to answer questions and withdraw from the study at any time. They were advised that consenting to the inquiry was entirely voluntary and withdrawing from the study did not influence the care provided by the homes.

3. Patterns of decision-making and influences on residents

Based on the case analyses of the three homes, distinct patterns of decision-making and the influences on the residents' approach to decision-making could be delineated. The processes by which residents were facilitated or hindered from decision-making were strongly influenced by the pattern of decision-making that predominated in the homes. **Table 2** summarizes the three processes and six elements that were identified to capture the subtleties of the process of decision-making for residents that unfolded from entry into the homes to how they continued to make decisions to adjust to the living environment.

Residents proceeded through a fairly logical approach and had varying degrees of involvement in decision-making. These processes demonstrated how residents settled into the home by becoming familiar with it and then becoming more involved in the decisions that influenced their lives. As residents moved through these decision-making processes that were practiced in the homes, the degree of negotiation that was possible determined the extent to which they were able to negotiate successful, less successful and unsuccessful decisions. As residents engaged in these processes the extent to which the family and staff ensured that decisions were successfully negotiated to meet needs or needs were not met were also highlighted. In comparing the similarities and differences in these processes across the three homes, three decision-making patterns were identified as negotiated, partially-flexible and constrained patterns of decision-making. Through the interactions between the participant groups, negotiations and/or compromises occurred that either facilitated or hindered residents' involvement

Processes	Elements
Making the unknown familiar	• Being accompanied and supervised
	• Being told and observing
Finding out what I can do and want	• Trial and error testing
	• Asking and questioning
Negotiating-compromising the past to fit the present	• Suggesting and negotiating
	• Compromising

Table 2. Decision-making processes matched against its elements.

in decision-making. Participants' decision-making patterns and how they shaped the three processes of adjustment to decision-making will be discussed below.

3.1. Negotiated patterns of decision-making

Residents from home one undertook most negotiation in decision-making. Some residents from home two were also allowed to practice this approach provided that decisions did not disrupt the smooth running of the home. This approach was less evident in home three and, when it did occur, it caused conflict resulting in the resident terminating their stay.

3.1.1. Making the unknown familiar

During the settling-in period, residents' abilities and desires were revealed through the processes of 'being accompanied and supervised', and 'being told and observing'. Staff were predominately identified as key people in the process of getting to know the resident's concerns, health condition, personality and personal preferences on which to base decision-making later on. As the weeks passed, the exchanges with accompanying and supervising staff allowed residents to gradually understand the operation of daily practices affecting their lives. Of concern to residents at this time was the ways in which baths were planned:

> Staff arrange baths for me. I do not bath on my own. I know the time to bath. If I bath today, I bath the day after tomorrow so I can prepare myself. But there's nothing for me to get ready 'cause they do it all for me. (POAH, elder, E5A).

This process also enabled most staff to claim that they knew about 70–80% of the resident's personal habits and preferences. The remaining 20–30% was attributed to the limited knowledge about family composition and support to give to them. This information was important in making a judgment about resident's abilities to make decisions. Information about the resident's mobility, level of independence and self-care abilities, capabilities, mental state, motivation to do own things, beliefs in one's ability to do it, and ability to make sensible suggestions were helpful. When they were perceived to be unable to mobilize safely, negotiating to do tasks independently were often rejected by staff. This was frustrating for some:

> You need a clear mental state, or else how can you do the task? I can make decision whenever I need to. You cannot deceive me on anything. You cannot ignore what I am saying. The only thing is that I cannot walk on my own and this is killing me (POAH, elder, E5A).

The process of being told and observing the daily routines enabled residents and families to learn the roles of staff and their expectations. Some residents quickly settled into a pattern of letting staff do things for them:

> *They are good to me. I do not have to do anything. I am over 90. Staff help to prepare everything for me. They do not need me to do anything.* (POAH, elder, E6A).

The importance of families in maintaining relationships with the residents was emphasized by the staff from the outset. Families played a central role during this transitional period by providing supplementary baseline information to the staff about their relative's condition and usual habits that shaped the level of supervision needed and improved understanding of the resident. Indeed, the superintendents and staff, especially in home one, initiated contact with the families each time they visited. The family's contribution in this process was to make regular visits to observe and get to know the home, and what was happening in the resident's daily life, and what was acceptable to do. Families were keen to lend a helping hand and to reassure the residents that they had not been abandoned. Families also learned from staff and observed them to see whether their requests were followed up.

3.1.2. Finding out what I can do and want

The processes of 'trial and error testing' and 'asking and questioning' marked the beginning of negotiation in the decision-making experiences of residents. These processes were largely triggered by the discrepancies arising from what was being told and observed about the home's operation and from the people around them. They wanted to 'trial and error test' and 'ask and question' about the possibility of doing things by themselves.

In homes one and two, the process of trial and error testing was usually observed in physical care decisions, although the processes differed slightly. These decisions were examples of major initial concerns, such as who performed the hygiene care, or decisions about meal choices were requested by the residents or families. Of concern to residents were asking to change the order of taking baths and who performed it. Bathing routines tended to prioritize those whom staff felt were most pressing (e.g. wound dressing or medical appointments). On the spot requests like 'I want to be first today' without a 'good' reason were not entertained. In home one, an upfront request to bath alone was made by the residents to the superintendents and, if staff agreed, the level of supervision needed was assessed. In reality staff felt constrained by the need to rush through baths and safeguard those who bathed alone. Residents spoke of the embarrassment of asking for help:

> *They do not really need to take care of me. If they do not call me (to help me), I bath myself. It's safe and simple. No need to ask others to help with things I can do. If I ask for too much help, I feel embarrassed and useless* (POAH, elder, E8B).

The main reason for wanting to regain independence and control over bathing was the dissatisfaction directed at staff for being too busy and rushing through the procedure. Instead of moaning, they proactively dealt with the problem:

> *They bathed me and did not completely wash away the soap. I kept it a secret, or the seniors will condemn them. I told them I could bath myself, and thanked them for helping me. They said to call them if I could not handle it.* (SH, elder, E4B).

Some residents (influenced by roommates) initiated plans to bath alone, without telling the staff. Experimenting cleansing in secret led them to become confident to persuade staff to let them do it under supervision:

They bathed me the first 2 weeks. How can you bath without them knowing? I saw a resident bathing alone so I bathed secretly a few times. I could do it. I did not know that before. They found out, scolded, observed me. Now I do it myself. (SH, elder, E11A).

Families' views of residents' abilities to make physical care decisions were welcomed. There was a general agreement to allow them to partake in 'basic' daily life decision-making when they were capable and they were not too disruptive to staff or families. Indeed, while some families promoted such decision-making, they also believed that residents should only make decisions on things that were within their capability, even if they could do this slowly.

3.1.3. Negotiating-compromising the past to fit the present

The processes of 'suggesting and negotiating' and 'compromising' with staff and families about creating a way of life that was reasonably familiar and comfortable for residents marked the continuation of the negotiated decision-making process. The process of suggesting-negotiating arose after residents, who were successful in making some changes, continued to ask and question, and were more likely to discuss and further explore their needs: Everyday it's I see what I can do. I depend on myself all the time. (POAH, elder, E2A).

In both homes one and two, an activity enjoyed by residents was the ability to go out alone, and not to be supervised by anyone. Undoubtedly, the ability to go outdoors independently was a rule determined by the home's management and was made known to residents and families on admission. Although residents were able to maneuver freely around the grounds of the home, granting them the freedom to leave the home grounds as they pleased depended on their physical capability, mental alertness and independence. Such requests were carefully negotiated with the family who had to sign a consent form to accept responsibility. The freedom and independence to go outdoors was highly valued, although the outskirts of home one was an industrial area and it was potentially dangerous for elders to be out alone. They therefore spent time walking along the streets, in front of the home. Whilst this created administrative work homes one and two believed that residents should be given freedom to connect with the community, and encouraged to go out freely, providing it had been approved beforehand.

Another example of the process of negotiating-compromising pertained to food choices. This was a longstanding and difficult problem that was not easy to solve. Over time, the food served and timing of meals were not entirely suitable. Some residents questioned the food textures and tastes, and made requests for a change. As there were no resident meetings in home one, the matter was discussed with the residents on an individual level. Avoiding foods the majority disliked was the preferred practice in communal living, as opposed to boosting food tastes for the few who raised it as a concern. With the help of families and approval of staff in both homes, this was resolved by allowing residents to purchase small bottles of soy sauce, pickle onions or shredded pickle to enhance the tastes of foods. Other food issues were not always easily resolved.

As most families were in full-time work and visited during the weekends, they got to know about the residents' decision-making capabilities through the staff who took initiative to tell them about the daily happenings. They were delighted to know that residents were taking care of themselves and finding things to occupy their time. Negotiating about care that went beyond the usual home practice (e.g. preparing packets of drinks or snacks families have brought), and exploring items to purchase for bed unit) were some topics that were successfully discussed by the family on behalf of the residents.

3.2. Partially flexible patterns of decision-making

This approach was most apparent in home two, and sometimes evident in home one due to the constraints of staff and facilities. Few residents from home three wanted to let staff know their needs because they were reluctant to confront the rigid culture of the home.

3.2.1. Making the unknown familiar

Compared with home one, the processes of accompanying and supervising elders was not as closely monitored by staff in home two, while the processes of telling and observing was given greater emphasis. The processes of accompanying and supervising involved staff helping residents to become familiar with the routine and physical care, particularly how they fitted in with the baths, meals and sleeping arrangements. Being a larger home, these processes identified issues that could potentially cause unharmonious relationships such as room- and table-sharing, and being prepared to minimize conflicts should they arise:

> The idea of decision-making depends on reciprocal relationship of elders to respect each other. It's communal living. You are not in a single room. Issues like over-using or not letting others use the air-conditioning and fans in the bedrooms, or asking to live on a specific floor. (SH, social worker, S8).

Residents and families were not fully told about the roles of staff (due to many staff) and the pattern of work. Instead families were told of an appointed social care staff and to approach the care staff on each floor for enquiries. They only needed to be observant, oblige and accept what they had been told. Indeed, residents learnt more by observing other resident's behaviour and attitudes of staff towards them, particularly towards room-sharing and how they formed friendships. Unlike home one where residents had single rooms, a major issue in home two was the resident's uncertainties about forming relationships in a large home.

Here families' visits to the residents were confined mostly to the weekends, and there were less daytime/evening visits to lend a helping hand, because of work and family commitments. Families found out about the home's routines largely through talking to the resident, the majority in this home being cognitively intact. The opportunity to move freely around and outside the home, without the operation of a rigid documentation procedure, was viewed with initial surprise by families, although they liked the freedom it gave:

> The rules for taking residents out are a bit loose. I thought it was strange when no one asked me questions (visited biweekly). The home likes to give freedom and convenience to resident and families, and prevents a feeling of imprisonment. (SH, daughter, R8).

3.2.2. Finding out what I can do and want

A policy that became more flexible in home two was a result of female residents' determined efforts to launder their own clothes (not an established home policy) by not approaching the staff first to ask for permission. There was considerable dissatisfaction with the laundry service that often produced creased clothes that were impossible to wear. Instead of openly expressing their dissatisfaction, residents chose to launder light clothing and balanced this by complying with the rules to let the home launder larger garments. Once it was clear that this did not cause major disruption, staff turned a blind eye and provided floor mats, fans and mops to ensure safety:

> I wash my clothes and hang them in the bathroom. I do not disturb the others. All elders in my room do their washing. Staff know it. It's no secret. We look after each other and consider safety. Dry the floor and turn on the fan if the bathroom is wet. (SH, elder, 6B).

Home two had the most choice of social activities (e.g. small groups of elders with dementia playing mahjong, or in large group of 100 to 130 residents). Such activities required staff to make decisions about scheduled indoor activities, including group size, target groups, purpose, and venues. Residents learned about these activities when staff informed them in person, or roommates discussed these activities among themselves. Through these activities, some residents realized their abilities and developed new interests and friends. They preferred activities that taught them to learn new skills such as singing, writing Chinese characters, and the physiotherapy sessions. Activities that required them to communicate had low enrolment. Indeed, it was those residents who were cooperative and obeyed the rules that seemed to be allowed more personal requests. For example, residents who had befriended other residents would group together to ask staff's permission first before engaging in mahjong gatherings. Some residents with difficulties in mobilization aspired for more outdoor activities, or to be trained to walk or use the wheelchair, and were finding ways to make this happen without being seen as troublesome:

> I seldom go outside. It's what you can do when you go outside. I do not know how to use the wheelchair. They do not have activities to allow people in wheelchair to go out and sit under the sun. All the activities are indoors. (SH, elder, 3A).

To increase resident's participation, special arrangements were facilitated by staff to maximize frail and less able residents to participate in different activities:

> We choose suitable time and venue for the residents. We know some residents come out and have their tea so activities are arranged at those times (SH, welfare worker, S5).

Despite visiting less often than in home one, families still provided close support and encouragement in the course of decision-making. While families became concerned about safety, they supported resident's decisions to launder own clothes by offering to take larger-sized clothes home to wash, but thought it was unnecessary to intervene with the home's practices when the solution to deal with the issue was not entirely inconvenient.

3.2.3. Negotiating-compromising the past to fit the present

The processes of 'suggesting and negotiating' and 'compromising' with staff and families occurred in such a way that allowed requests to be considered before coming to a final decision. Like home one, residents with prior successes in negotiation continued to make requests, however they were persuaded to take advice from staff, which was considered to be in their best interest, and thereby sometimes had to compromise their own expectations. For example, residents were highly influenced by the advice of their family members. Some residents were happy not to go outdoors unless accompanied by relatives. In such situation, they would not bargain with the staff. They would choose to wander in the home's premises and remain in the garden, which were acceptable alternatives:

> *I will not go outdoors by myself. There're rules. I cannot go out whenever I want without telling them.*
> *I say, "I'm going to the garden. If someone wants me I'll be there." That's already good enough for me.*
> (SH, elder, E6A).

Some alert residents with physical limitations compromised by sacrificing outdoor activities they had previously enjoyed due the burden they felt would be placed on others to help them. The choice of outdoor activities was limited to those that required no companion:

> *I have not joined the trips. I cannot walk. I need others to push me (on wheelchair), and it's hot outside.*
> *I join activities that do not need others' help. They said if my family can push me, I can go. I do not want*
> *to bother my family so I do not join.* (SH, elder, E8B).

Indeed, a resident's state of health seemed to be the determining criterion for having wishes granted. Staff were rather flexible and allowed negotiations when managing residents who insisted, for example, to go against relatives who forbid them from going outdoors. As this home had easy access to the shops, when such circumstances occurred, it was managed individually and flexibly by re-assessing the situation with the resident and family and coming to a new consensus that provided instructions for staff on the provision of care.

In principle home two was in agreement that residents should be accorded the freedom to do things for themselves, however there were contradictory policies that restricted their freedom. Continuing with the example of going outdoors, residents who wanted to go for a walk after dinner would be limited by the regulation to return by a certain time, and therefore limiting true freedom. Although it was difficult to check on the flow of people moving around the home, this issue was not addressed by confining residents to remain indoors to ensure their safety. Instead, strategies were developed to react positively to the resident's situations and still continue to keep the main entrance open to avoid feelings of being in jail or locked up.

In home one, while staff tried to maintain the resident's prior lifestyle of allowing them to keep hold of money and make decisions about small purchases, staff in home two did not fully facilitate this practice, although they welcomed appropriate purchases by the family provided there was minimal interference to the running of the home. Although some residents could keep a little money they had to negotiate help from families if they wished to purchase anything, and staff did not help to make any purchases. For residents with no relatives, money matters were handled by the resident until their health deteriorated and a guardian would be appointed.

The data highlighted that the type of decisions families made were guided by the expressed needs of the resident. Families would react in the best interest of these residents, who were less able to express personal preferences and tended to fit in with the majority. Families were also found to support residents to cooperate with the home's decisions and arrangements.

Some found themselves trying to reduce residents' dissatisfaction when they were prohibited from doing things. In the course of incorporating residents' preferences and exploring the best option to address their needs, the data revealed that families and staff had to first agree and, if necessary, compromise their own expectations before deciding on the best action to take to meet the residents' interests. For example dealing with residents' concerns such as returning home for a few days and purchasing accessories highlighted that an agreement between families-staff could be negotiated based on the resident's capabilities and provided that it did not unduly disrupt the home's routines. Indeed, only a minority got to go home to stay during the weekends, with the majority perhaps going home for a few hours. For others, going home to stay a few days was never discussed for fear that the elder would refuse to come back.

3.3. Constrained patterns of decision-making

This decision-making pattern was found across all the homes to varying degrees, but largely dominated life in home three.

3.3.1. Making the unknown familiar

Like the other two homes, home three shared similar practices in the way that information was provided to the residents and families during the early days of admission. Some staff believed that residents should be fully involved in decision-making. In reality, they tended to closely supervise elders and not allow them to take risks:

> When residents have health problems, will their decisions bring maximum benefit? It'll be difficult to ask them to make a correct decision. I'll consider the requests of those in good physical and psychological health. Why 'consider'? They might have done it in a certain way for many years, does it mean it's free of risk? Yes, we should respect them, but we should provide adequate supervision. (NSH, RN, S10).

As in home two, a key message disseminated to residents and families was the need to comply with the routines that dominated communal living. The processes of 'being accompanied and supervised' rather than 'being told and observing' was more evident in this home. Although the other two homes used these processes to enable newly-admitted residents to know how to 'behave' in the new home, and to acquire knowledge about the routines, home three continued to use these processes from admission and thereafter to strictly supervise residents, allowing far less involvement in the decision-making processes.

Close surveillance was welcomed by residents whose reason for admission was to have staff around to call them for help. However, for many, the level of supervision went too far. For instance, getting up from a chair to fetch a cane to try walking to the toilet was immediately supervised by a staff, who sat them on the toilet, only to return to help as soon as they had finished. Indeed, residents generally understood that close surveillance by staff was part of their training and way of doing things:

> It's their responsibility. They are taught not to allow residents to walk alone. They hold my arms, hold my clothes and go into the toilet with me. (NSH, elder, E5A).

Although the efforts of staff to get to know and listen to new residents were noted, generally residents soon learned to accept and conform to the norm:

> Care staff walk around to see if we are eating safely, and collect feedback about the meals. As the social care staff is responsible for the kitchen, she'll keep walking around the tables to see residents' eating condition – how much is eaten and tastes of foods. When they complain about the dry and tasteless meat, we explain that meals are healthier and low salt, of course, it's tasteless (laughs). (NSH, RN, S1).

However, very little effort was made to get to know the residents as individuals and communication with families was limited and often superficial:

> I rarely speak to the staff. I seldom have any problems. When I come, I greet them. They do not tell me about his condition. They are not fussy. I do not expect them to tell me. I have nothing to say. What else is there to talk about? (NSH, wife, R1).

Consequently, the process of settling-in at home three involved far less open exchange of information and was an instrumental process based on informing residents-families about what was expected of them, as opposed to exploring their needs.

3.3.2. Finding out what I can do and want

Unlike the other homes, the residents rarely undertook their own physical care as bathing alone was totally discouraged, even if they were capable. Only three residents engaged in some negotiations about baths after declaring a clear need:

> I bath myself. I can do it myself. I do not need to ask for help with bathing if I can do it. If I cannot do it, there's nothing I can do except to ask for help. If I can manage for myself, I do it on my own. I am safe. (NSH, elder, E7B).

Another resident made a strong request to bath alone but this was not granted because she believed that her independent nature was a threat to staff authority. This elder stayed less than 2 months and left because she could not fit in with the home's expectations. The above excerpt highlights the resident's generally obliging attitude towards fitting in with the constraints of communal living and following the schedule. It seemed that only personal requests that had no impact on the home were considered:

> They cannot completely make their own decisions. If it's dinner time and they want to bath, this cannot happen. They need to follow our arrangements. What I can do is to meet their personal requests, if it's not over-exaggerated and is sensible, we let them have their way, like exercising and going to church. (NSH, health worker, S9).

Another attempt made by residents to find out their own capabilities was in relation to developing relationships with residents and learning how to pass the day. Unlike home two which had many social activities to draw residents together, in-house group social activities in home three (e.g. bingo and beach ball games) were not particularly enjoyable. Whilst these activities helped to 'pass the time' they did not help to form any meaningful relationships. As opportunities to develop meaningful relationships were limited, residents valued any opportunities to engage in activities that would help them to pass the time and the more able residents did much to try and encourage more options. Other activities were more therapeutic and enabled residents to either make the effort to keep in good health or to choose to maintain contacts with the outside community. There was a high enrolment in the few in-house exercise sessions available and many of the residents made a conscious decision to include physical therapy sessions into their week to stay in good health.

In the constrained atmosphere of home three, families initiated and supported residents in the rehabilitation process and helped them to realize the capabilities by arranging elders to attend additional physical/acupuncturist sessions and organized private transport to take them. Indeed involvement of the family, whilst valued in all the homes, was especially appreciated in home three. As families became well-aware of their duties to visit and take residents out for meals, the phone calls lessened as their visit became a weekend activity:

> She does not want a lot – only asks when we'll take her out to have meals and dim sum. It's reasonable. She's stuck in the home every day and has nothing to do. (NSH, son, R4).

Regardless of their abilities, residents were strictly prohibited from going out alone and moving beyond the vision of staff. Some families found this reassuring:

> They have a door bell and the code to enter the home. I totally agree with this arrangement. If not, they'll escape from the home. (NSH, son, R4).

However such regulations and the general attitude among staff to do things for residents made some feel useless and ashamed:

> I feel ashamed when others help me to wash my face and brush my teeth. I am not very old. One brings me into the toilet on a wheelchair. One twists a towel for me. One holds the mouth wash cup for me. I feel useless. Now, I can only pull a blanket over myself. (NSH, elder, E6A).

3.3.3. Negotiating-compromising the past to fit the present

Only the able and articulate residents could engage in efforts to negotiate/comprise and even then opportunities were limited. Indeed, action was limited even when a group of them joined forces and raised shared concerns. This is described below and highlights something approaching a sense of relative helplessness in the face of limited action by staff and the absence of realistic alternatives:

> A naughty resident always disturbs us with a stick when we are sleeping. She does not sleep and walks around with her stick. She keeps the five of us awake by playing with the remote control that raises and lowers the beds. What can we do? I do not want to change rooms – what if there's another naughtier resident? Staff have done nothing, only told her not to disturb us. What can they do? This is an aged home. If we are healthy, we will not be here. (NSH, elder, E6A).

Another issue that elicited suggestions from residents related to food choices. Some comments about what to eat were sought in a resident meeting, which enabled the few 'smart and well-spoken' residents the liberty to express their food preferences and tastes. But the existence of structures to seek views at this home did not mean that action followed and the need for safety and conformity seemed to prevail.

> Do you think they have the right to choose what they eat here? Meals are set in advance. They suggest food they cannot eat. It's only their desires. We think of safety, difficulties eating it, and can others eat it, too. (NSH, health worker, S2).

The monthly resident meeting (with low attendance) was a regular activity bringing together superintendent, social worker, nurses and families. But these were largely symbolic rather than actively managed to ensure optimal attendance and a contribution from all. Over time, families learned to recognize and approach individual staff with whom residents had forged relationships on a one-to-one level to get updates about the resident's daily care. While staff believed that families must be told of the resident's current lifestyle and condition, there was a perception among staff that building relationships with families was difficult because they were very busy people with little time to spend wanting to know about the home. In fact, to the contrary, some families were highly interested in what went on at the home, and took the limited opportunities to interact with the staff:

> I want to know what's happening here and its development, whether it'll build 10 more floors or cut the manpower. There's no channel to converse with them. (NSH, son, R2).

Generally families were in agreement that residents should make their own decisions with the families' role being to present opinions and offer different choices to them:

> You must rely on yourself and make your own decision. The decisions are still made by the elders. Apart from meal times, things like resting, getting up, brushing teeth and washing face can be decided by him. (NSH, wife, R1).

Overall, and despite the obvious limitations, especially in home three it was felt that the resident should still be given choice to make decisions:

> He can make many decisions and do things for himself. It's just the physical functioning of his upper and lower limbs are degenerating. There's no problem with his ability to be reason and think logically. When you give him choices, he can still make a decision on what choice he wants. (NSH, son, R2).

In reality, there were few opportunities for discretionary choice in home three and despite the constrained-rigid leadership style that enforced staff to regularly report the resident's progress to families blunders did occur that affected family-staff relationships and impacted the families' level of confidence in staffs' decision-making. Unlike the other two homes which were praised for providing families with reassurance, unsatisfactory blunders in handling the residents' health and medical concerns, including mismanagement of follow-up appointments and communication breakdown among staff, were beginning to surface at home three and resulted in families becoming dissatisfied. Misunderstanding often arose when messages about the resident's care were not always correctly conveyed. Moreover, as families were not formally informed about different staff members' roles, they formed their own perceptions of staff's job responsibilities that were not always correct. This could result in further confusion and misunderstanding.

4. Discussion: decision-making processes and patterns of residents

The findings generated served to provide an in-depth understanding of the decision-making experiences of older people residing in residential care homes in HK, and the roles and level of involvement family members and care providers in supporting them, or not, to meet their wishes and preferences. Based on the vivid accounts of experiences that were described by the participants, the patterns of decision-making in the homes were shaped by three processes and six elements. This provided an understanding of how daily life decisions were made, from entry into the home to continuing to be involved in decision-making after becoming familiar with the homes. At the heart of the findings lies the extent to which residents were able to negotiate daily decisions in their life or whether they were required to compromise their needs and accept the routines of the home itself.

Across the homes the decision-making processes and related patterns of Chinese residents revealed the influence of staff and family members, as opposed to residents solely making autonomous decisions. This supports the definition of Circielli [17], who defined decision-making as 'a process where individuals … make them (decisions) with others in dyads or groups' (p. 33). This was true for most of the residents in this study. Residents proceeded through three decision-making processes: 'making the unknown familiar', 'finding out what I can do and want', and 'negotiating-compromising the past to fit the present' to become familiar with the home first before becoming involved in daily life decisions.

'Making the unknown familiar' was the first process concerned with assisting residents and families to settle in by using strategies to accompany, supervise, tell and observe. It marks the process of learning from staff to become familiar with the routines, rules and policies of what was possible and allowed. While this provided limited opportunities for residents to participate in decision-making, it was important in laying the grounds for different decision-making patterns that developed when residents were engaged in later decision-making. Practices across the homes were in place to facilitate the processes of telling and observing the residents. Whilst they varied somewhat across the homes, these systems were intended to enable more staff to know about the residents' health condition, personality, preferences, and desires to be involved, and thereby begin to form judgments of the resident's decision-making ability and potential, and the degree of supervision/help to provide. These systems emphasized interaction with the residents to get to know their needs. However, especially in the early period discussion and information exchange tended to be brief and superficial as both staff and residents described the challenges of finding time to talk in the busy regime. Indeed rather than focusing on individual needs processes served to reinforce the importance of group living and forming reciprocal relationships with everyone to maintain harmony and cooperation. It was in this interaction that the balance between negotiation, partial and total compromise emerged. It was not surprising for residents, especially in home three and to a lesser in extent in home two, to perceive that decision-making was primarily made by staff and there was no longer a need to make major decisions now that they were institutionalized. As families were new to the setting, like the residents they had to settle in, and relied on staff to tell them the 'rules'.

There is relatively more literature concerning the process of 'making the unknown familiar' compared with the other two processes, with literature highlighting the need to ease the transition to a care home for newly-admitted residents [36–39]. These studies emphasize that the pressure and losses surrounding the move into the home should be offset by providing appropriate information and support to enable residents and families to play a full and active role in the life of the home. In easing the transition, O'May [38] mentions being able to 'maintain ownership of decisions about the future', although says little about what these decisions can include. She suggests that residents and families should be involved in initiatives to consider the homes as a positive choice, such as facilitating trial visits. Clearly this did not happen in the present study.

Of some resonance to this current study, but taking a different approach to 'familiarity' is the work by Reed and Payton [40] which described 'constructing familiarity' as an active process undertaken by residents to adapt to the new home environment over a six-month period. Based on the sparse information that was usually obtained on arrival, residents were found to actively create their own knowledge of the home and focused their efforts on constructing relationships with fellow residents in order to make the home less strange. The authors suggest that 'constructing familiarity' is a potential useful strategy for dealing positively with a major disruption in a person's life; in this case, moving into the homes. The findings were limited to a consideration of residents' knowledge of the physical locality of the home and residents who lived there, with other aspects of adjustment to daily life such as physical needs not being considered. In contrast to this study, gaining familiarity in the homes was primarily concerned with an overall understanding of their daily operation and its influence on all aspects of the resident's life, from which residents could begin to examine their own decision-making potential.

Clearly 'familiarity' is a potentially important concept that needs more careful elucidation as to its meaning and how this unfolds over time. This study focused on the period immediately following admission up until 3 months. The process of gaining familiarity may, as already noted, begins before entry and continues beyond 3 months. The literature would suggest that familiarity is important in a time period varying from a few weeks prior to a move to up to 6 months post-move [41–42]. There are benefits in involving residents earlier and becoming familiar with the home before becoming a resident.

'Finding out what I can do and want' was the second process in exploring residents' capabilities, expectations, and preferences in making some decisions through the processes of 'trial and error testing' and 'asking and questioning'. The processes of trial and error marked the onset of negotiation. While residents were still settling into the home, negotiating and compromising did not feature in the earlier processes of 'observing', 'being told' and 'trial and error testing'. Therefore, the key processes of negotiating-compromising emerged when they began 'asking and questioning'. An interesting finding was that not all residents had expectations to make changes, but they all aspired to find out their capabilities and when would they be able to perform activities alone, and when supervised assistance was needed. This suggested that it was less important for residents to make decisions solely on their own, but rather by knowing the possibilities they could make a choice about whether to pursue independent action or to let staff do things for them. The main activities residents liked was the opportunity to perform alone or with minimal supervision related to physical care, and making personal possessions/purchases. Only when residents had a chance to trial an activity and were absolutely sure of their competence, would they consider proceeding to negotiate with staff. In situations when they were less competent to go it alone or did not think that they would be allowed to do so, they allowed staff to intervene and compromises were made. Little is known in the existing literature about how these negotiations occur and the findings from this study have important implications for those involved in determining resident's decision-making abilities and potential following entry to residential care homes. These findings challenge beliefs from other studies in HK that all residents are willing to accept help from staff, and are happy being passive recipients of care, and to conform to the dependent role [43]. This perception is in consistent with Confucian ethics and moral obligations to assist and take good care of chronically ill Chinese older people in old age [44–45]. This did not seem appropriate to many residents in this study. Indeed, only those residents in home three were seen to be less active in seeking to perform personal tasks and apparently wanted to be cared for. But this may primarily have been the result of their early learning about the strict 'regime' implemented in this home. An exploratory study by Low et al. [46] had already indicated that many Chinese residents were using their own efforts to support themselves in the homes. Yet, there is again a tension here between residents wanting to maintain privacy in their lives and the Chinese cultural belief in maintaining balance and harmony in relationships. Such findings shed new insights into the creation of social identity and acceptable behaviors for older people in care homes within a Chinese cultural context.

In understanding resident's decision-making potential and abilities, findings of this current study demonstrate the delicate processes of negotiation and compromise necessary in order to successfully 'negotiate-compromise the past to fit the present' so as to create a way of life that would be familiar and comfortable for the residents. The actions of the resident, family and staff enacted within the dominant pattern of decision-making in the home shaped the extent to which the resident's wishes were either accommodated or compromised. Residents challenged boundaries of the rules and policies of the home to enable them to make judgments about how much flexibility and control they could have over aspects of their lives. In many circumstances, efforts were abandoned as they complied with the prevailing practice of the home. This often followed a process of negotiating and compromising with their requests until an agreed decision was reached. Findings from this current study revealed that when homes operated a rigid-constrained regime, discussions and negotiations were minimal and after experiencing early failure no more efforts were made by the residents to suggest further changes to their lifestyle. This raises important questions about the extent to which residents can operate with a degree of independence or whether in reality the needs of the 'home' will largely always hold sway.

A number of studies have explored the experiences and well-being of the resilient older person who is relatively active in retaining their unique identity when faced with major threats in later life [47–50]. Among older people receiving long-term community care, Janssen et al. [49] identified sources of strengths to buffer against stressful situations. These are:

- Individual domain: refers to a person's qualities (e.g. beliefs about own competence, efforts to exert control, capacity to understand own situation),

- Interactional domain: refers to an older person's cooperation and interaction with others to achieve personal goals, and.

- Contextual domain: refers to political-societal level (e.g. accessibility to care and available material resources).

The first two domains are of particular relevance to residents in the homes as they capture the dynamic interaction between individual and interactional elements of negotiation/compromise found in this study. An important consideration is the implicit dilemma of when to hold on and retain control of the situation and when to relinquish that control to others. Paying sensitive attention to understanding an individual person's personal qualities and attributes may be necessary to help assess resilience capabilities and enable residents to continue maintaining a degree of independence [49]. Home staff could learn much from this.

Similar to the results from this study Cook [47] concludes that 'participants (are) engaged in deliberate decision-making and careful planning to influence their life in the home' (p. 271); for example, modifying their own space, and introducing personal items. Whilst continuing to participate in the daily life in care homes, she revealed how frail residents tried to actively reconstruct their life to do the things that were important to them in order to retain their unique identity to 'live meaningful, purposeful and enjoyable lives' (p. 270). In the process of reconstructing a new home life, they implemented three resident-led strategies:

- Resident-initiated/resident implemented strategies: the person identifies what is needed to influence their life and takes action to achieve them.

- Resident initiated/other executed strategies: the person identifies what needs to take place and seeks support from staff, family and friends.

- Resident negotiation to identify possibilities for living in the home and ways to achieve these: the person participates in decision-making processes such as care planning and resident committees with staff to influence their home life.

These strategies above resonate with the decision-making patterns emerging from this study but in the Hong Kong context there appeared to be more emphasis on the second set of strategies. Cook [47] mentions that residents may know their needs, but their influence in meeting them may be reduced, and therefore there is a reliance on others to help them to follow up on the negotiated issue or to compromise their decisions. Conversely, in situations where residents were less competent to go it alone, they allowed staff to intervene and compromises were made.

5. Conclusion

The wider literature on decision-making highlights the analytical deductive or the intuitive decision-making approaches to reaching decisions [51]. While the intuitive approach is a quicker, relies on non-analytical reasoning, and makes association with prior learning/memory of similar situations that is context based, the analytical deductive approach is in contrast slower, rule based, systematic logical thinking and context-free [52]. Findings of this study identified that daily lifestyle decisions were residents' main concerns and that in reality decisions involved a combination of both approaches. Residents have to learn the new 'context', compare it with similar experiences (usually often limited) as well as becoming familiar with the rules, both implicit and explicit operating in the homes. If things are to improve there is a need for far greater awareness among families and staff of the delicate processes at play. It is to be hoped that this study has begun to provide just some insights for instigating future improvements in residential care homes for older people.

Acknowledgements

I wish to sincerely thank my supervisors, Professor Mike Nolan and Dr. Sue Davies who fully supported and encouraged me from a long-distant. It was their endearing patience, passion, enthusiasm and energy that drove me to the finishing line.

Conflict of interest

No conflicts of interest.

Author details

Lisa Pau Le Low

Address all correspondence to: lisalow@cihe.edu.hk

School of Health Sciences, Caritas Institute of Higher Education, Tseung Kwan O, N.T., Hong Kong

References

[1] Dellasega C, Nolan M. Admission to care: Facilitating role transition amongst family carers. Journal of Clinical Nursing. 1997;**6**:443-451

[2] Fiveash B. The experience of nursing home life. International Journal of Nursing Practice. 1998;**4**:166-174

[3] Lee DTF. Residential care placement: Perceptions among elderly Chinese people in Hong Kong. Journal of Advanced Nursing. 1997;**26**:602-607

[4] Edwards H, Courtney M, Spencer L. Consumer expectations of residential aged care: Reflections on the literature. International Journal of Nursing Practice. 2003;**9**:70-77

[5] Liukkonen A. Life in a nursing home for the frail elderly: Daily routines. Clinical Nursing Research. 1995;**4**(4):358-371

[6] Griffith-Kenney JW, Christensen PJ. The Nursing Process: Application of Theories, Frameworks and Models. St. Louis: Mosby; 1986

[7] Moore PA. Decision making in professional practice. British Journal of Nursing. 1996; **5**(10):635-640

[8]   Bohinc M, Gradisar M. Decision-making model in nursing. Journal of Nursing Administration. 2003;**33**(12):627-629

[9]   Schaefer J. The interrelatedness of the decision-making process and the nursing process. American Journal of Nursing. 1974;**74**(10):1852-1855

[10] Banning M. A review of clinical decision making: Models and current research. Journal of Clinical Nursing. 2008;**17**(2):187-195

[11] Bolmsojö I, Sandman l, Anderson E. Everyday ethics in the care of elderly people. Nursing Ethics. 2006;**13**(3):249-263

[12] Benner P. From Novice to Expert. California: Addison-Wesley, Menlo Park; 1984

[13] Benner P, Tanner C. Clinical judgment: How expert nurses use intuition. American Journal of Nursing. 1987;**87**(1):23-31

[14] Buckingham CD, Adams A. Classifying clinical decision-making: A unifying approach. Journal of Advanced Nursing. 2000;**32**:981-989

[15] Schon D. From technical rationality to reflection in action. In: Dowie J, Elstein A, editors. Professional Judgment: A Reader in Clinical Decision Making. Cambridge: Cambridge University Press; 1983. pp. 21-75

[16] Dreyfus SE, Dreyfus HL. A Five-Stage Model of Mental Activities Involved in Direct Skill Acquisition. Washington, DC: Storming Media; 1980

[17] Circielli VG. Family Caregiving: Autonomous and Paternalistic Decision-Making. Newbury Park, California: Sage; 1992

[18] Davies S, Wilson-Brown C. Shared decision-making in care homes. In: National Care Home Research and Development Forum, editor. My Home Life: Quality of Life in Care Homes - a Review of the Literature. London: Help the Aged; 2007. pp. 85-95

[19] Rowles GD, High DM. Family involvement in nursing home facilities. A decision-making perspective. In: Stafford PB, editor. Gray Areas: Ethnographic Encountered with Nursing Home Culture. New Mexico: School of American Research Press; 2003. pp. 173-202

[20] Tversky A, Kahneman D. The framing of decisions and the psychology of choice. Science. 1981;**211**:453-458

[21] Johnson R, Popejoy LL, Radina ME. Older adults' participation in nursing home placement decisions. Clinical Nursing Research. 2010;**19**:358-375

[22] Chow NWS. The practice of filial piety among the Chinese in Hong Kong. In: Chi I, Chappell NL, Lubben J, editors. Elderly Chinese in Pacific Rim Countries: Social Support and Integration. Hong Kong: Hong Kong University Press; 2001. pp. 125-136

[23] Chow N. Asian value and aged care. Geriatrics and Gerontology International. 2004; **4**:S21-S25

[24] Hong Kong Government (2006). The 2005-2006 policy address: Policy agenda. Hong Kong: Hong Kong Government Printer. Retrieved 6 February, 2006, from http://www.policyaddress.gov.hk/05-06/eng/news.htm

[25] Low LPL. The determinants of a quality home life for older people in Hong Kong. Hong Kong Journal of Nursing. 1997;**33**(1):4-9

[26] Low LPL. Dependency of elders in residential care homes - preliminary findings from older women. 6th European Doctoral Conference in Nursing Science (p. 54), Maastricht, Netherlands, 29 September–1 October; 2005

[27] Baltes MM. The Many Faces of Dependency in Old Age. Cambridge: Cambridge University Press; 1996

[28] Rodwell MK. Social Work Constructivist Research. London: Garland; 1998

[29] Charmaz K. Constructing Grounded Theory. A Practical Guide through Qualitative Analysis. London: Sage; 2006

[30] Charmaz K. Grounded theory: Objectivistic and constructivist methods. In: Denzin N, Lincoln Y, editors. Handbook of Qualitative Inquiry. Thousand Oaks, California: Sage; 2000. pp. 509-535

[31] Patton MQ. Qualitative Evaluation and Research Methods. 2nd ed. Newbury Park, California: Sage; 1990

[32] Warren CAB. Qualitative interviewing. In: Gubrium JF, Holstein JA, editors. Handbook of Interview Research: Context and Method. C.A: Thousand Oaks; 2002. pp. 83-101

[33] Schreiber RS, Stern PN. Using Grounded Theory in Nursing. New York: Springer Publishing; 2001

[34] Charmaz K. Qualitative interviewing and grounded theory analysis. In: Gubrium JF, Holstein JA, editors. Handbook of Interview Research: Context and Methods. Thousand Oaks, California: Sage; 2002. pp. 675-694

[35] Glaser B. Theoretical Sensitivity. Mill Valley, California: Sociology Press; 1978

[36] Davies S, Nolan M. 'Making the best of things': Relatives' experiences of decisions about care-home entry. Ageing and Society. 2003;**23**:429-450

[37] Davies S, Nolan M. 'Making the move': Relatives' experiences of the transition to a care home. Health and Social Care in the Community. 2004;**12**(6):517-526

[38] O'May F. Transition into a care home. In: National Care Homes and Research and Development Forum. editor, My Home Life: Quality of Life in Care Homes – A Review of the Literature. London: Help the Aged; 2007. pp. 42-50

[39] Reed J, Payton V, Bond S. Settling in and moving on: Transience and older people in care homes. Social Policy and Administration. 1998;**32**:151-165

[40] Reed J, Payton V. Constructing familiarity and managing the self: Ways of adapting to life in nursing and residential homes for older people. Ageing and Society. 1996;**16**:543-560

[41] Knight C, Haslam A, Haslam C. In home or at home? How collective decision making in a new care facility enhances social interaction and wellbeing amongst older adults. Ageing and Society. 2010;**30**:1393-1418

[42] Reed J, Payton V. Working to Create Continuity: Older People Managing the Move to the Care Home Setting. Report No. 76. Centre for Health Services Research: University of Newcastle, Newcastle Upon Tyne; 1996

[43] Lee DTF. A review of older people's experiences with residential care placement. Journal of Advanced Nursing. 2002;**37**:19-27

[44] Holroyd EE. Hong Kong Chinese family caregiving: Cultural categories of bodily order and the location of self. Qualitative Health Research. 2003a;**13**(2):158-170

[45] Holroyd EE. Chinese family obligations toward chronically ill elderly members: Comparing caregivers in Beijing and Hong Kong. Qualitative Health Research. 2003b; **18**(3):302-318

[46] Low LPL, Lee DTF, Chan AW. An exploratory study of Chinese older people's perceptions of privacy in residential care homes. Journal of Advanced Nursing. 2007;**57**(6):605-613

[47] Cook G. Older people actively reconstructing life in a care home. International Journal of Older People Nursing. 2008;**3**(4):270-373

[48] Cook G. Ensuring older residents retain their unique identity. Nursing and Residential Care. 2010;**12**(12):290-293

[49] Janssen BM, Regenmortel TV, Abma TA. Identifying sources of strength: Resilience from the perspective of older people receiving long-term community care. European Journal of Ageing. 2011;**8**:145-156

[50] Moyle W, Clarke C, Gracia N, Reed J, Cook G, Klein B, Marais S, Richardson E. Older people maintain mental health well-being through resilience: An appreciative study in four countries. Journal of Nursing and Health Care of Chronic Illness. 2010;**2**:113-121

[51] Hammond KR. Intuitive and analytical cognition: Information models. In: Sage A, editor. Concise Encyclopedia of Information Processing in Systems and Organizations. Oxford: Pergamon Press; 1990. pp. 306-312

[52] Croskerry P, Norman G. Overconfidence in clinical decision-making. American Journal of Medicine. 2008;**121**(5A):S24-S29

5

Cognitive Aging

Neyda Ma Mendoza-Ruvalcaba,
Elva Dolores Arias-Merino,
María Elena Flores-Villavicencio,
Melina Rodríguez-Díaz and
Irma Fabiola Díaz-García

Abstract

The study of cognitive function in gerontology is considered relevant because it is an important risk factor for other pathologies in the old age, such as physical disability and dependence, depression, and frailty, mainly because of early pathological changes in cognitive function which are considered a preclinical state that may progress to dementia. In this chapter, cognitive functioning and the dimensions that are included in it (attention, memory, meta-memory, processing speed, executive functions, visuospatial skills, and language) are conceptualized. Additionally, the current evidence is analyzed regarding age-associated changes that are experienced during cognitive aging. These changes, or cognitive decline, are distinguished from those that are part of cognitive pathologies, the most common mild cognitive impairment and dementia. Such pathologies are conceptualized based on the current diagnostic criteria, and controversies and challenges are discussed. Additionally, we analyze the risk factors for cognitive functioning in aging, both modifiable and nonmodifiable ones. A review of the main nonpharmacological intervention techniques used from the gerontology approach is made. It includes the cognitive training in the case of age-related decline or techniques of stimulation and cognitive rehabilitation in the case of mild cognitive impairment or dementia. Finally, we conclude with an analysis of the current state of this topic in the field of gerontology and its relevance in professional practice.

Keywords: cognitive aging, age-related decline, mild cognitive impairment, dementia, cognitive intervention

1. Introduction

Population aging is a global reality that is happening in a gradual and unavoidable manner, as a result of the low birth rate and mortality in the population, and at the same time, due to the increase in life expectancy. However, aging is not only a population phenomenon but also an individual reality [1], which involves a series of changes in people at biological, psychological and social levels. In the psychological field, changes in the domains related to personality, affectivity, emotions, emotional control, and interpersonal relationships have been reported [2].

Regarding cognitive functioning, the changes that occur during aging are of increasing interest for gerontology because of the implications they could have in case they finally appear in their most pathological form: dementia.

Historically, the research of cognitive functions has its epistemological origin in the studies carried out by the philosopher Galenus, who argued that in the ventricles of the brain, the consciousness of the human being was found as a set of different capacities: perception, intellect, and memory. From the philosophy of Rene Descartes (1596–1650) arises the neurophysiological theory, which defined the relationship between body and spirit and tried to find the explanation of mental function in the ventricles as the basis of psychic functions, later setting the pineal gland as related to mental disorders.

Later, Flourens (1794–1867) argued that all neural tissues are involved in the different cognitive functions. But it was until Gall's studies (1758–1828) with his Frenology theory, that on one side, cognitive functions were associated with structures by examining the skull, and on the other side, the role of the cerebral cortex in relation to cognitive functions was presented. It was until the nineteenth century, with the establishment of the neuropsychology, when the correlation of anatomo-clinical structures with the alterations in cognitive functions was clearly set up [3, 4].

During the nineteenth century, the first stage of neuropsychology was established. Its study object is the relationship between the cerebral organization and the behavior in its broadest sense: actions, emotions, motivations, and social relations. The unit of analysis of neuropsychology is the individual, including his personal history, and his social and cultural environment. The founders of this approach are Luria, Vygotsky, and Leontiev, with the concern of locating psychological functions within circumscribed parts of the brain, defined higher mental human functions as complex reflex-like processes of social origin whose functioning is both conscious and voluntary and are possible due to their structure and functioning [5]. Later, in 1981, Luria proposed that cognitive functioning analysis should be done by looking for what is located outside the individual, the place where the origins of conscious activity are found. He also developed the idea that several macroanatomical areas and brain regions help each other to ensure control of the so-called human cognitive functions [6]. The cognitive psychology perspective studies the cognitive functioning as the way to know the world, through the construction of reality guided by experience. From there, the cognitive structure is formed and the concept of a cognitive scheme arises [7].

Piaget's theory can be found under this perspective, where the study of structures is left aside to focus on the development of cognitive functioning and its schemes, from a constructive approach of knowledge that at the same time disproves empiricists and innatists theories, based on a psychogenetic perspective [8].

Neuropsychology is a discipline with an integrative view, which today contributes decisively to our knowledge about how the brain and the alterations of its functioning work, focused on the cognitive development in relation to sociocultural factors.

The conceptualization of cognitive functioning functions had several meanings.

Cognitive functioning has been defined as an evolutionary process in which individuals are immersed, which begins in fertilization and ends in death. In this process, both the organism in general and the nervous system in particular experience a series of changes that, in interaction with the environment, enable the development and maturation of both the nervous system itself and the behavior [9].

A more integrative view of mind-brain relationships defines the cognitive functions as functional interactions within and among cortical networks, which in turn are distributed throughout the cerebral cortex as memory, attention, perception, language, and intelligence; all sharing the same structure [4].

From another perspective, cognitive functions come from the information processing activity in neural networks distributed along the cortex and represent past and future schemes of action. This perspective suggests that temporal organization affects perceptual processes, action, and cognition within a sequence designed to achieve a goal [10].

From a psychopedagogical framework, complex cognitive functions consist of the organizing and sequencing of plans, the ability to respond to various stimuli at the same time, cognitive flexibility, the ability to respond according to the context, resistance to distraction, and inhibition of inappropriate behaviors [11].

From Piaget's theoretical position, cognitive functions are considered as the mechanisms of information processing, which main function is to transform the internal and external stimuli into inputs for development and, in addition, to provide the individual with tools to face the positive entropy, and also the trend to exhibit states of thermodynamic equilibrium [12].

From the point of view of the structural cognitive modifiability theory, the cognitive functions are classified as perceptual thinking (basic functions), strategic (executive functions), analogical (educational functions), and reflexive (meta-cognitive functions) according to the last generation of the constructivism paradigm [13].

Finally, from the neuropsychology perspective, the different components of cognitive functions are defined as the abilities developed by brain structures that allow them to work with the information that is acquired from the environment. These cognitive abilities are divided into two groups: those known as basic cognitive functions such as sensation, perception, memory, attention and concentration; and higher cognitive functions such as thought, language, and intelligence, which are considered complex systems and also group different functions [14].

2. Age-associated changes

During the last decades, several scientific efforts have been focused on the study of normal cognitive aging. This has resulted in agreements, as well as numerous discrepancies around the topic, mostly regarding the use of different research methodologies, as well as the little control of other variables that are considered to be closely related to cognitive functioning.

In addition, finding differences between normal cognitive aging and a cognitive impairment involving pathology is clinically difficult, since the limits of diagnosis are not precise.

This task becomes even more complicated if these differences are also associated with other variables such as age, schooling, and other population differences [15].

The concept of cognitive functioning in normal aging has been defined as "the functioning of the cognitive system, either in adaptation or alteration, which can generate a regression or successful management of the functions of daily life in older adults" [16].

The study of the changes that occur in the cognitive domains has found a close relationship between the physiological and social aspects. On one hand, research focused on the study of the human brain through different techniques (brain mapping, electroencephalogram and cerebral magnetic resonance among others) has reported that the mechanism behind successful cognitive aging may be the preservation of the hippocampal function combined with a high responsiveness in the frontal area [17].

Likewise, studies developed with electroencephalogram and neuropsychological tests found a reduction in age-dependent cerebral electrical power in cortical areas such as the parietal, temporal, and occipital lobes, causing a decline in functions such as memory, attention, visuospatial skills, and processing speed, concluding that the physiological aging of the brain is characterized by a loss of synaptic contacts and neuronal apoptosis that causes a dependent decline in sensory aspects, processing, motor performance, and some cognitive functions.

On the other hand, Steffener et al. [18] conducted a study which reported that cognitive changes during normal aging are due to the slow decrease across different ages of cerebral blood flow and the gray matter volume, mainly in areas such as the prefrontal cortex and the temporal convolutions of the putamen and occipital regions. On the other hand, the social aspects that have been described in different longitudinal studies and were related to the changes of the cognitive functioning in older adults are the schooling, the good health, the social participation, the lifestyle, and the genetic factors [17, 18].

It should be pointed out that socioenvironmental variables can contribute to an individual's cerebral aging and therefore modify his cognitive and behavioral profile. This causes that while some of these factors can affect negatively, precipitating cognitive deterioration in normal aging, others can soften or even slow their effects.

To recognize which cognitive functions normally decline in older adults and when they occur is a complicated task, however, research has agreed that the domains generally involved in it are attention, verbal memory, visuospatial and visuoconstructive skills, processing speed and some of the executive functions such as inhibition, working memory and mental flexibility, while functions such as semantic memory and language are preserved, and even the latter can improve over the years [19–21].

Attention is a complex, dynamic, multimodal, and hierarchical functional system that makes easier the processing of information, selecting the relevant stimuli to perform a certain sensory, cognitive, or motor activity [21]. According to data, cognitive changes are particularly difficult for older adults, mainly in activities that involve orienting them between several elements or constantly changing between different successive testing options, due to the decrease in selective visual attention, which in part is due to the degradation of sensory processing.

It is important to emphasize that attention control is related to other cognitive functions such as processing speed, which suggests that older adults are less involved in tasks of anticipatory attentional resources due to the slower reaction time during aging [22].

Changes associated with age have been studied from the different domains of cognitive functioning.

Memory is a neurocognitive function that allows us to record, encode, consolidate, retain, store, retrieve, and evoke information [21]. This cognitive function has a sequence of three types of memory, from sensory to short-term (which is a transitory, fragile and sensitive storage to interfering agents) to long term memory (responsible for the more permanent storage of information and involves a process of consolidation); each have their own particular mode of operation but they all cooperate in the process of memorization and can be seen as three necessary steps in forming the lasting memory. There are also three main processes involved in the human memory: encoding, storage and recall (retrival) [23].

Memory is one of the most studied cognitive domains because it is a frequent complaint that older adults make during normal aging. Kral's research since 1962 has led to evidence of the existence of a slowly progressing memory loss characterized by the inability to remember, sometimes relatively unimportant parts of the experiences of the past. The affectation of this domain in its processes of acquisition, consolidation, and spontaneous evocation is related to the cerebral biological functioning that will depend on variables such as quality of life.

Regarding the different types of memory, aging has a significant effect, on one hand, on the decline of immediate and episodic memory rather than on semantics and, on the other hand, on evocation rather than consolidation. Aging also affects the codification of new information, especially when strategic processing is needed [24].

Perception is the mental capacity that allows us to integrate and recognize through our senses. It allows us to recognize those objects to which we pay attention and to create our own knowledge patterns. In that sense, there must be an encounter between the sensorial information and the memory files that leads to the perception or interpretation of reality.

It is often difficult to dissociate spatial skills from constructional ones, being the latter defined as the ability to integrate elements into an organized whole (examples of these skill are copying geometric figures and the construction with cubes), since it requires the handling of space. According to the Pan-American Health Organization, changes in these cognitive functions in aging are due to the decline of visual acuity and processing, which causes problems of sensitivity to illumination and vision difficulties in poorly lit places, problems to distinguish colors, to focus at different distances and deficits related to spatial perception in general.

The executive functions (or meta-cognitive processes) would be those processes involved in the planning and supervision of cognitive processing. The term "executive" encompasses a series of cognitive processes, including updating and tracking information and inhibiting responses [24].

This kind of functions could be understood as a set of high-level operations that sequence and control the basic operations and, at the same time, make decisions in the moments of choosing among alternatives. Because they are linked with other cognitive functions, it is difficult to evaluate them in a specific way. At the same time, it is more complicated to find tasks that refer only to the performance of each one of them.

Some of the tasks that have been considered as executive functions are the working memory, the majority of everyday cognitive tasks that require the establishment of goals, the implementation and follow-up of the operations to reach those goals, and both the checkup of each one of these operations and of the fulfillment of the final purpose; their relevance could be used as evidence of the importance of executive functions in the lives of people [25]. In normal aging, it has been found that changes in executive functions are mainly observed in: working memory, when keeping information available for a short period of time; in inhibition, because over the years, more problems to concentrate on relevant information are experienced and inhibit attention to irrelevant aspects, in addition inhibitory processes are less efficient to allow the initial entry of information into the operational memory and in mental flexibility [26].

Processing speed has been defined as the reaction time that produces a global effect on cognition [27]. It is one of the functions in which a decline has been found as part of normal aging, and it has even been associated with the cause of cognitive changes in other domains such as care and executive functioning.

Moreover, as a cognitive task becomes more complex, older adults may not have the necessary resources of mental operations to carry out the later phases of it because cognitive functioning is slower and sometimes does not allow them to complete some mental operations that are needed for a correct final task performance [28]. Other studies compared two groups, one of young adults and other of older adults, and applied neuropsychological tasks to measure executive functioning and found a lower performance in inhibitory control, abstraction, and working memory but not the rest of this kind of functions [29].

The subjective perception of adults about their cognitive functioning (also called meta-memory) is another factor that significantly influences the activities of daily living (ADL) during aging, a recent study showed that a third of the evaluated population reported memory problems, thinking skills, and their ability to reason, all of them associated with their overall health [30].

Finally, it is important to note that the cognitive changes that occur in normal aging are presented as a slight decline and do not interfere with the level of independence during aging; if these changes appear in the opposite way, it is possible to suspect deterioration or cognitive change related to a pathology.

3. Mild cognitive impairment and dementia

In cognitive aging, there is a decline which is considered normal. Some cognitive functions remain stable while others decline as part of normal aging. These cognitive changes associated with age occur to people who do not have pathologies that affect memory or cognitive abilities, and these changes do not interfere with the ability to participate in everyday activities. However, cognitive changes in aging can have a wide range, from those that are normal to those that are pathological, and between these there may be a series of intermediate changes. This transition state is known as Mild Cognitive Impairment (MCI) [31].

The construct of Mild Cognitive Impairment (MCI) has been extensively used worldwide, both in clinical and in research settings, to define the gray area between intact cognitive functioning and clinical. The MCI intends to identify this intermediate stage of cognitive impairment that is often, but not always, a transitional phase from cognitive changes in normal aging to those typically found in dementia [32]; in this sense, MCI is considered a predemential syndrome [33].

In 2013, the American Psychiatric Association (APA) proposed new criteria for dementia in the fifth edition of the Diagnostic and Statistical Manual for Mental Disorders (DSM-5) and recognizes the predementia stage of cognitive impairment [34]. The condition, which has many of the features of MCI, is known as mild neurocognitive disorder (NCD). Mild NCD recognizes subtle features of cognitive impairment that are different from aging but do not represent dementia. Furthermore, mild NCD focuses on the initial phases of cognitive disorders and precedes major NCD that is analogous to the previous diagnosis of dementia.

There are several subtypes of MCI, which differ according to the type and number of impaired cognitive abilities, the most common is the amnesic which mainly involves memory problems, while in the nonamnesic, memory operation is not compromised. Likewise, when only one dimension of cognitive functioning is affected, it is called DCL of a domain or multidomain if more than one cognitive ability (e.g., memory, reasoning, executive functions, etc.) is affected [32]. These MCI subtypes are usually related to different pathological processes, for example, it has been found that people with amnestic DCL are more likely to progress to Alzheimer's disease (AD) [35, 36], while people with nonamnestic MCI are more likely to develop Lewy Body Dementia [36].

According to this definition, MCI is operationalized based on clinical data of changes in cognitive abilities (see **Table 1**). The subjective cognitive complaint needs to be confirmed by objective cognitive measures, such as neuropsychological test batteries. Objective cognitive impairment is defined as a poor performance in one or more cognitive measures, which suggests deficits in one or more cognitive areas or domains. There is no gold standard to specify which neuropsychological test battery to use, but it is important that all the main cognitive areas are examined. Typically, executive functions, attention, language, memory, and visuospatial skills are taken into account. Functional abilities are investigated by means of a thorough interview with the person and with the next of kin and registered in terms of activities of daily living (ADL) and instrumental activities of daily living (IADL) scales [32].

According to this definition, MCI is operationalized based on clinical data of changes in cognitive abilities (see **Table 1**). The subjective cognitive complaint needs to be confirmed by objective cognitive measures, such as neuropsychological test batteries. Objective cognitive impairment is defined as a poor performance in one or more cognitive measures, which suggests deficits in one or more cognitive areas or domains. There is no gold standard to specify which neuropsychological test battery to use, but it is important that all the main cognitive areas are examined. Typically, executive functions, attention, language, memory, and visuospatial skills are taken into account. Functional abilities are investigated by means of an in-depth interview with the person and with the person's next of kin and registered in terms of both activities of daily living (ADL) and instrumental activities of daily living (IADL) scales [32].

It has been shown that a significant proportion of people with MCI progresses to dementia in periods of 1–2 years and approximately 50% progresses toward dementia over a 5-year period [37].

	Normal aging [31]	Mild cognitive impairment [32]	Dementia DSM-IV [41]	Major neurocognitive disorder DSM-5 [34]
Memory	Absence or presence or memory complaints Normal objective memory according to age. Memory problems are gradual, do not worsen suddenly	Subjective cognitive complaint, raised by the patient or an informant, or observations made by the clinician	A1. Memory impairment	A. Evidence of significant cognitive decline from a previous level of performance in one or more cognitive domains: • Learning and memory • Language • Executive function • Complex attention • Perceptual-motor • Social cognition
Other cognitive functions	Normal cognitive functioning according to age	Objective cognitive impairment in one or more cognitive domains preferably relative to appropriate normative data for that individual	The course of deterioration is characterized by a gradual onset and a continuous cognitive impairment. A2. At least one of the following: • Aphasia • Apraxia • Agnosia • Disturbance in executive functioning	Evidence of decline is based on: Concern of the individual, a knowledgeable informant, or the clinician that there has been a significant decline in cognitive function; and a substantial impairment in cognitive performance, preferably documented by standardized neuropsychological testing or, in its absence, another quantified clinical assessment.
Activities of daily living (ADL)	Preservation of functional independence	Preservation of functional independence	B. The cognitive deficits in A1 and A2 each cause significant impairment in social or occupational functioning and represent a significant decline from a previous level of functioning	B. The cognitive deficits interfere with independence in everyday activities. At a minimum, assistance should be required with complex instrumental activities of daily living
Associated pathologies	No dementia	No dementia	C. The cognitive deficits do not occur exclusively during the course of delirium	C. The cognitive deficits do not occur exclusively in the context of a delirium D. The cognitive deficits are not better explained by another mental disorder

Table 1. Comparison of the different diagnostic criteria in normal aging, mild cognitive impairment and dementia (according to DSM-IV and DSM-5).

Dementia is a NCD that usually begins gradually and has a progressive course. It can be variable, and there is often a long period of time between the occurrence of the first signs of cognitive impairment and the moment they meet the criteria for the dementia diagnosis [38].

The American Psychiatric Association (APA) introduced in 2013 the term "Major neurocognitive disorder" replacing the term "dementia," defined as a decline in mental ability severe enough to interfere with independence and daily life [34]. However, not all the care professionals and organizations are likely to use the new term. Currently, the Alzheimer's Association, for example, uses the term *dementia* instead of *neurocognitive disorder*. See criteria in **Table 1**.

Globally, around 47 million people have dementia, with nearly 60% living in low- and middle-income countries, and there are 9.9 million new cases every year; Alzheimer's disease is the most common cause of dementia and may contribute to 60–70% of cases. The estimated proportion of the general population aged 60 years and over with dementia at a given time is between 5 and 8 per 100 people. The total number of people with dementia is projected to near 75 million in 2030 and almost triple by 2050 to 132 million. Much of this increase is attributable to the rising numbers of people with dementia living in low- and middle-income countries [39]. The most common forms of dementia are Alzheimer's disease and vascular dementia (VD) [40]. **Table 1** shows a comparison of diagnostic criteria in normal aging, mild cognitive impairment, and dementia.

4. Risk factors for mild cognitive impairment and dementia

Science has gradually shown which risk factors (RF) for MCI and dementia can be currently considered. The knowledge of RF for these pathological processes plays an important role in its prevention. Ideally, prevention strategies should target people who are not even symptomatic [42]. Prevention of dementia is a public health priority [43].

In the health sciences field, a RF is the probability of suffering a certain disease, having a complication or dying [44]. In this paper, we will present some of the most recognized RF, classifying them according to their origin in social, biological, and psychological and by their nature in modifiable and nonmodifiable (see **Table 2**).

4.1. Biological factors

4.1.1. Vascular disorders

Regarding blood pressure (BP), both high and low BP have been linked to cognitive impairment and dementia [45]. The role of cerebral blood vessels in the wide spectrum of pathologies underlying cognitive impairment highlights the importance of vascular structure and function in brain health [46]. The pathophysiology of the relationship between BP and cognition

Risk factors	Modifiable	Nonmodifiables
(A) Biological	Vascular disorders	Genetic
	Metabolic disorders: diabetes mellitus	Brain injuries
(B) Psychological	Depression	—
(C) Social	Education	Age
	Intellectual commitment	Sex

Table 2. Risk factors for MCI and dementia.

is unclear, but hypoperfusion and neurodegeneration have emerged as potential underlying mechanisms [45, 47]. Results from a longitudinal study as part of the Kungsholmen Project [48] showed that low diastolic pressure predicted the risk of dementia among very old people. In the study, blood pressure showed a substantial decrease for approximately 3 years before the dementia syndrome became clinically evident [45].

In contrast, cohort studies have found that elevated blood pressure levels in the middle age may increase the risk of dementia in advanced age. As a result, the exposure to four risk factors related to BP: smoking, hypertension, high cholesterol, and diabetes in the middle age increased the risk of dementia in old age compared to only having one of the risk factors [49]. This relationship between blood pressure and the risk of dementia may depend on the age of patients when blood pressure is measured, as well as the time interval between blood pressure and dementia assessments [50, 51].

4.1.2. Metabolic disorders: diabetes mellitus

Diabetes mellitus (DM) is associated with a dementia risk of 1.5–2.5 times higher among old adults in the community. DM is a significant risk factor not only for vascular dementia but also for Alzheimer's Disease. The mechanisms that support this association are unclear but may be multifactorial in nature, such as cardiovascular risk factors, glucose toxicity, changes in insulin metabolism, and inflammation [52].

Both hyperglycemia and hyperinsulinemia, as part of the metabolic process leading to DM type 2 (DM2), are associated with cognitive dysfunction and dementia due to stroke. This is often accompanied by other mental function disorders, such as depression or anxiety [53]. An epidemiological study showed that the incidence rates of hospitalization for VD in adult aged 70 years and over were twice as high in patients with DM2 as in those who did not presented it [54].

4.1.3. Genetic factors

Genetics clearly plays a role in AD, both in early and late onset. Early-onset AD or beginning before age 65 years can be caused by one of the more than 200 sequence variants in the genes of the beta amyloid precursor protein, presenilin 1 (PSEN1), or presenilin 2 (PSEN2) [55, 56]. Despite the consistent genetic basis for AD, significant variability in onset age has been observed, suggesting an important role of environmental factors or genetic modifiers in determining the onset age [56]. Late-onset AD is also heavily influenced by genetics, although the Mendelian pattern of inheritance is often unclear. There are several factors that could explain this, even if causal mutations exist [57]. Late-onset AD is complex, and apolipoprotein E is the only genetic risk factor unanimously accepted for its development. Several genes involved in AD have been identified using advanced genetic technologies; however, there are many additional genes that have not been identified [58].

Related to this, a long research that analyzed the Genealogical Index of Familiarity up to 14 generations showed that the pairs of people with family ties who died of AD were significantly related. The relative risk for AD death among the relatives of individuals who died of AD increased significantly for close and distant relatives [57].

4.1.4. Previous brain injuries

A new area of interest involves understanding the effect that head trauma has on the behavior and cognitive abilities of brain aging. This issue becomes even more important as the geriatric population grows [59].

Traumatic brain injury (TBI) is an injury in which effects could be devastating often resulting in lifetime cognitive deficits [60]. More than 70% of people with TBI report memory deficits [61]. Contact sports are a source of recurrent TBI. Athletes whose last concussion was in early adulthood (more than 30 years before examination) were reported to have poorer episodic memory and poorer response inhibition, as well as significantly reduced movement speeds in neuropsychological tests, when compared with same-age athletes without a history of concussion [62]. Regarding the cognitive aging process, the evidence showed that cognition problems exhibited by young adults after severe TBI are similar to many cognitive weaknesses in attention deficit and poor working memory of an elderly population with no neurological history. There is evidence that TBI can result in decreased cognitive reserve that can accelerate the cognitive decline normal process, leading to premature aging, potentially increasing the risk of dementia [63].

4.2. Psychological factors

4.2.1. Depression

Depression can affect cognitive functions and may emulate cognitive impairment. It can be considered comorbidity, a prodromal factor or a consequence of vascular cognitive impairment, more than a factor that specifically alters vascular physiology or neural health, leading to cognitive impairment [64]. Some studies have concluded that depressive symptoms are associated with cognitive impairment; however, the mechanisms underlying the association between these two common conditions need further exploration. It is unclear whether cognitive impairment over time can be explained by depression or it is just a sign of an incipient dementia [65].

4.3. Social factors

4.3.1. Age and sex

Through studies results, the age and sex of the individuals have been considered as risk factors of mild cognitive impairment and dementia. Some studies have reported that the prevalence of dementia increases exponentially with age [66] and doubles every 5 years after the age of 65 years. Several studies showed an increasing prevalence among the older age groups [67, 68]. In higher income countries, prevalence is 5–10% among those over 65 years [68]. Regarding sex, there are results in which dementia is higher in women than in men [68, 69]. One possible explanation for this is that women live longer than men [68]. However, recently, another cohort study reported that both the prevalence and the incidence were higher in men [69, 70].

4.3.2. Education and intellectual commitment

Dr. James A. Mortimer was one of the first to propose a relationship between years of formal education and risk of dementia. He suggested that education can be a protective factor against dementia, raising the level of "intellectual reserve." Regarding this, a systematic review of the literature on the relationship between education and dementia in the last 25 years concluded that lower education was associated with an increased risk of dementia in many but not all studies.

Education associated with the risk of dementia showed different results according to the population, and the years of education did not uniformly reduce the risk of dementia. It seems that a more consistent relationship with dementia occurred when the years of education reflected cognitive ability, suggesting that the effect of education on the risk of dementia can be better assessed in the context of a life development model [71].

In addition to this, occupations performed during lifetime that did not require complex cognitive processes or stimulants seem to be associated with an increased risk of dementia. For example, when studying a group of nuns (average 54 years of age), a strong association was found between low educational and occupational levels with dementia. The risk of dementia increased in those participants with poor education, without professional training and who had never been in charge of a leadership position. These findings support the hypothesis of the benefits of having a cognitive reserve capacity against the consequences of brain diseases [72]. In this sense, it was reported that university preparation represented a lower risk of dementia among five categories, where illiterates showed the highest proportion of individuals with dementia, while the lowest proportion was found in university students [73].

5. Intervention in cognitive aging

Broadly speaking, research on cognitive aging shows a gradual decline scenario, which may or may not be normative, and is associated with age and previously identified risk factors. The progression from normality to pathology is a concern in the health sciences field due to the negative implications that mild cognitive impairment and dementia have on people's lives.

This is why gerontology has focused on the study of nonpharmacological intervention techniques that promote the improvement or maintenance of cognitive functioning at a level that allows people to lead a functional and disability-free life associated with cognitive pathologies. The main conceptual basis for nonpharmacological intervention on cognitive functioning in aging focuses mainly on the concepts of brain plasticity, brain reserve, and cognitive reserve.

Under the concept of brain plasticity [74], in the last 25 years, evidence has been presented to support the idea that the brain is far more flexible in structure and function than it was previously believed. Brain plasticity refers to the extraordinary ability of the brain to modify its own structure and function following changes within the body or in the external environment. Although it is stronger during childhood, it remains the fundamental and significant lifelong property of the brain during aging. Brain plasticity is implicated in learning abilities and plays a fundamental role in degenerative brain disorders. Recent research suggests that the pathology of the Alzheimer's disease, for example, is associated with the loss of plasticity.

The brain reserve is related to neurobiological aspects and it has a more passive approach, since it refers to the size and number of neurons that a person has after a brain injury.

Finally, the cognitive reserve has been defined as the adaptation of the brain to an injury situation using pre-existing cognitive processing resources or compensation resources through the activation of neural networks [75]. The cognitive reserve allows better tolerance of the effects of the disease associated with dementia, supporting a greater amount of neuropathologies before reaching the symptoms of the disease. The cognitive reserve influences the manifestation of the symptoms of cognitive impairment and, at least partially, in its development toward dementia [76]. People with MCI and low reserves show a steeper decline early in the process of deterioration, compared to the high level of reserve this marked deterioration would have at the end of the process, due to the protective role of this reserve [77].

The intervention for the optimization of cognitive functions is based on these concepts to implement nonpharmacological treatments, in order to overcome the challenges of cognitive changes associated with aging, prevent pathologies such as MCI and dementia, and, finally, if it is necessary, alleviate their effects.

According to the British Psychological Society [78], there are a variety of nonpharmacological treatments and interventions which can help people to maintain good mental health, especially after diagnosis of MCI or dementia. Psychosocial interventions can help the diagnosis of dementia, reducing stress and improving mood (such as anxiety or depression), improving and maintaining cognitive functioning, and promoting quality of life in general. Specifically, treatments for improving and maintaining cognitive functioning in aging are Cognitive Training, Cognitive Stimulation Therapy, and Cognitive Rehabilitation that have significant differences in terms of their purpose, target population, duration, and management.

The Cognitive Training, also called Brain Training, involves specific aspects of memory and other cognitive skills. Since it is not personally tailored, regular pastimes such as crosswords, Sudoku, games, or exercises on a computer would also count as cognitive training. Cognitive training is for anyone who wants to keep his brain active and enjoys brain training games and puzzles, including people living with dementia. Exercises are designed to train specific functions, such as memory of words, logic and reasoning, attention, problem solving, and mathematics. Training could be a regular activity done continuously and can be self-administered [78].

Cognitive Stimulation Therapy (CST) is a group therapy that is used to help strengthen personal communications skills, thinking, and memory. CST groups run for a limited number of sessions (usually 12–14, one or two per week). As a complement, the maintenance cognitive stimulation therapy (MCST) groups continue indefinitely and aim to maintain the benefits that CST groups provide. CST and MCST are suitable for people with diagnosis of mild cognitive impairment or dementia in mild-to-moderate stages. A typical CST session lasts for 1 hour and may involve games, singing, applying reminiscence therapies, sharing stories, discussing current events, practicing arts, and making crafts. CST has shown to be beneficial for cognition and quality of life, and it is also cost-effective. Additionally, if CST is followed by MCST, it offers a significant improvement in cognitive function providing long-term benefits [79].

On the other side, cognitive rehabilitation is an approach to manage the impact that dementia-related difficulties, such as problems with thinking and memory, can have on everyday life. It is recommended for people who have early-onset dementia. Cognitive rehabilitation is not about curing or reducing dementia-related difficulties with thinking and memory, instead it is about learning ways of compensating these difficulties or managing them better. Many cognitive rehabilitation programs could involve families and careers. Usually, it is implemented by gerontologists, occupational therapists, clinical psychologists or clinical neuropsychologists [78]. Cognitive rehabilitation mainly focuses on identifying and addressing individual needs and goals, which may require strategies for taking in new information or compensatory methods such as memory aids, and has provided preliminary indications of its potential benefits in improving activities of daily living in people with mild Alzheimer's disease [80].

Any kind of cognitive intervention should be based on a previous diagnosis, including two types of assessment. The first should be a screening (usually with the Mini-Mental State Examination), and the second is an in-depth evaluation (with standardized tests in the socio-cultural context, according to age and schooling) of the performance of the individual in different cognitive tasks. From the diagnosis results if the person shows a "normal" or intact performance, meaning that he preserves his cognitive functions as expected to his age and schooling in their context; or it presents a significantly inferior performance that can be classified as slight cognitive impairment and in case of suspected dementia. This previous evaluation is needed to take the decision of whether an intervention is necessary and what kind is required, what aspects should be developed on and what capacities should be promoted [81].

The objectives of intervention programs based on training and/or cognitive stimulation are generally set out in terms of "improving, maintaining, strengthening, and restoring." While in programs based on cognitive rehabilitation, the objectives are defined in terms of "compensate."

Once the type and purpose of the treatment have been selected, during the planning of the cognitive intervention, basic methodological aspects must be considered, in order to systematize the steps involved in the process. These guidelines include [82]: (1) Systematic organization of the session and its activities, (2) progression, starting with easy and continue with difficult activities, (3) intensity, with a suitable and adapted rhythm, (4) logic and sense, with meaning and actual sequence, (5) the activities should be interesting, (6) motivation, curiosity, and desire to learn, (7) the activities should be gratifying, (8) personal and emotional involvement, the elements of the process should have a pleasant and emotional sense, (9) the elements of the process should promote the interpersonal relationships of people with their environment.

As a basic guideline during the intervention work, it is recommended to maintain a routine through a structured session, in this sense, as part of the training and/or cognitive stimulation a session scheme is proposed. It includes the following elements, not necessarily in this order:

1. Orientation to reality (personal, spatial and temporal) [81].

2. Attention/concentration technique.

3. Relaxation technique.

4. Psycho-educational technique, knowledge and theoretical information promote the improvement of the perception of memory.

5. Practical training in the use of mnemonic strategies adapted to the needs of the person (see **Table 3**).

6. Feedback and closure. Always ask: How does this help me in everyday life?

Strategies	Technique	Definition and examples
Internal	Organization/categorization	It consists of establishing categories of data or information grouping it based on their common characteristics. (e.g., grocery lists according to the type of food, color, location in the kitchen)
	Visualization	Based on the ability to recreate visual mental images. (Ex: visually imagine a photo or movie where all the elements that want to be remembered are found)
	Mental associations	Relate items that want to be remembered (e.g., associate the name of a person with a physical characteristic)
	Mental hooks	Associate elements linked to the imagination and location, which can mentally link data that can be easily located in the mind
	Story technique	Organize a story with data from a list of items or events that want to be remembered (e.g., to create a story that includes the planned activities during the day)
	Itinerary method	It is about making mental associations of an image in a specific place. To achieve this, a mental journey or an itinerary should be made, setting in certain places the elements to remember (e.g., in the different rooms of the house)
	Mental maps	It involves creating a panoramic view of a situation in order to remember both general and specific data
External	Memory aids	These are aids located in the context or near the person's environment. In this situation a person or object promotes the memory (e.g., change the ring from one finger to another, carrying a schedule, diary, calendar, etc. Ask a person to remind me of an activity)

Table 3. Mnemonic strategies and techniques that can be used as part of training and cognitive stimulation programs.

Mnemonic strategies are used for improving memory processes and with it ensuring that important information is available when needed in our daily lives. Memory strategies can be distinguished according to their origin, whether they are external or internal. The first involves using aids that are outside our body to help us remember things, while internal strategies are mental activities that engage the person in remembering information [31] (**Table 3**). Both types of strategies are effective ways of learning and retaining information and are widely used as part of training and cognitive stimulation programs in the aging process.

On the other hand, interventions based on cognitive rehabilitation, designed for people with mild to severe dementia, should be highly personalized to fulfill the requirements regarding both to the potential and deterioration of the person, so it is difficult to design sessions with rigid schemes. However, this does not imply that the work should not be systematized. In a review of interventions targeting people with Alzheimer's disease or related dementia, a diversity in the types of interventions was found which consisted mainly of memory training, reminiscence therapy, validation therapy, and life review techniques [83].

6. Final remarks

Cognitive changes associated with aging can range from subtle to severe, those related to normal aging are generally mild and do not interfere with the ability to participate in normal daily activities. On the other hand, cognitive pathologies, such as dementia, affect a person's ability to live independently and are overwhelming for the families of affected people. Physical, emotional, and economic pressures can cause great stress to families, and support is required from the health, social, financial, and legal systems [39]. Mild cognitive impairment falls between these extremes. In MCI, cognitive changes are more substantial than those seen in normal aging but not severe enough to cause disability. Both MCI and dementia are pathological conditions, caused by underlying brain disorders or conditions that are not part of the normal aging process [31].

In the study of the age-associated changes, declines in memory, attention, perception, speed processing, and some executive functions have been reported; however, there is considerable inconsistency in the results. Limitations of the studies should be analyzed in order to identify bias associated with methodology, differences in the assessment tools, and diagnostic and performance criteria. The optimal approach to study the age-related cognitive decline involves the longitudinal examination of population-based aging cohorts [84]. Despite this, researching on cognitive decline in normal aging is very relevant in the gerontology field, due to the possibility that it may represent a less severe but similar process to that in dementia [85]. Moreover, as decline in cognitive functioning and the onset of dementia are associated with older age, the study of social, environmental, and individual risk factors is also needed.

Estimating the burden of the disease and its proportion due to the major risk factors of mild cognitive impairment and dementia allows effective preventive measures to be taken, especially against those risk factors that are modifiable and highly dependent on lifestyles. The cardiovascular and DM2 risk decrease with healthy eating, physical exercise, and therapeutic control. On the other hand, continuous learning that stimulates lifelong cognitive training and leisure activities that represent intellectual challenges can also reduce the risk of cognitive impairment; also, depression symptoms could be successfully treated.

Besides the study of cognitive change in aging, the progress toward the pathologies and risk factors, the field of study of the gerontology involves the challenge to develop effective intervention programs for promoting cognitive health in aging and old age. In this sense, it has largely shown that loss of function in cognitive domains is partly preventable and controllable, since it is susceptible to training through strategies of cognitive stimulation and rehabilitation. Despite the heterogeneity and variety in interventions and outcomes, that limit generalizability, the role of nonpharmacological interventions targeting MCI is promising, and must studies found a benefit with the intervention [86].

Finally, population aging coincides with other converging and interdependent global trends that are shaping our collective future, regarding the epidemiological transitions the past decades have witnessed a major transformation in the profile of diseases that are the principal causes of disability and mortality. Today, chronic, noncommunicable diseases are the major cause of death and disability, and the rates are rising. The vast majority of older people have chronic conditions, and many have multiple conditions [87]. Mental diseases related to cognitive functioning are in the spotlight, specifically the dementia, considered as a public health priority [39]. The full impact of the pathologies in cognitive aging, mean mild cognitive impairment, or dementia is resonating throughout society. The economic costs of these pathologies impact families, health-care systems, businesses, and social structures. The emotional, psychological, and physical burdens of cognitive pathologies in aging impact individuals, his/her family, as well the formal support networks that provide assistance [83].

From Gerontology, the challenge entails rethinking the life course, to make aging a positive and disability-free individual experience. In this sense, the World Health Organization has proposed as a key element the active aging [88], also called "successful" [89] or "healthy" [90]. In any case, this type of ideal aging requires that the person can maintain an autonomous cognitive ability, which allows the functionality and control of his own life, for which it is necessary to preserve healthy cognitive functions.

Acknowledgements

Funded by the National Council of Science and Technology (CONACYT), México. Project: 256589.

Author details

Neyda Ma Mendoza-Ruvalcaba[1]*, Elva Dolores Arias-Merino[2],
María Elena Flores-Villavicencio[2], Melina Rodríguez-Díaz[1] and Irma Fabiola Díaz-García[2]

*Address all correspondence to: nmendoza_ruvalcaba@yahoo.com.mx

1 University of Guadalajara CUTONALA, Tonalá, Jalisco, Mexico

2 University of Guadalajara CUCS, Mexico

References

[1] Fernández Ballesteros R, Robine MA, Walker A, Kalache A. Active aging: A global goal. Current Gerontology Geriatrics Research. 2013;**2013**:1-4. http://dx.doi.org/10.1155/2013/298012

[2] Fernández-Ballesteros R, Moya RM, Iñiguez J, Zamarrón MD. Qué es la psicología de la vejez. Madrid: Biblioteca Nueva; 2009

[3] Maestú F, Quesney-Molina F, Ortiz-Alonso T, Campo P, Fernández-Lucas A, Amo C, Campo P. Cognición y redes neurales: una nueva perspectiva desde la neuroimagen funcional. Revista de Neurologia. 2003;**37**(10):962-966

[4] Villa-Rodríguez MA. Definición y breve historia de la Neuropsicología. México: UNAM; 2009. Available from: www.villaneuropsicologia.com/uploads/1/4/4/5/14457670/definicion_e_historia_de_la_neuropsicologia.pdf

[5] Luria AR. La alteración de las funciones corticales superiores en presencia de lesión en los sectores frontales. Las funciones corticales superiores del hombre. Habana: Editorial Orbe La; 1977. pp. 260-373

[6] Coelho Rebelo Mala LA, Fernández Da Silva C, Ribeiro Correia C, Perea-Bartolomé MV. EL modelo de Alexander romano Vich Luria (revisitado) y su aplicación a la evaluación neuropsicológica. Revista Galego-Portuguesa de Psicoloxía e Educación. 2006;**11-12**(13): 155-194

[7] Romo M. Teorías implícitas y creatividad artística. Arte, individuo y Sociedad. Vol. 10. Madrid: Servicio de Publicaciones, Universidad Complutense; 1998. pp. 11-28

[8] Martí E. La perspectiva piagetiana de 10s años 70 y 80: de las estructuras al funcionamiento. Anuario de Psicología. 1990;**44**:19-45

[9] Lapuente FR, Sánchez Navarro JP. Cambios neuropsicológicos asociados al envejecimiento normal. Anales de Psicología. 1998;**14**:1427-1443. Available from: http://udg. redalyc.org/articulo.oa?id=16714104. [Fecha de consulta: September 8, 2017]

[10] Tirapu-Ustárroz J, García-Molina A, Luna-Lario P, Roig-Rovira T, Pelegrín-Valero C. Modelos de funciones y control ejecutivo (II). Revista de Neurologia. 2008;**46**(12):742-750

[11] Pistoia M, Abad-Mas L, Etchepareborda MC. Abordaje psicopedagógico del trastorno por déficit de atención con hiperactividad con el modelo de entrenamiento de las funciones ejecutivas. Revista de Neurologia. 2004;**38**(Supol 1): S149-S155. (1086-1094). DOI: https://doi.org/10.1016/j.neurobiolaging.2013.10.095

[12] Fontaines RT, Rodríguez Y. Estructuras e interacciones en la construcción del conocimiento: Una propuesta a partir de los planteamientos teóricos de Piaget y Vigotsky. Laurus Revista de educación. 2008;**14**(28):97-121

[13] Duque AV. Funciones cognitivas. Prolegómenos de aprendizaje en estudiantes de Trabajo Social. Revista Eleuthera. 2013;**10**:160-181

[14] Correia R. Cambios cognitivos en el envejecimiento normal: Influencias de la edad y su relación con el nivel cultural y sexo. Curso Humanidades y Ciencias Sociales de la Universidad de ña Laguna España; 2012. Available from: http://riull.ull.es/xmlui/handle/915/3392 ISBN 978-84-15287-27-8

[15] Montes J, Gutiérrez L, Silva J. Perfil Cognoscitivo de Adultos Mayores de 60 Años Con y Sin Deterioro Conoscitivo. Revista Chilena Neuropsicología. 2012;**7**:121-126. DOI: 10.5839/rcnp.2012.0703.05

[16] Pereira J. Actividad Fisica y Capacidad Cognitiva en el Envejecimiento Humano [thesis]. España, Spain: Universidad de Granada; 2011

[17] Pudas S, Persson J, Luna X, Nilsson L, Nyberg L. Brain characteristics of individuals resisting age-related cognitive decline over two decades. The Journal of Neuroscience. 2013;**20**:8668-8677. DOI: 10.1523/JNEUROSCI.2900-12

[18] Steffener J, Brickman A, Habeck C, Salthouse T, Stern Y. Cerebral blood flow and gray matter volume covariance patterns of cognition in aging. Human Brain Mapping. 2013;**34**:3267-3279. DOI: 10.1002/hbm.22142

[19] Ballesteros S, Mayas J, Reales JM. Cognitive function in normal aging an in older adults with mild cognitive impairment. Psichotema. 2013;**1**:18-24. DOI: 10.7334/psicothema2012.181

[20] Salthouse TA. When does age-related cognitive decline begin? Neurobiology of Aging. 2009;**30**:507-514. DOI: 10.1017/S1355617709990385

[21] Potellano JA. Introducción a la neuropsicología. Madrid, Spain: McGraw Hill, México; 2005

[22] Pierre M, Ibañez V, Missonnier P, Rodriguez C, Giannakopoulos P. Age-associated modulations of cerebral oscillatory patterns related to attention control. NeuroImage. 2013;**82**:531-546. DOI: doi.org/10.1016/j.neuroimage.2013.06.037

[23] Atkinson RC, Shiffrin RM. Human memory: A proposed system and its control processes. In: Spence KW, Spence JT, editors. The Psychology of Learning and Motivation. New York: Academic Press. 1968. pp. 89-195

[24] Duda B, Puente A, Miller S. Cognitive reserve moderates relation between global cognition and functional status in older adults. Journal of Clinical and Experimental Neuropsychology. 2014;**4**:368-378. DOI: 10.1080/13803395.2014.892916

[25] Villar F. Capítulo 6. Psicología Cognitiva y procesamiento de la información. In: Psicología Evolutiva y Psicología de la Educación. 2003. pp. 308-372

[26] Luo L, Craik F. Aging and memory: A cognitive approach. La Revue Canadienne de Psychiatrie. 2008;**6**:346-353

[27] Salthouse TA. The processing-speed theory of adult age differences in cognition. Psychological Review. 1996;**103**:403-428

[28] Park DC. Cognitive Aging: A Primer. New York: Psychology Press; 2012

[29] Silver H. Executive fuctions and normal aging: Selective impairment in conditional exclusion compared to abstraction and inhibition. Dementia and Geriatric Cognitive Desordes. 2011;**31**:53-62

[30] Ficker L, Lysack C, Mena H, Lichtenberg A. Perceived cognitive impairment among African American elders: Health and functional impairments in daily life. Aging & Mental Health. 2013;**4**:471-480. DOI: 10.1080/13607863.2013.856859

[31] Anderson N, Murphy K, Troyer A. Living with Mild Cognitive Impairment. New York: Oxford University Press; 2012

[32] Petersen RC, Caracciolo B, Brayne C, Gauthier S, Jelic V, Fratigliono L. Mild cognitive impairment: A concept in evolution. Journal of International Medicine. 2014;**275**:214-228. DOI: 10.1111/joim.12190

[33] Petersen RC. Mild cognitive impairment as a diagnostic entity. Journal of Internal Medicine. 2004;**256**:183-194

[34] American Psychiatric Association. Diagnostic and Statistical Manual of Mental Disorders. 5th ed.. (DSM-5). Arlington, VA: American Psychiatric Association; 2013

[35] Fischer P, Jungwirth S, Zahetmayer S, Weissgram S, Hoenigschnabl S, Gelpi E, Krampla W, Tragl KH. Conversion from subtyper of mild cognitive impairment to Alzheimer dementia. Neurology. 2007;**68**(4):288-291

[36] Ferman T, Smith G, Kantarci K, Boeve B, Pankratz V, Dickson D, Graff-Radford N, Wszolek Z, Gerpen J, Uitti R, Pedraza O, Murray M, Aakre J, Parisi J, Knopman D, Petersen R. Nonamnestic mild cognitive impairment progresses to dementia with Lewy bodies. Neurology. 2013;**81**(23):2032-2038

[37] Tuokko H, Frerichs R. Cognitive impairment with no dementia (CIND): Longitudinal studies, the findings, and the issues. The Clinical Neuropsychologist. 2000;**14**(4):504-525

[38] Perminder SS, Brodaty H, Reppermund S, Kochan NA, Trollor JN, Draper B, Slavin M, Crawford J, Kang K, Broe GA, Mater KA, Lux O. Risk profiles of subtypes of mild cognitive impairment: The Sydney memory and ageing study. Journal of the American Geriatrics Society. 2012;**60**:24-33. DOI: 10.1111/j.1532-5415.2011.03774.x

[39] World Health Organization. 2017. Available from: http://www.who.int/mediacentre/factsheets/fs362/en/ [Accessed: September 11, 2017]

[40] Ortiz GG, Pacheco-Moisés FP, Flores-Alvarado LJ, Macías Islas MA, Velázquez-Brizuela IE, Ramírez-Anguiano AC, Torres-Sánchez ED, Morales-Sánchez EW, Cruz-Ramos JA, Ortiz-Velázquez GE, Cortés-Enriquez F. Alzheimer disease and metabolism. In: Zerr, editor. Understanding Alzheimer's Disease. Croatia: Technical Editor; 2013

[41] American Psychiatric Association. Diagnostic and Statistical Manual. 4th ed. Washington, DC: APA Press; 1994

[42] Geda YE. Mild cognitive impairment in older adults. Current Psychiatry Reports. 2012;**14**:320-327. DOI: 10.1007/s11920-012-0291-x

[43] Reisberg B, Prichep L, Mosconi L, John ER, Glodzik-Sobanska L, Boksay I, et al. The pre-mild cognitive impairment, subjective cognitive impairment stage of Alzheimer's disease. Alzheimers Dementia. 2008;**4**(Suppl 1):S98-S108. DOI: 10.1016/j.jalz.2007.11.017

[44] Álvarez-Cáceres R. Estadística aplicada a las ciencias de la salud. España: Ediciones Díaz de Santos; 2007. p. 107

[45] Qiu C, Winblad B, Fratiglioni L. Low diastolic pressure and risk of dementia in very old people: A longitudinal study. Dementia and Geriatric Cognitive Disorders. 2009;**28**:213-221. DOI: 10.1159/000236913

[46] Ladecola C. Neurovascular regulation in the normal brain and in Alzheimer's disease. Nature Reviews. Neuroscience. 2004;**5**:347-360. DOI: 10.1038/nrn1387

[47] Rose KM, Couper D, Eigenbrodt ML, Mosley TH, Sharrett AR, Gottesman RF. Orthostatic hypotension and cognitive function: The atherosclerosis risk in communities study. Neuroepidemiology. 2010;**34**:1-7. DOI: 10.1159/000255459

[48] Fratiglioni L, Viitanen M, von Strauss E, Tontodonati V, Herlitz A, Winblad B. Very old women at highest risk of dementia and Alzheimer disease: Incidence data from the Kungsholmen project, Stockholm. Neurology. 1997;**48**:132-138

[49] Whitmer RA, Sidney S, Selby J, Johnston SC, Yaffe K. Midlife cardiovascular risk factors and risk of dementia in late life. Neurology. 2005;**64**:277-281. DOI: 10.1212/01.WNL.0000149519.47454.F2

[50] Qiu C, Winblad B, Fratiglioni L. The age-dependent relation of blood pressure to cognitive function and dementia. Lancet Neurology. 2005;**4**:487-499. DOI: 10.1016/S1474-4422(05)70141-1

[51] Li G, Rhew IC, Shofer JB, Kukull WA, Breitner JC, Peskind E, et al. Age-varying association between blood pressure and risk of dementia in those aged 65 and older: A community-based prospective cohort study. Journal of the American Geriatrics Society. 2007;**55**:1161-1167. DOI: 10.1111/j.1532-5415.2007.01233.x

[52] Ninomiya T. Diabetes mellitus and dementia. Current Diabetes Reports. 2014;**14**:487. DOI: 10.1007/s11892-014-0487-z

[53] Lu FP, Lin KP, Kuo HK. Diabetes and the risk of multi-system aging phenotypes: A systematic review and meta-analysis. PLoS One. 2009;**4**:e4144. DOI: 10.1371/journal.pone.0004144

[54] Muñoz-Rivas N, Méndez-Bailón M, Miguel-Yanes JM, Hernández-Barrera V, Miguel-Díez J, Jimenez-Garcia R, et al. Observational study of vascular dementia in the Spanish elderly population according to type 2 diabetes status: Trends in incidence, characteristics and outcomes (2004-2013). BMJ Open. 2017;**7**:e016390. DOI: 10.1136/bmjopen-2017-016390

[55] Van Cauwenberghe C, Van Broeckhoven C, Sleegers K. The genetic landscape of Alzheimer disease: Clinical implications and perspectives. Genetics in Medicine. 2016;**18**:421-430. DOI: 10.1038/gim.2015.117

[56] Lopera F, Ardilla A, Martínez A, Madrigal L, Arango-Viana JC, et al. Clinical features of early-onset Alzheimer disease in a large kindred with an E280A presenilin-1 mutation. Journal of the American Medical Association. 1997;**277**:793-799. DOI: 10.1001/jama.277.10.793

[57] Kauwe JS, Ridge PG, Foster NL, Cannon-Albright LA. Strong evidence for a genetic contribution to late-onset Alzheimer's disease mortality: A population-based study. PLoS One. 2013;**8**:e77087. DOI: 10.1371/journal.pone.0077087

[58] Giri M, Shah A, Upreti B, Rai JC. Unraveling the genes implicated in Alzheimer's disease. Biomedical Reports. 2017;**7**:105-114. DOI: 10.3892/br.2017.927

[59] Young JS, Hobbs JG, Bailes JE. The impact of traumatic brain injury on the aging brain. Current Psychiatry Reports. 2016;**18**:81. DOI: 10.1007/s11920-016-0719-9

[60] Zaloshnja E, Miller T, Langlois JA, Selassie AW. Prevalence of long-term disability from traumatic brain injury in the civilian population of the United States, 2005. Journal of Head Trauma Rehabilitation. 2008;**23**:394-400. DOI: 10.1097/01.HTR.0000341435.52004.ac

[61] Lew HL, Poole JH, Guillory SB, Salerno RM, Leskin G, Sigford B. Persistent problems after traumatic brain injury: The need for long-term follow-up and coordinated care. Journal of Rehabilitation Research and Development. 2006;**43**:7-10

[62] De Beaumont L, Theoret H, Mongeon D, Messier J, Leclerc S, Tremblay S, et al. Brain function decline in healthy retired athletes who sustained their last sports concussion in early adulthood. Brain: A Journal of Neurology. 2009;**132**:695-708. DOI: 10.1093/brain/awn347

[63] Wood RL. Accelerated cognitive aging following severe traumatic brain injury: A review. Brain Injury. 2017;**7**:1-9. DOI: 10.1080/02699052.2017.1332387

[64] Steffens DC, Otey E, Alexopoulos GS, Butters MA, Cuthbert B, Ganguli M, et al. Perspectives on depression, mild cognitive impairment, and cognitive decline. Archives of General Psychiatry. 2006;**63**:130-138. DOI: 10.1001/archpsyc.63.2.130

[65] Ganguli M, Du Y, Dodge HH, Ratcliff GG, Chang CC. Depressive symptoms and cognitive decline in late life: A prospective epidemiological study. Archives of General Psychiatry. 2006;**63**:153-160. DOI: 10.1001/archpsyc.63.2.153

[66] Jorm AF, Jolley D. The incidence of dementia: A meta-analysis. Neurology. 1998;**51**:728-733

[67] Qiu C, Kivipelto M, Von Strauss E. Epidemiology of Alzheimer's disease: Occurrence, determinants, and strategies toward intervention. Dialogues in Clinical Neuroscience. 2009;**11**:111-128

[68] Ward A, Arrighi HM, Michels S, Cedarbaum JM. Mild cognitive impairment: Disparity of incidence and prevalence estimates. Alzheimers Dementia. 2012;**8**:14-21. DOI: 10.1016/j.jalz.2011.01.002

[69] Petersen RC, Roberts RO, Knopman DS, Geda YE, Cha RH, Pankratz VS, et al. Prevalence of mild cognitive impairment is higher in men. The Mayo Clinic study of aging. Neurology. 2010;**75**:889-897. DOI: 10.1212/WNL.0b013e3181f11d85

[70] Roberts RO, Geda YE, Knopman DS, Cha RH, Pankratz VS, Boeve BF, et al. The incidence of MCI differs by subtype and is higher in men: The Mayo Clinic study of aging. Neurology. 2012;**78**:342-351. DOI: 10.1212/WNL.0b013e3182452862

[71] Sharp ES, Gatz M. Relationship between education and dementia an updated systematic review. Alzheimer Disease & Associated Disorders. 2011;**25**:289. DOI: 10.1097/WAD.0b013e318211c83c

[72] Bickel H, Kurz A. Education, occupation, and dementia: The Bavarian school sisters study. Dementia and Geriatric Cognitive Disorders. 2009;**27**:548-556. DOI: 10.1159/000227781

[73] Sharifi F, Fakhrzadeh H, Varmaghani M, Arzaghi SM, Alizadeh Khoei M, Farzadfar F, et al. Prevalence of dementia and associated factors among older adults in Iran: National Elderly Health Survey (NEHS). Archives of Iranian Medicine. 2016;**19**:838-844. DOI: 0161912/ AIM.005 Available from: https://www.ncbi.nlm.nih.gov/pubmed/?term=Taheri%20 Tanjani%20P%5BAuthor%5D&cauthor=true&cauthor_uid=27998158

[74] Kolb B. Robbin Gibb. Searching for the principles of brain plasticity and behavior. Cortex. 2014;**58**:251-260

[75] Stern Y. Imaging cognitive reserve. In: Stern Y, editor. Cognitive Reserve: Theory and Applications. Philadelphia, PA: Taylor & Francis; 2007. pp. 251-263

[76] Stern Y. The concept of cognitive reserve: A catalyst for research. Journal of Clinical and Experimental Neuropsychology. 2003;**25**:589-593

[77] Lojo-Seoane C, Facal D, Juncos-Rabadán O. "Previene la actividad intellectual el deterioro cognitivo" Relaciones entre la reserva cognitiva y deterioro cognitivo ligero. Revista Española de Geriatría y Gerontología. 2012;**47**(6):270-278. DOI: 10.1016/j.regg.2012.02.006

[78] British Psychological Society. A Guide to Psychosocial Interventions in Early Stages of Dementia. London: British Psychological Society; 2014

[79] Aguirre E, Spector A, Hoare Z, Streater A, Woods B, et al. Maintenance cognitive stimulation therapy (MCST) for dementia: A single-blind, multi-centre, randomised controlled trial of maintenance CST vs. CST for dementia. British Journal of Psychiatry. 2014;**204**(6):454-461

[80] Bahar-Fuchs A, Clare L, Woods B. Cognitive training and cognitive rehabilitation for persons with mild to moderate dementia of the Alzheimer's or vascular type: A review. Alzheimer's Research & Therapy. 2013;**5**(4):35-49

[81] Yanguas JJ, Leturia FJ, Leturia M, Uriarte A. Intervención psicosocial en gerontología: Manual práctico. 2nd ed. Madrid, Spain: Cáritas; 2002

[82] Point Geiss P, Carroggio R. Ejercicios de motricidad y memoria para personas mayores. Paidotribo: España; 2011

[83] Sanders S, Morano C. Alzheimer's disease and related dementias. In: Cummings S, Kropf N, editors. Handbook of Psychosocial Interventions with Older Adults. Evidence Based Approaches. New Yok: Routledge; 2009

[84] Sachdev et al. COSMIC (cohort studies of memory in an international consortium): An international consortium to identify risk and protective factors and biomarkers of cognitive ageing and dementia in diverse ethnic and sociocultural groups. BMC Neurology. 2013;**13**:165. DOI: 10.1186/1471-2377-13-165

[85] Cullum S, Huppert FA, McGee M, Dening T, Ahmed A, Paykel E, Brayne C. Decline across different domains of cognitive function in normal ageing: Results of a longitudinal population-based study using CAMCOG. International Journal of Geriatric Psychiatry. 2000;**15**:853-862

[86] Horr T, Messinger-Rapport B, Pillai JA. Systematic review of strengths and limitations of randomized controlled trials for non-pharmacological interventions in mild cognitive impairment: Focus on Alzheimer's disease. Journal of Nutrition, Health and Aging. 2015 February;**19**(2):141-153. DOI: 10.1007/s12603-014-0565-6

[87] International Longevity Centre Brazil. Active Aging: A Policy Framework in Response to the Longevity Revolution. Rio de Janeiro, Brazil: ILC-BR; 2015

[88] World Health Organization. Active Aging. A Policy Framework. Geneva, Switzerland: WHO; 2002

[89] Rowe JW, Kahn RL. Successful aging. The Gerontologist. 1997;**37**(4):433-440. DOI: https://doi.org/10.1093/geront/37.4.433

[90] World Health Organization. Global Strategy and Action Plan on Aging and Health (2016-2020). Geneva, Switzerland: WHO; 2016

6

The Elderly in the Emergency Department

Alexander Morales Erazo

Abstract

The evaluation, treatment, and prognosis of the elderly hospitalized in an emergency service are different from the adult patient, and it is necessary to know their particularities to provide optimal care.

Keywords: emergency service, geriatric patient, biological aging, fragility

1. Introduction

Aging can be defined as a decline in functional properties at cellular, tissue, and organic levels, with the consequent loss of homeostasis and adaptability to internal and external noxas, increasing vulnerability to disease and death [1].

As a result of the increase in the number of elderly people, their health problems have increased significantly. Parallel to the demographic change that conditioned population aging, the "epidemiological transition" appeared that modified the profile of prevalent diseases, chronic noncommunicable diseases being the core of attention. All these conditions present frequent exacerbations and relapses, making the elderly require repeatedly assessment in an emergency service. However, it is clear that the care models in the emergency services are not adapted to the geriatric patient [2].

The demand in the attention to the emergency services has been growing progressively in the last years, and this increase is more noticeable in the population of older adults. Older people have differential features, in relation to younger age groups, starting from the biological point of view with not only physiological changes related to aging but also functional, psychological, and social changes, all of which lead to a decrease or narrowing of the homeostatic responses to the different noxas, placing them in a state of greater vulnerability, which has an effect of greater comorbidity, loss of autonomy, disability, sensory alterations, cognitive deterioration, and a social-familiar problematic that can occur simultaneously, determining a special difficulty for their evaluation and treatment and, many times, altering its prognosis adversely [3].

In this way, the concept of biological aging is important, understood as the state of an individual resulting from the wear and tear associated with age plus its conditions of illness, functionality, mental well-being, and social support. This biological aging is very different among the elderly, regardless of their chronological age and condition differences in the functional capacity [4].

In a recent Spanish study, it was established that older patients had a higher priority in the care by severity, had more complementary tests taken, had a longer average stay, had a higher probability of hospital admission and of being exitus, and needed assessment by the social services. In addition, it requires more complex evaluations, more consultations with other specialists, and a higher percentage of readmissions [5]; however, they attend in a justified manner and with a significantly used pattern different from young adults. Therefore, the progressive aging of the population may seriously affect the dynamics and functioning of the hospital emergency services.

In young patients admitted to an emergency department, it has been determined that there are undoubtedly clinical factors related to the acute disease, which decisively influence the outcome. However, this is not so clear in the elderly, and the characteristics that go beyond the severity of the acute disease modify the prognosis. More specifically, these conditions refer to the functional, emotional, and cognitive states, the level of comorbidity, the degree of polypharmacy, and the social support networks. Due to their condition of high vulnerability or fragility, in the elderly patients, the health problems are explained in the multicausality model, and the resolution of these does not derive from the attention of a single cause, but from a comprehensive identification and treatment of all related factors that affect the prognosis [6].

Hospitalization alone is already a negative factor in the outcome of elderly patients. Survival decreases by the mere fact of being reduced to a hospital bed, immobilized, both in men and women, but above all in the older groups (>80 years) [7]. Even if you take into account that the emergency services are noisy, in constant movement and lack of privacy, which can be disconcerting for the elderly and enhance their deterioration in relation to hearing, vision, attention, and understanding.

In general, the elderly patients have a longer stay in the emergency department, requiring more time for medical assessment and nursing care, and alarmingly they have a higher frequency of readmissions, generating a great assistance pressure on the professionals that attend these services [8].

The lack of knowledge of the elements that affect the prognosis of the elderly patients in the emergency services is still notorious, which results in diagnostic errors and what is more serious therapeutic errors, affecting adversely the outcome; the aim of this paper is to provide knowledge that leads to the identification of these factors and may lead to earlier and more successful intervention lines.

2. Epidemiology

Recent studies have shown a progressive increase in emergency visits, which is much more noticeable in the elderly population. In fact, some studies mention that up to 25% of all emergency visits correspond to elderly patients. In general, they represent more than 15% of all consultations and almost 50% of all admissions to intensive care units. Therefore, some authors mention that "the emergency units are aging" [9].

In the United States, the Centers for Disease Control and Prevention (CDC) report that between 1993 and 2003, there was an increase in the absolute number of visits to the emergency department, with the group of people over 65 years of age, who had the highest frequency of visits (an increase of 26%). If this trend is maintained, it is expected that the frequency of emergency consultations in the elderly will double from 6.4 million to 11.7 million by 2013 [10]. Elderly patients are four to six times more likely to be admitted to an emergency unit than a non-elderly patient.

3. Conditions that can alter the evolution and prognosis of the elderly in the emergency department

3.1. Physiological response to stress

The organic response to different acutely unbalanced pathologies is altered in some elderly, especially in the fragile ones [11]. Among the most relevant physiological changes associated with age are mentioned:

- Alteration in the homeostasis of intercellular junctions and the production of the second messengers, which causes some adrenergic receptors to be internalized, decreasing the effectiveness of catecholaminergic responses.

- Presbycardia or cardiac aging conditioned by the increase in cardiac stiffness with a decreased diastole capacity and greater dependence on atrial contraction, which results in less tolerance to increased extravascular volume and lower tolerance to tachyarrhythmias.

- The physiological changes of lung aging make it more difficult to adapt to situations that generate hypoxemia. Among them are an increase of the rib cage rigidity, decrease in the forces of elastic retraction of the lung parenchyma, and decline in the strength of the respiratory muscles. All this generates changes in pulmonary dynamics with an increase in residual volume, decrease in tidal volume, and decrease in FEV1 associated with age. The effectiveness of protective airway reflexes is also altered. The alveoli flatten and the gaseous exchange surface decreases. In general, all these changes produce a decrease in the PO_2, for which one must be cautious when interpreting the arterial gases in an older adult and apply a formula to correct them by age.

- The most important changes that affect the aged kidney are a reduction in size, decreased renal blood flow, and a drop in the glomerular filtration rate. Therefore, older adults have difficulty managing water loads, either in hypervolemia or in dehydration states, as well as regulating plasma osmolarity.

- Deregulation of the immune system, low-grade inflammation, and alteration of acquired immunity make the responses to infections less effective.

- There is desensitization of the vascular mechanoreceptors with alteration of the vasoconstrictive responses upon hypotension states.

- Endocrine changes with pancreatic aging, islets decrease, and insulin resistance increases, causing an increase in fasting plasma glucose. There is also an alteration in the production of counter-regulatory hormones.

3.2. Characteristics of the disease as it ages

The disease presentation in the elderly makes it difficult to approach it, due to situations such as:

- Multipathology

- Complex medication regime

- Atypical presentation

- Frequent Iatrogenic

- Multiple consultations

3.3. Laboratory tests

Although laboratory tests are an invaluable aid, in the elderly they cannot get altered in the presence of disease or have higher rates of false positives, related to physiological changes [12]. The following are worthy of mention:

- In the elderly the erythrocyte sedimentation rate is not a reliable indicator of the presence of inflammation. C-reactive protein (CRP) is more sensitive, with the disadvantage that it can take up to 12–24 h to rise after a bacterial aggression and maintain its levels even days after healing. Recently, it has been published in a systematic review that PCR accuracy decreases as the patient's age increases. Procalcitonin maintains a good diagnostic capacity in this patient profile, and a value of >0.5 ng/ml is significantly associated with greater mortality at 30 days [13].

- Serum creatinine does not reflect renal function, if one considers that it is a protein of muscular origin and the sarcopenia associated to age.

- It is common to find in the elderly of the community (20%) and institutionalized patients (50%) the presence of asymptomatic bacteriuria, which should not be misinterpreted as a urinary infection and even less should be given an antibiotic treatment.

- The readings of hemoglobin and hematocrit in the elderly are the same as for the adult population. The myth of the so-called anemia of aging is false.

- The same applies for the serum sodium values, being these from 135 to 145 mosm/Lt and being an error to believe that the elderly tolerate hyponatremia better; in fact, studies have shown an increase in cognitive alterations, falls, and acute coronary mortality, with values less than 135 mosm/Lt.

3.4. Pharmacological response

When using drugs in the elderly, it is necessary to know some changes that can alter the responses to medications [14]:

- In general terms, there is no alteration in the absorption of oral medications, and this remains one of the choices.

- There is a decrease in liver size, hepatic blood flow, and liver microsomal enzymes, which alter the metabolism of some drugs.

- The free fraction of drugs that travel bound to albumin or alpha-2-microglobulin, which are variably decreased with age, increase and so does toxicity.

- With aging, there is a greater proportion of body fat and less water and lean mass, which changes the bioavailability of drugs.

- Greater toxicity of some molecules associated with decreased renal function.

- Specific pharmacodynamic alterations for some molecules due to changes in the quantity or sensitivity of receptors at the cellular level.

4. Most frequent pathologies in the elderly at the emergency department

Next, emphasis will be placed on the most frequent pathologies in an emergency department and their differential characteristics in the elderly.

4.1. Hypertension in the emergency room in the geriatric patient

In the past, it was controversial to define the readings for normal blood pressure in the elderly and when to administer pharmacological treatment. Today, it is clear that the normal readings correspond to those of the adult population and that the benefit of administering pharmacological management is evident, even at very advanced ages. However, the latest studies (SPRINT, PURE) have put confusion regarding the goals. In the emergency department, it is important to differentiate between emergency and hypertensive emergencies, due to the implications in defining the speed and route of treatment.

Key points

- Rule out pseudo-hypertension at very advanced ages.

- During the measurements, the patient must be in a controlled environment and in an appropriate position, with an adequate technique and the minimum possible stress.

- Always evaluate the underlying comorbidities that alter the prognosis of the current decompensation.

- In a hypertensive emergency, the blood pressure readings should not be lowered abruptly, as it generates more morbidity and mortality.

- As an adequate physiological goal in elderly hypertensive patients, a pulse pressure between 50 and 60 mm Hg is recommended.

- In hypertensive emergencies use medication orally. It is a mistake to use the sublingual route because of its unpredictable effects and because the drugs were not designed for this route. In emergencies, use the intravenous way, and transfer the patient to an intermediate or intensive care room.

- In the elderly, no drugs with adrenergic blocking effect such as clonidine or prazosin are the first choice, because of their excessive hypotensive effects and, in the case of clonidine, its sedative and anticholinergic effects.

4.2. Acute coronary syndromes in the elderly

It is estimated that 60–65% of all heart attacks occur in people older than 65 years and 80% of the deaths due to this cause affect this population. They are one of the most frequent causes of emergency consultation, where more mistakes are committed, both in diagnosis and in the therapeutic decision-making.

Key points

- Only 57% of those over 80 have chest pain. In octogenarians, the main presenting symptom is dyspnea. Syncope, dizziness, delirium, and falls are also frequent. This leads to frequent delays in diagnosis and treatment.

- In relation to age, there are more incidences of tachyarrhythmias.

- An elderly person is more likely to show a non-ST-segment elevation myocardial infarct (STEMI) than with an ST-segment elevation myocardial infarct (STEMI), given the phenomenon of ischemic preconditioning.

- NT-proBNP levels are associated with short-term mortality in the elderly population treated in emergency services.

- Long-term mortality and morbidity are increased compared to younger patients, either with medical or intervention management. Heart failure, bleeding, and reinfarction rates are more frequent. However, the benefit of the treatment remains.

- In part, the poor results in the elderly are explained by the decrease in the use of treatments because of toxicity fear. The protocols must be applied strictly and not to discriminate the age. Consider the general state of health, life expectancy, functional status, and cognitive status.

- The intervention strategy has shown greater benefits in the elderly compared with thrombolysis.

- Always provide the patient with cardiac and functional rehabilitation.

4.3. Pulmonary thromboembolism in the elderly

Although it is not clear whether advanced age is an independent risk factor for thromboembolism, elderly patients have a high incidence of risk factors for clot formation. Venous stasis, commonly caused by immobility, has been found to be the most common risk factor.

Key points

- The diagnosis is notoriously difficult at all ages. In 70% of the cases in which the patient dies of a pulmonary embolism, there was no antemortem suspicion of the diagnosis.

- The rule in the elderly is that the pulmonary embolism occurs in a subtle and atypical way. Acute dyspnea, pleuritic chest pain, tachypnea, tachycardia, and hemoptysis are less frequent. Syncope and hemodynamic instability increase in frequency.

- D-dimer decreases its utility with advancing age because the values rarely fall below the negative predictive threshold.

- As aging is related to a decrease of the oxygen partial pressure and an increase in the alveolar-arterial gradient, gasometrical changes can be difficult to be interpreted in the elderly.

4.4. Geriatric patient with cerebrovascular disease in the emergency department

Neurovascular disease is the major cause of disability and death in the elderly. The aging brain is less resistant to physiological stress: the cerebral blood flow gradually decreases with age, the collateral circulation is diminished, the cerebrovascular barrier is less efficient, the cerebral self-regulation is altered, and the neuronal oxidative metabolism decreases. All this makes an ischemic event more pronounced, and the time threshold for effective interventions lowers.

Key points

- Twenty-one percent (21%) of elderly patients with cerebral ischemia have a normal physical examination.

- Always look for common risk factors: atrial fibrillation, carotid atherosclerosis, myocardial infarction, valvular disease, and dyslipidemia.

- The approach by an interdisciplinary group is important to improve the functional prognosis.

- Thrombolysis in cerebrovascular disease has shown full benefits up to the 75 years. In older patients there is evidence of benefit, coming from clinical trials with a small number of patients or case reports. Therefore, there is no contraindication for age. The key is to choose the patient properly, based on parameters of functionality, comorbidity, and strict application of the protocols.

- The use of ASA plus clopidogrel has not improved the final results, but it does increase the risk of intracranial bleeding.

- Start the integral rehabilitation therapy early once the patient stabilizes.

- Avoid all cost prostration or immobility.

4.5. Infections in the elderly at the emergency department

The incidence of infectious processes in patients older than 75 years who attend the emergency services has increased significantly in the last 10 years (from 24.8% to 31.7%), as well as the severity of their clinical presentation and short-term mortality (30 days). This is explained by the summing effect of immunosenescence plus fragility [15].

Key points

- The criteria of systemic response syndrome are not always present in the infected elderly and decrease its usefulness to stratify the risk in this age group.

- The most accepted criterion for fever in the elderly is an increase of 1.2°C based on the basal temperature or higher than 37.2 (sensitivity 83%).

- Several studies have documented the absence of fever, as traditionally defined, in the presence of serious infections. The cut point of 38.2° centigrade loses sensitivity (40%).

- It is common that there is no leukocytosis in the elderly, as part of the infectious response. The cutoff point of the greatest sensitivity for infection is an absolute count of 14,000.

- Tachycardia may not occur.

- The respiratory rate greater than 24 is conserved as part of the inflammatory response.

- In cases of bacteremia, it is more difficult to identify the source.

- The only independent predictors of bacteremia in the elderly are the altered mental state (odds ratio [OR] 2.88; 95% CI 1.52–5.50), vomiting (OR 2.63; 95% CI 1.16–6.15), and the presence of bands in the leucogram greater than 6% (OR 3.50; 95% CI 1.58–5.27).

- The etiology is multimicrobial in 5–17% of patients.

- The presence of a Barthel index less than 60, systolic blood pressure less than 90 mm Hg, and serum lactate >4 mmol/l are significantly associated with short-term mortality.

4.6. Urinary tract infection in the elderly in the context of emergencies

Key points

- Tendency to overdiagnosis due to high prevalence of asymptomatic bacteriuria. 52.2% of urinary tract infections are misdiagnosed.

- Do not attribute a septic picture in an elderly person to a urinary infection first, until carefully ruling out other causes.

- Treating asymptomatic bacteriuria does not improve mortality but increases the side effects of antibiotics and the rates of infection by resistant germs.

- The presence of symptoms is less clear in the elderly with cognitive impairment or the use of probes to stay in those who prevail atypical presentations (delirium, falls, functional decline, etc.).

- If in doubt, focus on the blood picture or PCR.

4.7. Pneumonia in the elderly

The incidence of community-acquired pneumonia (CAP) increases with age and is associated with high morbidity and mortality due to physiological changes associated with aging and a greater presence of chronic diseases. Pneumonia is the fifth cause of death in the United States among those over 65 years. It results in 600,000 hospitalizations and almost 60,000 deaths [16].

Key points

- There is an increased risk of pneumonia due to deglutition disorder, neurological disease, functional decline, malnutrition, use of sedatives, comorbidity, chronic neuropathies, smoking, heart failure, and institutionalization.

- *Streptococcus pneumoniae* remains, as in other ages, as the most frequent etiological agent. However, with aging the microorganisms colonize the oropharynx change, with an increase in Gram-negative and anaerobic germs; consequently, these increase as causal agents. The state of the denture also influences.

- The diagnosis is complicated by the absence of classic symptoms, there is fever in only 26% of cases when compared with young people, and 44% have cough, fever, and dyspnea due to clinical history. In institutionalized patients, alterations of the mental state are more frequent.

- The CURB-65 is an index that has been validated adequately in the elderly and allows to decide the appropriate level of care to administer the treatment.

- To stratify the risk and possible complications in elderly patients with pneumonia who enter the emergency department, it is useful to classify them as fragile and non-fragile.

- Lack of fever, absence of hypoxia, and altered mental state are associated with therapeutic delay.

- Studies have shown a decrease in mortality in the elderly, related to the rapid administration of the appropriate antibiotic treatment.

- Pneumonia in institutionalized patients and pneumonia associated with health care are related with higher comorbidity, poor functional status, and higher mortality.

- Patients with risk factors such as institutionalization in nursing homes, hospitalization for more than 2 days in the last 90 days, wound care in the last 30 days, high frequency of resistance to antibiotics in the community, infusion of home medications, dialysis, a member of the family with resistant germs and diseases, or immunosuppressive therapy should be covered for resistant germs (*Pseudomonas*, *Klebsiella*, *Acinetobacter*, and *Staphylococcus* resistant to methicillin).

- Remember the importance of vaccination against influenza and pneumococcus to the impact on mortality and hospitalizations in the ICU, respectively.

4.8. Approach of abdominal pain in the elderly patient at the emergency department

If in the young man, the acute abdomen becomes a diagnostic challenge, in the elderly it is a real mystery. It is frequent that a nonspecific pain and a soft abdomen without many signs conceal a true abdominal catastrophe. Total mortality for an elderly man who enters with abdominal pain complaint exceeds 10% [17].

Key points

- In the "surgical abdomen of the old man," the atypical presentation of the different entities is usual.

- There is difficulty in the interrogation (dementia, basic pathology, loss of senses).

- Fever and leukocytosis are not constant.

- The decrease of the myenteric receptors in the viscera modifies the perception of pain, making it diffuse and badly defined, with the absence of the so-called signs of peritoneal irritation, which increases the false-negative rate.

- The use of NSAIDs masks peritonitis and increases the risk of peptic ulcer.

- Normotensions are synonymous with hypotension in patients with abdominal infection and who are chronically hypertensive.

- Prolonged presentation time, normothermia or hypothermia, and leukopenia are synonyms of severe intra-abdominal infections.

4.9. Psychiatric emergencies in the elderly

Emergency physicians frequently fail to identify and focus on psychiatric disorders, either as a primary reason for consultation or concomitant to the index disease, although they adversely and independently affect the prognosis [18].

Key points

- It is essential, upon the appearance of new psychiatric symptoms in the elderly, to rule out organicity: infections, metabolic disorders, tumors of the central nervous system, reactions to drugs, etc.

- Discard substance abuse.

- Investigate mistreatment of the elderly.

- Depression is the most frequent psychiatric disorder in the elderly, with subsyndromal depression being the most common. It must be clarified that depression is not a natural consequence of aging and must always be treated.

- The most common entities within the "late-onset psychosis" (older than 60 years) are as follows in order: dementias, delirium, affective disorders, schizophrenia, and schizophreniform disorders.

- Delirium: acute alteration of the state of consciousness, fluctuating, with difficulty to maintain the attention, alteration of the sleep-wake pattern, alteration of the perception. Always look for the triggering factor.

- Dementia: cognitive disorder of long duration without alteration of the conscience. It contributes to 16–23% of psychotic symptoms in aging.

- The elderly has the highest rate of death by suicide compared to all age groups.

- Fundamental: good clinical history and functional and neurological examination.

- In the agitated elderly patient, the use of mechanical restrictions produces greater complications.

5. Forecast of the elderly in the emergency service

The early detection of the high-risk adult patient is essential to avoid new admissions and visits in the emergency room and to improve the level of physical and cognitive function. In adults, prognostic assessment methods are based on the clinical characteristics of severity of the index event. But the older adult cannot be seen under the traditional biomedical gaze that the unifactorial analysis of patients tends to. The complexity of the disease in the elderly is preferable to approach it from a biopsychosocial approach through multidimensional analysis, which identifies how the demographic, clinical, psychological, functional, and social factors influence the acute disease in the elderly and alter its forecast [19]. At the emergency environment, we need brief, simple, and validated tools that help us detect problems in different areas. However, currently there are few prognostic indices used in clinical practice that include these variables typical of the elderly baseline condition.

Having clear prognostic variables to help the quick detection of the patient at high risk of this outcome helps to decide which patients should be considered for aggressive interventions, treatments with curative purposes, support treatments, or treatments only for palliative purposes.

Currently, there are models of structured triage in the emergency services, being the most prominent: the Australian model (Australasian Triage Scale (ATS)), the Canadian scale of triage and gravity for emergency services (Canadian Emergency Department Triage and Acuity Scale (CTAS), the Manchester Triage System (MTS), the Emergency Severity Index (ESI), and the Andorran model of triage (Model Andorra of Triage (MAT)); however, these are not suitable for use in elderly patients.

When referring to the young and adult population, there are known instruments that try to predict the short-term prognosis of critical hospitalized patients, such as the APACHE III used in the intensive care units (ICU); the SUPPORT, to establish the 6-month prognosis of hospitalized patients both inside and outside the ICU; and more recently the short version of the EORTC QLQ-30 for use in palliative care. The drawback of these evaluations is that they overestimate age a priori as an element of risk, without considering that there are also "robust" elderly or with successful aging, in which the chronological age alone does not weigh as a negative factor.

The scales "Identification of Seniors at Risk" (ISAR) and the "Triage Risk Screening Tool" (TRST) have been published for use in the elderly, which allow assessing the risk of complications at release of the service and classifying the degree of fragility [20].

The prognosis of the diseases in geriatric patients is frequently influenced by the basal health condition of the elderly, which is determined by the nutritional status, the mental state, and the functional capacity (level of independence for the activities of daily life), variables that are not contemplated in the scales of habitual use in adults. In this sense, it has been shown that the deterioration of each of these areas can be an independent factor of mortality in the elderly.

The multidimensional geriatric assessment is an evaluation carried out by an interdisciplinary team to identify the problems and establish a care plan to improve the functionality and quality of life of the geriatric patient. It offers an integral and holistic view of the elderly adult patient, in which the clinical condition is evaluated, but psychological, functional, and social evaluation is also included. In fact, having knowledge of the instruments used in daily practice in geriatric care is extremely useful. Different scales and protocols are used and duly validated. Several authors have proposed to stratify the risk of the geriatric patient in the emergency department based on a model of comprehensive geriatric assessment, adapted to this service [21].

6. The frail senior in the emergency room

The frail senior is the one who has his homeostatic reserves to the limit, with a high probability of suffering a deleterious outcome. The detection of this patient is fundamental in the emergency services, since in this scenario it is where there is more risk of entering the cascade of functional decline and dependence. It is interesting how the acute disease acts as a trigger, unmasking the frailty picture. Studies have shown how frail senior people in the emergency room have higher rates of hospitalization, functional deterioration, readmissions, and short-term mortality, when compared with non-frail elderly. For the screening of frail elderly people in the emergency department, the ISAR, TRST, deficit accumulation index (DAI), and comprehensive geriatric assessment are recommended in selected patients defined as high risk. Identifying frail elderly allows designing a special care plan, which has shown a decrease in the number of admissions in residence at 30 days, an increase in patient satisfaction, less functional deterioration, fewer readmissions, and without increasing costs. No impact on mortality or institutionalization has been demonstrated [22].

7. Decision-making

It is common to observe how some interventions are systematically denied to the elderly, arguing as the only reason age. This produces gross errors, since chronological age alone does not provide enough information to make the best decision. They are the multidimensional parameters that include basal functionality, comorbidities, and emotional-cognitive and social support, which together reflect biological aging and support the relevance or not of the proposed treatment [23].

8. Conclusion

The diagnostic approach and the therapeutic approach of the elderly, in the emergency department, should be framed in a deep knowledge of their physiological alterations, a careful anamnesis, and therapeutic prudence. Because of the diminished homeostatic reserve of the elderly, the time to establish adequate treatment is shorter.

Conflict of interest

I declare not having any conflict of interest in the elaboration of this paper.

Author details

Alexander Morales Erazo[1,2,3,4,5]*

*Address all correspondence to: alexandermoraleserazo@gmail.com

1 Internal Medicine and Geriatrics, Caldas University, Manizales, Caldas, Colombia

2 CES University, Medellín, Antioquia, Colombia

3 Cooperative University of Colombia, Pasto, Colombia

4 Nariño Departamental Hospital, Pasto, Nariño, Colombia

5 COMETA Foundation, Pasto, Nariño, Colombia

References

[1] Fedarko NS. The biology of aging and frailty. Clinics in Geriatric Medicine. 2011;**27**:27-37

[2] Hwang U, Morrison S. The geriatric emergency department. Journal of the American Geriatrics Society. 2007;**55**(11):1873-1876

[3] Baztán J, Rangel O, Gomez J. Deterioro funcional, discapacidad y dependencia en el anciano. En: Fundamentos de la atencion sanitaria a los mayores. 1a ed. Madrid: Elservier; 2015. pp. 372-382

[4] Morales A, Ocampo J. Valoración geriátrica integral. En: Texto de medicina Interna: aprendizaje basado en problemas. 1a ed. Distribuna; 2013. pp. 2019-25

[5] Sanz N, Martel J, Sanchis-Bayarri V, Castellano E. Factores pronósticos en pacientes pluripatológicos de edad avanzada en un hospital de asistencia a crónicos de media y larga estancia (HACMLE). Anales de Medicina Interna. 2006;**23**(11):529-532

[6] Bermudez M, Guzman G, Fernadez M. Impacto del paciente anciano en los servicios de urgencias hospitalarios. Revista Española de Geriatría y Gerontología. 20180101, Issue: Preprints. (ISSN: 0211139X. Número de acceso: ejs42992624)

[7] Strange GR, Chen EH. Use of emergency departments by elder patients: A five-yearfollow up study. Academic Emergency Medicine. 1998;**5**(12):1157-1162

[8] Martín-Sanchez FJ, Merino C, Fernandez Alonso C. El paciente geriátrico en urgencias. Anales Sis San Navarra. 2010;**33**(1):163-172

[9] Moya Mir MS. Epidemiología de las urgencias del anciano. Monografías Emergencias. 2008;**2**:6-8

[10] McKay RD. Increasing rates of emergency department visits for elderly patients in the United States. Annals of Emergency Medicine. 2008;**51**:769-774

[11] Duaso E, Lopez-Soto A. Valoracion del paciente fragil en urgencias. Emergencias. 2009; **21**:362-369

[12] LLorente S, Arcos PI, Alonso FM. Factores que influyen en la demora del enfermo en un servicio de urgencias hospitalarias. Emergencias [Internet];**12**(3) Disponible en: http://www.semes.org/revista_EMERGENCIAS/

[13] Gómez-Cerquera JM, Daroca-Pérez R, Baeza-Trinidad R, Casañas-Martínez M. Validity of procalcitonin for the diagnosis of bacterial infection in elderly patients. Enfermedades Infecciosas y Microbiología Clínica. 2015;**33**:521-524

[14] Mattu A. Geriatric emergency medicine. Emergency Medicine Clinics of North America. 2006;**24**:13-14

[15] Julian-Jimenez A, Gonzales J, Martinez M. Short-term prognostic factors in the elderly patients seen in emergency departments due to infections. Enfermedades Infecciosas y Microbiología Clínica. 2017;**35**(4):215-219

[16] Gonzales J, Linares P, Menedez R. Guidelines for the management of community acquired pneumonia in the elderly patient. Revista Española de Quimioterapia. 2014;**27**(1):69-86

[17] Cardenas A. Criterio de los estudiantes de Medicina y de expertos sobre el diagnóstico del abdomen agudo quirúrgico en el anciano. Educación Médica Superior. 2014;**28**(4):643-651

[18] Valencia C, Heredia R, Moreno A. Envejecimiento y delirium: un viejo conocido en el Departamento de Urgencias. Meduis. 2014;**27**(2):85-92

[19] Morales A, Cardona D. Factores pronósticos de mortalidad temprana en ancianos ingresados en un servicio de urgencias. Revista Española de Geriatría y Gerontología. 2017;**52**(5):257-260

[20] Aranguren E, Capel JA. Estudio de la validez pronóstica de la recepción, acogida y clasificación de pacientes en el área de urgencias en un hospital terciario. Anales Sis San Navarra. 2005;**28**(2):177-188

[21] Calle A, Marquez MA. Valoración geriátrica y factores pronósticos de mortalidad en pacientes muy ancianos con neumonía extrahospitalaria. Archivos de Bronconeumología. 2014;**50**(10):429-434

[22] Martin-Sanches J, Fernandez C, Gil P. Puntos clave en la asistencia al anciano frágil en Urgencias. Medicina Clínica. 2013;**140**(1):24-29

[23] Gomez JF, Curcio CL. Salud del anciano: Valoracion. 1st ed. Blanecolor; 2014. 870 p

7

Aging Process and Physiological Changes

Shilpa Amarya, Kalyani Singh and
Manisha Sabharwal

Abstract

Ageing is a natural process. Everyone must undergo this phase of life at his or her own time and pace. In the broader sense, ageing reflects all the changes taking place over the course of life. These changes start from birth—one grows, develops and attains maturity. To the young, ageing is exciting. Middle age is the time when people notice the age-related changes like greying of hair, wrinkled skin and a fair amount of physical decline. Even the healthiest, aesthetically fit cannot escape these changes. Slow and steady physical impairment and functional disability are noticed resulting in increased dependency in the period of old age. According to World Health Organization, ageing is a course of biological reality which starts at conception and ends with death. It has its own dynamics, much beyond human control. However, this process of ageing is also subject to the constructions by which each society makes sense of old age. In most of the developed countries, the age of 60 is considered equivalent to retirement age and it is said to be the beginning of old age. In this chapter, you understand the details of ageing processes and associated physiological changes.

Keywords: ageing, physiological changes, elderly health, sensory changes, geriatrics

1. Introduction

The term 'Elderly' is applied to those individuals belonging to age 60 years and above, who represent the fastest growing segment of populations throughout the world. The percentage of elderly in developing countries tends to be small, although numbers are often large. In the year 1990, there were more than 280 million people belonging to the age 60 years or over in developing regions of the world, and 58% of the world's elderly were living in less-developed regions [1].

According to World Population Prospects (1950–2050), the proportion of elderly in developing countries is rising more rapidly, in comparison with developed ones [2]. The report published by the US Department of Health and Human Services shows that more developed nations have had decades to adjust to this change in age structure (**Figures 1** and **2**). As we see in **Figure 1**, it has taken more than a century for France's population aged 65 or older to rise from 7 to 14%, whereas many developing countries are growing rapidly in number and percentage of older individuals [2].

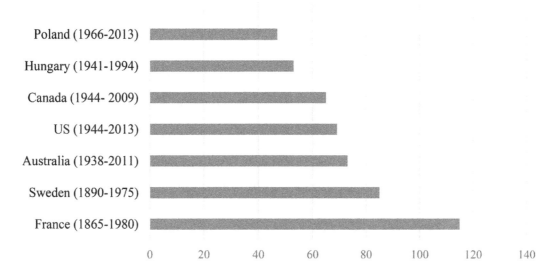

Figure 1. Speed of population ageing in developed countries. Source: U.S. Census Bureau [3]; Kinsella & Gist [4].

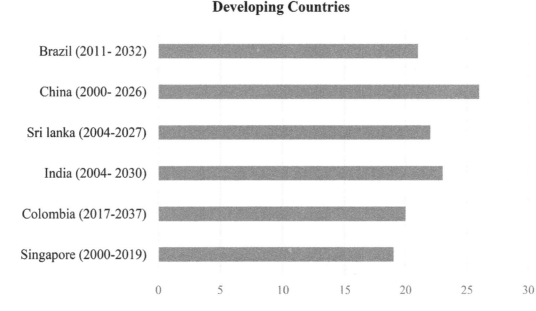

Figure 2. Speed of population ageing in developing countries. Source: U.S. Census Bureau [3]; Kinsella & Gist [4].

It is expected that by the year 2020, 70% of the world's elderly population will be in developing countries, with the absolute number exceeding 470 million which is double the number of the developed world [5]. The main factor responsible for this changing pattern of population ageing includes a rapid decline in both fertility and premature mortality [6]. Decline in fertility is particularly apparent in some developing countries like China, Cuba and Uruguay, although the fertility level in other developing countries such as Kenya, Zaire and Bangladesh remains high [7].

2. Ageing process and physiological changes

2.1. Changes in nervous system

Ageing is associated with many neurological disorders, as the capacity of the brain to transmit signals and communicate reduces. Loss of brain function is the biggest fear among elderly which includes loss of the very persona from dementia (usually Alzheimer's disease). Multiple other neurodegenerative conditions like Parkinson's disease or the sudden devastation of a stroke are also increasingly common with age [8].

Alzheimer's and Parkinson's diseases are the progressive neurodegenerative diseases associated with ageing [9]. Alzheimer's is characterised by progressive cognitive deterioration along with a change in behaviour and a decline in activities of daily living. Alzheimer's is the most common type of pre-senile and senile dementia. This disease causes nerve cell death and tissue loss throughout the brain, affecting nearly all its functions. The cortex in the brain shrivels up and this damages the areas involved in thinking, planning and remembering. The shrinkage in a nerve cell is especially severe in the hippocampus (an area of the cortex that plays a key role in the formation of new memories) as well as the ventricles (fluid-filled spaces within the brain) also grow larger. Alzheimer's disease causes an overall misbalance among the elderly by causing memory loss, changes in personality and behaviour-like depression, apathy, social withdrawal, mood swings, distrust in others, irritability and aggressiveness [10, 11].

Nearly, 33 million Indians have neurological disorders, and these occur twice as often in rural areas [12]. According to the World Health Organisation (WHO) [13], nearly 5% of men and 6% of women aged 60 years or above are affected with Alzheimer's-type dementia worldwide. In India, the total prevalence of dementia per 1000 elderly is 33.6%, of which vascular dementia constitutes approximately 39% and Alzheimer's disease constitutes approximately 54% [14].

Stroke is another common cause of mortality worldwide [13]. However, in India, the prevalence rate of stroke among elderly is reported to be very low compared to Western countries [15–17].

2.2. Cognition

A mild decline in the overall accuracy is observed with the beginning of the 60s that progresses slowly, but sustained attention is good in healthy older adults. Cognitive function declines and impairments are frequently observed among the elderly. Normally, these changes occur as outcomes of distal or proximal life events, where distal events are early life experiences such as cultural, physical and social conditions that influence functioning and cognitive development [17].

Cognition decline results from proximal factors (multiple serial cognitive processes) including processing speed, size of working memory, inhibition of extraneous environmental stimuli and sensory losses. This is a threat to the quality of life of those affected individuals and their caregivers [18].

Impaired cognition among elderly is associated with an increased risk of injuries to self or others, the decline in functional activities of daily living and an increased risk of mortality [19–21]. Mild cognitive impairment is increasingly being recognised as a transitional state between normal ageing and dementia [22, 23].

2.3. Memory, learning and intelligence

According to various studies [24–26], the effect of normal ageing on memory may result from the subtly changing environment within the brain. The brain's volume peaks at the early 20s and it declines gradually for rest of the life. In the 40s, the cortex starts to shrink and people start noticing the subtle changes in their ability to remember or to do more than one task at a time. Other key areas like neurons shrink or undergo atrophy and a large reduction in the extensiveness of connections among neurons (dendritic loss) is also noticed. During normal ageing, blood flow in the brain decreases and gets less efficient at recruiting different areas into operations. The whole group of changes taking place in the brain with ageing decreases the efficiency of cell-to-cell communication, which declines the ability to retrieve and learn [27]. It also affects the intelligence, especially fluid intelligence (problem-solving with a novel material requiring complex relations) declines rapidly after adolescence. Perceptual motor skills (timed tasks) decline with age [28].

2.4. Special senses

2.4.1. Vision

Ageing includes a decline in accommodation (presbyopia), glare tolerance, adaptation, low-contrast activity, attentional visual fields and colour discrimination. Changes occur in central processing and in the components of the eye. These numerous changes affect reading, balancing and driving [29].

2.4.2. Hearing

Ageing causes conductive and sensory hearing losses (presbycusis); the loss is primarily high tones, making consonants in speech difficult to discriminate [30].

2.4.3. Taste acuity

Losing sense of taste is a common problem among adults [31]. Taste acuity does not diminish but salt detection declines. Perception of sweet is unchanged and bitter is exaggerated. The salivary glands get affected, and the volume and quality of saliva diminish. All changes combine to make eating less interesting [32]. Studies show that the physiological decline in the density of the taste acuity and papillae results in a decline of gustatory function [33]. In fact, studies done on taste dysfunction show that ageing-associated changes in the density of taste acuity may affect taste function differently in different regions of the tongue [34]. Taste perception declines during the normal ageing process. A study done on the healthy elderly shows that after about 70 years of age, taste threshold begins to increase resulting in dysgeusia [34]. Chewing problems associated with loss of teeth and use of dentures also interfere with taste sensation and cause reduction in saliva production [32].

2.4.4. Smell

As we get older, our olfactory function declines [35]. Hyposmia (reduced ability to smell and to detect odours) is also observed with normal ageing [36]. The sense of smell reduces with an increase in age, and this affects the ability to discriminate between smells. A decreased sense of smell can lead to significant impairment of the quality of life, including taste disturbance and loss of pleasure from eating with resulting changes in weight and digestion [36].

It has been reported that more than 75% of people over the age of 80 years have evidence of major olfactory impairment. Many long-term studies show the evidence of a decline in olfaction considerably after the seventh decade [37]. Another study found that 62.5% of 80–97-year-olds had olfactory impairments [38]. However, it is widely accepted that taste disorders are far less prevalent than olfactory losses with age [38]. Ageing also causes atrophy of olfactory bulb neurons. Central processing is altered, resulting in a decreased perception and less interest in food [39].

2.4.5. Touch

As we age, our sense of touch often declines due to skin changes and reduced blood circulation to touch receptors or to the brain and spinal cord. Minor dietary deficiencies such as the deficiency of thiamine may also be a cause of changes [40]. The sense of touch also includes awareness of vibrations and pain. The skin, muscles, tendons, joints and internal organs have receptors that detect touch, temperature or pain [41].

A decline in the sense of touch affects simple motor skills, hand grip strength and balance. Studies have shown that muscle spindle (sensory receptors within the muscle that primarily detects changes in the length of this muscle) and mechanoreceptor (a sense organ or a cell that responds to mechanical stimuli such as touch or sound) functions decline with ageing, further interfering with balance [42].

3. Changes in musculoskeletal system

Normal ageing is characterised by a decrease in bone and muscle mass and an increase in adiposity [43, 44]. A decline in muscle mass and a reduction in muscle strength lead to risk of fractures, frailty, reduction in the quality of life and loss of independence [45]. These changes in musculoskeletal system reflect the ageing process as well as consequences of a reduced physical activity. The muscle wasting in frail older persons is termed 'sarcopaenia'. This disorder leads to a higher incidence of falls and fractures and a functional decline. Functional sarcopaenia or age-related musculoskeletal changes affect 7% of elderly above the age of 70 years, and the rate of deterioration increases with time, affecting over 20% of the elderly by the age of 80 [46]. Strength declines at 1.5% per year, and this accelerates to as much as 3% per year after 60 years of age [47]. These rates were considered high in sedentary individuals and twice as high in men as compared with those in women [48]. However, studies show that on an average, men have larger amounts of muscle mass and a shorter survival than women. This makes sarcopaenia potentially a greater public health concern among women than among men [48].

Skeletal muscle strength (force-generating capacity) also gets reduced with ageing [45, 46] depending upon genetic, dietary and, environmental factors as well as lifestyle choices. This reduction in muscle strength causes problems in physical mobility and activity of daily living. The total amount of muscle fibres is decreased due to a depressed productive capacity of cells to produce protein. There is a decrease in the size of muscle cells, fibres and tissues along with the total loss of muscle power, muscle bulk and muscle strength of all major muscle groups like deltoids, biceps, triceps, hamstrings, gastrocnemius (calf muscle), and so on. Wear and tear or wasting of the protective cartilage of joints occurs. The cartilage normally acts as a shock absorber and a gliding agent that prevents the friction injuries of the bone. There are stiffening and fibrosis of connective tissue elements that reduce the range of motion and affect the movements by making them less efficient. As part of the normal cell division process, telomere shortening occurs. DNA is more exposed to chemicals, toxins and waste products produced in the body. This whole process increases the vulnerability of cells.

With ageing, toxins and chemicals build up within the body and tissues. As a whole, this damages the integrity of muscle cells. Physical activity also decreases with age, due to a change in lifestyle. Somehow, the physiological changes of the muscles are aggravated by age-related neurological changes [49]. Most of the muscular activities become less efficient and less responsive with ageing as a result of a decrease in the nervous activity and nerve conduction.

A study was done by Williams et al. [50], who evaluated the muscle samples from both elderly and young adults and suggested that limb muscles are 25–35% shorter and less responsive in elderly healthy individuals when compared to young adults. In addition, the overall fat content of muscles was also higher in elderly population, suggesting transformation in the normal remodelling with age. Age-related musculoskeletal changes are much more prominent in fast-twitch muscle fibres as compared to slow-twitch muscle fibres. With ageing, the total water content of the tissue decreases and loss of hydration also adds to the inelasticity and stiffness. Alterations in the basal metabolic rate and slowing metabolism (as part of the physiological ageing process) result in muscle changes. This leads to the replacement of proteins with fatty tissue (that makes muscle less efficient).

Hormonal disorders can affect the metabolism of bones as well as muscles. Research suggests that menopause in women marks the aggravation in the deterioration of musculoskeletal changes due to lack of oestrogen that is required for the remodelling of bones and soft tissues. Certain systemic conditions like vascular disorders or metabolic disorders, in the case of diabetes, affect the remodelling of tissues as the rate or volume of nutritional delivery for the regeneration of cells is compromised. It is very important to control the pathological processes to optimise healing and repairing the potential of the musculoskeletal system. Essential vitamins like vitamin D and vitamin C play major roles in the functional growth of muscles and bones. Lack of certain minerals like calcium, phosphorus and chromium can be the result of age-related digestive issues. As such, it results in imbalance in the production of certain hormones like calcitonin and parathyroid that regulate the serum concentration of vitamins and minerals (due to tumours that are highly prevalent in elderly) or it causes a decreased absorption from the gut.

Age-related deterioration of muscular strength and balance control mechanisms has been associated with a reduced performance on functional tasks [51–53]. Comparing the isometric strength levels of the same muscle group, the loss of strength begins sooner among women than among men. It is reported that women are weaker than men in the absolute strength of various muscle groups in all stages of life. Various studies state that women have a longer life span, so the prevalence of disability among women is also more compared with men and it is marked with advancing age [54–56].

4. Body composition changes in old age

The human body is made up of fat, lean tissue (muscles and organs), bones and water. After the age of 40, people start losing their lean tissue. Body organs like liver, kidneys and other organs start losing some of their cells. This decline in muscle mass is associated with weakness, disability and morbidity [57, 58].

The tendency to become shorter occurs among the different gender groups and in all races. Height loss is associated with ageing changes in the bones, muscles and joints. Studies show that people typically lose almost one-half inch (about 1 cm) every 10 years after age 40 [59]. Height loss is even more rapid after age 70. These changes can be prevented by following a healthy diet, staying physically active and preventing and treating bone loss [60, 61].

Changes in the total body weight vary for men and woman, as men often gain weight until about age 55 and then begin to lose weight later in life. This may be related to a drop in the male sex hormone testosterone. Women usually gain weight until age 67–69 and then begin to lose weight. Weight loss later in life occurs partly because fat replaces lean muscle tissue and fat weighs less than muscle [60]. Studies have also shown that older people may have almost one-third more fat compared to when they were younger. Fat tissue builds up towards the centre of the body, including around the internal organs [60, 62, 63].

5. Obesity in elderly: prevalence

Today, as standards of living continue to rise, weight gain is posing a growing threat to the health of inhabitants from countries all over the world. Obesity is a chronic disease, prevalent in both developed and developing countries, and it is affecting all age groups. Indeed, it is now so common that it is replacing the more traditional public health concerns, such as infectious diseases and undernutrition, as the most common and significant contributors of ill health [64–67] (**Figure 3**).

As per World Health Organisation (WHO), globally, approximately 2.3 billion elderly people are overweight and more than 700 million elderly people are obese [68]. Most elderly belonging to the middle and high socio-economic groups are prone to obesity and complications related to obesity, due to sedentary lifestyles and a reduced physical mobility [69]. Obesity is considered as one of the major risk factors which causes the onset and increases the severity of non-communicable diseases (NCDs). It is a worldwide health problem, affecting elderly from both developed and developing countries. In elderly, obesity contributes to the early onset of chronic morbidities and functional impairments which lead to premature mortality [70].

5.1. Obesity among elderly: developed countries

The population in developed countries have proportionally a greater number of older adults living to older ages, and the prevalence of obesity is rising progressively, even among this age group [71].

The prevalence of obesity among elderly belonging to United States ranges from 42.5% in women to 38.1% in men, belonging to the age group 60–79 years. The prevalence differs for the elderly belonging to the age group 80 years and above, that is, 19.5% for females and 9.6% for males [72–74].

Comparatively, the prevalence of obesity in Europe is slightly lower but it is still a significant health issue. The prevalence of obesity among elderly in the United Kingdom is 22% among women and 12% among men aged 75 years or older [70, 75–77]. These statistics bode ill as the proportion of world's elderly population is growing rapidly (**Figure 4**).

In Australia, the percentage of weight gain has been so high that instead of losing weight with an increase in life, men and women aged 60–70 weigh more on average than they did when they were 20 years younger (**Figure 5**). Australian studies show that the prevalence of obesity

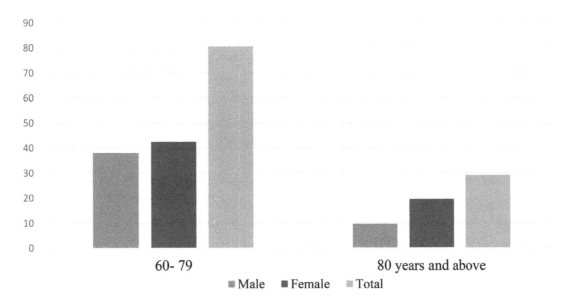

Figure 3. Prevalence of obesity among elderly aged 60 years and above, by sex: The United States, 2013. Source: [68].

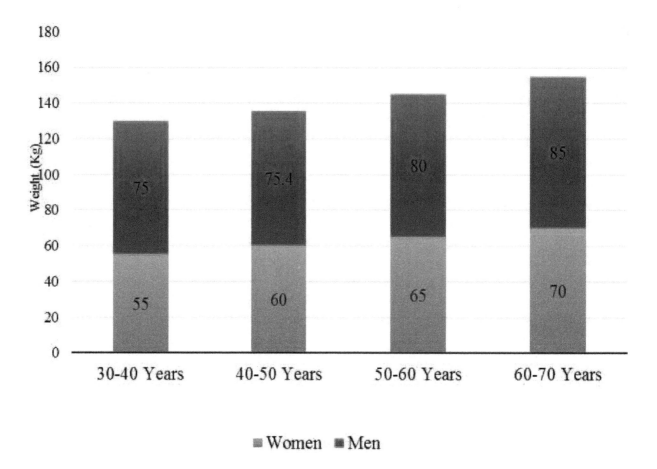

Figure 4. Trends in weight by age cohort, 1980–2000 (Australia). Source: Bennett et al. [81].

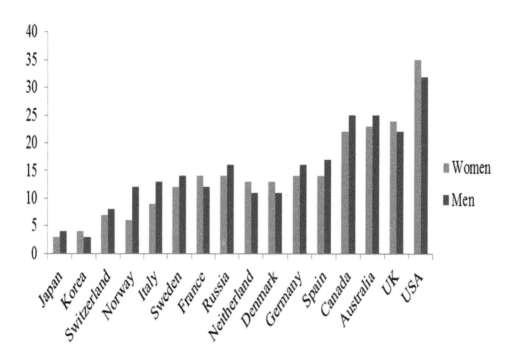

Figure 5. Worldwide prevalence of obesity among elderly women and men with BMI of ≥30 kg/m^2. Source: OECD [79]. Analysis of health survey data.

among elderly has increased in the age group of 60–69 years at about 24% for males and 30% for females, whereas it is less common among the elderly belonging to age group 80 years and above [78, 80]. Studies show that the percentage of Australian elderly reporting increased abdominal fat is markedly increasing over the years. Based on waist circumference, more than 30% of elderly males and 44% of elderly females in Australia are currently at a substantially increased risk of NCDs [78, 80, 81].

Studies from the Netherlands show that obesity was present in 18% of men and 20% of women belonging to the age group of 60 years and above [82]. Also, the increase in waist circumference ranged from 40% among males to 56% among females [82, 83].

In France, studies show that the prevalence of obesity among elderly was relatively stable during early years (1980–1991), 6.4–6.5% in males and 6.3–7.0% among females [83], but studies from recent years [84, 85] have highlighted a sharp increase in obese elderly, 19.5% for both males and females; this prevalence rate decreased gradually after 70 years of age, that is, from 19.5 to 13.2% [86]. The Scottish Health Survey shows that in 10 years (2003–2013), the prevalence of obesity has increased as the body mass index (BMI) continues to rise in people 60–70 years of age, especially among females [87]. In this same period, there was an increased curve shown for the waist circumference (5–10 cm) in both the sexes between 50 and 70 years of age. This inappropriate increase in waist circumference and a slight increase in BMI in the Scottish Health Survey may indicate a substantial gain in visceral fat mass and loss of lean tissue that predisposes to ill health in the obese elderly [88, 89].

In Spain, 35% of subjects aged 65 years or older suffered from obesity (30.6% of males and 38.3% of females) and 61.6% had an increased waist circumference (50.9% of males and 69.7% of females) [88].

5.2. Prevalence of obesity: developing countries

Over the past years, obesity among elderly was considered as a problem only in high-income countries, but the trend is changing now; excess weight, as well as obesity, is dramatically increasing in low-income and middle-income countries as well, particularly in urban settings [90]. Various studies show a significant change in the mean body weight, physical activity and diet along with progressive economic development in developing countries. Possibilities are high that obesity and its co-morbidities will continue to affect an increasing number of populations in these regions. Lifestyle and environmental factors are acting in a synergistic manner to fuel the obesity epidemic. As per WHO estimates, there is a decline in undernourished population across the world, whereas the overnourished population has increased to 1.2 billion [90]. A WHO report shows that more than 1 billion elderly are overweight and 300 million are obese. The problem of obesity is increasing in the developing world with more than 115 million people suffering from obesity-related problems [90]. The obesity rate has increased threefold or more since 1980 in the Middle East, the Pacific Islands and India [91, 92]. However, the prevalence of obesity is not as high in all developing countries, like China and some African nations [93].

As per the WHO report, the prevalence of overweight and obese elderly in China was 19.0 and 2.9%, respectively. However, the prevalence has increased over the past years; in the latest study, the prevalence of overweight and obesity among elderly was 21.0 and 7.4% [94, 95]. There was a slight increase in the prevalence of overweight and obesity among women than among men in China.

According to WHO estimates, among all Gulf regions, Kuwait ranked number one with the highest prevalence of overweight and obesity (78.8%) among elderly (60 years and above) [92]. Worldwide, Kuwait is ranked 11th, that is, the highest in obesity among the Arab countries and the Middle East [93, 96]. Studies from Sri Lanka show a prevalence rate of 25.2% for overweight and 9.2% for obesity. The prevalence of central obesity among elderly was highest at 26.2% [97, 98]. The prevalence of overweight and obesity in Brazil was 41.8% for females and 23.4% for males. According to the prevalence studies of obesity among elderly in Nigeria [99], overweight among elderly ranged from 20.3 to 35.1% and obesity ranged from 8.1 to 22.2%. WHO reported that the prevalence of obesity in Sub-Saharan African countries ranged between 3.3 and 18.0% and that obesity has become a leading risk factor for diabetes mellitus and cardiovascular diseases in the urban areas of Africa [93, 99]. The situation can get worse within a decade if the present trend continues and overweight could emerge as the single most important public health problem in adults. Overweight or obesity may not be a specific disease but it is certainly considered as a major contributory factor leading to various degenerative diseases in adult life. Prevention and control of this problem must, therefore, claim priority attention [100].

As per a study done in Delhi on urban elderly, nearly 14% of men and more than 50% of women belonging to what may be a higher-income group (HIG) were overweight (BMI >25) and obese (BMI >30) [101]. The prevalence of abdominal obesity among the elderly group was also reported as high. Assuming that the HIG in India number is around 100 million (half the number of the middle class), it may be computed that there are roughly 40–50 million overweight subjects belonging to the HIG in the country today. Visweswara et al. [102] studied females of Hyderabad (60 years and above) belonging to the high socio-economic status and reported the prevalence rate of obesity as 36.3%. Gopinath et al. [103] studied urban elderly in Delhi and reported the rate of prevalence of obesity as 33.4%. A study done in the Union Territory of Chandigarh showed an increase in BMI (>25) resulting in the high prevalence rate of overweight (33.14%) and obesity (7.54%) among elderly [104, 105].

6. Causes of obesity among elderly

The relationship between energy intake and energy expenditure is an important determinant of body fat mass. Obesity occurs when the consumption of calories is more than the calorie expenditure. The possible causes of obesity are depicted in **Figure 6**. Various studies indicate that how much we eat does not decline with advancing age; therefore, it is likely that a decrease in energy expenditure particularly in the beginning of old age (50–65 years) contributes to the increase in body fat as we age [62, 106]. At the age of 65 years and above, hormonal

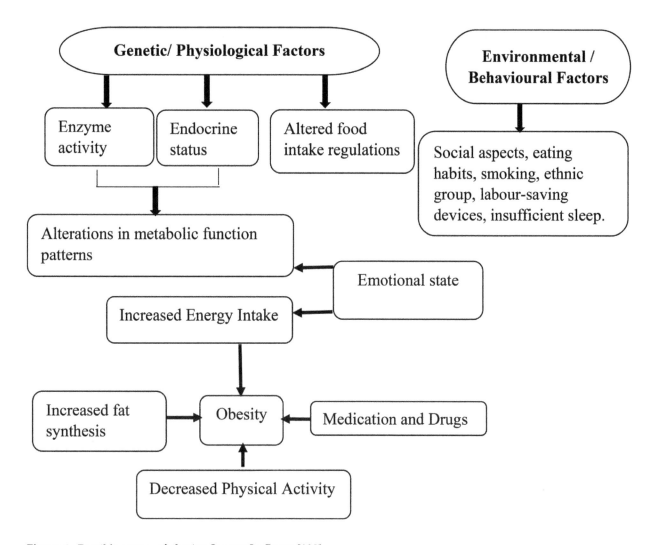

Figure 6. Possible causes of obesity. Source: La Berge [108].

changes cause an accumulation of fat. Ageing is associated with a decline in the secretion of growth hormone, serum testosterone, resistance to leptin and a reduced responsiveness to thyroid hormone [107]. Studies show that resistance to leptin could cause a decrease in the ability to regulate appetite downward [74]. Several other genetic, environmental and social factors contribute to obesity among elderly.

6.1. Genetic factors

Science does show a link between obesity and heredity [109]. Various studies indicate that obesity is related to the inherited genes and there is a link between obesity and heredity [110–113]. According to a study, visceral fat is more influenced by the genotype than subcutaneous fat [114].

6.2. Environmental and sociological factors

Like genetics, environment also has a major role to play in obesity. The food we consume, physical activity and lifestyle behaviour are all influenced by the environment. For example, the adoption of modern diet over traditional diet, the trend towards 'eating out' rather than preparing food in the home, the development of high-rise buildings that often lack sidewalks and a deficit of readily accessible recreation areas are some of the common environmental factors associated with obesity.

Poverty and low education level also appeared as a reason for obesity among elderly. Studies state that the lack of nutritional knowledge, purchase of low-cost fat and organ meat are also associated with overweight and obesity. Poor hygienic conditions also appeared as a major reason [114].

6.3. Other causes of obesity

Other health issues and illnesses that are associated with obesity and weight gain are hyperthyroidism, polycystic ovary syndrome, Cushing's syndrome and depression [2]. Obese elderly are more likely to report symptoms of depression, such as hopelessness, sadness or worthlessness [115]. Sleep plays a major role. Lack of sleep contributes to obesity [106]. Certain drugs, such as antidepressants and steroids, may stimulate appetite or cause water retention or reduce the metabolic rate [82], causing an increase in weight. Health issues like arthritis and joint pain decrease mobility and activity intolerance, contributing to obesity [116]. Joint pain decreases mobility, and activity intolerance may lead to weight gain because of a decreased activity. Older adults are more likely than younger adults to experience functional limitations associated with chronic illnesses that may begin a stress-pain-depression cycle that can result in lifestyle patterns leading to obesity [117]. Finally, the complex relationship between lifestyle pattern and functional ability merits attention as a contributor to obesity [93].

7. Conclusion

In developing countries, as compared to developed countries, gerontology has drawn comparatively lesser attention. This is because the increased life expectancy of elderly resulting in a demographic transition which developing countries are witnessing today has already been faced by developed countries, several decades back. However, in recent years with a rising percentage of elderly population, epidemiologists, researchers, demographers and clinicians have focussed their attention towards elderly care health issues and various problems associated with ageing and numerous implications of this demographic transition.

Elderly face various problems and require a multi-sectoral approach involving inputs from various disciplines of health, psychology, nutrition, sociology and social sciences.

Conflict of interest

There is no conflict of interest.

Author details

Shilpa Amarya*, Kalyani Singh and Manisha Sabharwal

*Address all correspondence to: shilpamarya@gmail.com

Lady Irwin College, University of Delhi, New Delhi, India

References

[1] World Health Organization and World Health Organization. Management of Substance Abuse Unit. Global Status Report on Alcohol and Health, 2014. World Health Organization; 2014

[2] Dobriansky PJ, Suzman RM, Hodes RJ. Why Population Aging Matters: A Global Perspective. National Institute on Aging, National Institutes of Health, US Department of Health and Human Services, US Department of State; 2007

[3] US Census Bureau. In: Commerce USDo, editor. Statistical Abstract of the United States: 2012. 2012. p. 111

[4] Kinsella K, Gist YJ. Older Workers, Retirement, and Pensions: A Comparative International Chartbook. Washington, DC: United States Bureau of the Census (IPC/95-2RP); 1995

[5] Resnikoff S, Pascolini D, Mariotti SP, Pokharel GP. Global magnitude of visual impairment caused by uncorrected refractive errors in 2004. Bulletin of the World Health Organization. 2008;86(1):63-70

[6] McNicoll G. Consequences of rapid population growth: An overview and assessment. Population and Development Review. 1984;Jun 1:177-240

[7] Cleland J, Bernstein S, Ezeh A, Faundes A, Glasier A, Innis J. Family planning: The unfinished agenda. The Lancet. 2006;368(9549):1810-1827

[8] McKhann GM, Knopman DS, Chertkow H, Hyman BT, Jack CR, Kawas CH, Klunk WE, Koroshetz WJ, Manly JJ, Mayeux R, Mohs RC. The diagnosis of dementia due to Alzheimer's disease: Recommendations from the National Institute on Aging-Alzheimer's association workgroups on diagnostic guidelines for Alzheimer's disease. Alzheimer's & Dementia. 2011;7(3):263-269

[9] Esopenko C, Levine B. Aging, neurodegenerative disease, and traumatic brain injury: The role of neuroimaging. Journal of Neurotrauma. 2015;32(4):209-220

[10] Das SK, Pal S, Ghosal MK. Dementia: Indian scenario. Neurology India. 2012;60(6):618

[11] Mayeux R, Stern Y. Epidemiology of Alzheimer disease. Cold Spring Harbor Perspectives in Medicine. 2012;2(8):a006239

[12] Muthane UB, Ragothaman M, Gururaj G. Epidemiology of Parkinson's disease and movement disorders in India: Problems and possibilities. Japi. 2007;**55**:719-724

[13] World Health Organization. Noncommunicable Disease Country Profiles, 2014. Geneva, Switzerland: WHO Document Production Services; 2014

[14] Mishra S, Palanivelu K. The effect of curcumin (turmeric) on Alzheimer's disease: An overview. Annals of Indian Academy of Neurology. 2008;**11**(1):13

[15] Das SK, Banerjee TK, Biswas A, Roy T, Raut DK, Mukherjee CS, Chaudhuri A, Hazra A, Roy J. A prospective community-based study of stroke in Kolkata, India. Stroke. 2007; **38**(3):906-910

[16] Nandi DN, Banerjee G, Mukherjee SP, Nandi PS, Nandi S. Psychiatric morbidity of a rural Indian community. The British Journal of Psychiatry. 2000;**176**(4):351-356

[17] Kapoor SK, Banerjee AK. Prevalence of common neurological diseases in a rural community of India. Indian Journal of Community Medicine. 1989;**14**(4):171

[18] Harada CN, Love MCN, Triebel KL. Normal cognitive aging. Clinics in Geriatric Medicine. 2013;**29**(4):737-752

[19] Bassuk SS, Wypij D, Berkmann LF. Cognitive impairment and mortality in the community-dwelling elderly. American Journal of Epidemiology. 2000;**151**(7):676-688

[20] Leiknes I, Lien UT, Severinsson E. The relationship among caregiver burden, demographic variables, and the clinical characteristics of patients with Parkinson's disease—A systematic review of studies using various caregiver burden instruments. Open Journal of Nursing. 2015;**5**(10):855

[21] Rowe JW, Kahn RL. Successful aging. The Gerontologist. 1997;**37**(4):433-440

[22] Tabert MH, Albert SM, Borukhova-Milov L, Camacho Y, Pelton G, Liu X, Stern Y, Devanand DP. Functional deficits in patients with mild cognitive impairment prediction of AD. Neurology. 2002;**58**(5):758-764

[23] Tuokko HA, Frerichs RJ, Kristjansson B. Cognitive impairment, no dementia: Concepts and issues. International Psychogeriatrics. 2001;**13**(S1):183-202

[24] Cabeza R, Moscovitch M. Memory systems, processing modes, and components: Functional neuroimaging evidence. Perspectives on Psychological Science. 2013;**8**(1):49-55

[25] Driscoll I, Hamilton DA, Petropoulos H, Yeo RA, Brooks WM, Baumgartner RN, Sutherland RJ. The aging hippocampus: Cognitive, biochemical and structural findings. Cerebral Cortex. 2003;**13**(12):1344-1351

[26] Balota DA, Dolan PO, Duchek JM. Memory changes in healthy older adults. The Oxford Handbook of Memory. 2000. pp. 395–409

[27] Besdine RW, Wu D. Aging of the human nervous system: What do we know? Medicine and Health Rhode Island. 2008;**91**(5):161

[28] Greve KW, Bianchini KJ, Mathias CW, Houston RJ, Crouch JA. Detecting malingered performance on the Wechsler adult intelligence scale: Validation of Mittenberg's approach in traumatic brain injury. Archives of Clinical Neuropsychology. 2003;**18**(3):245-260

[29] Salvi SM, Akhtar S, Currie Z. Ageing changes in the eye. Postgraduate Medical Journal. 2006;**82**(971):581-587

[30] Khullar S, Babbar R. Presbycusis and auditory brainstem responses: A review. Asian Pacific Journal of Tropical Disease. 2011;**1**(2):150-157

[31] Imoscopi A, Inelmen EM, Sergi G, Miotto F, Manzato E. Taste loss in the elderly: Epidemiology, causes and consequences. Aging Clinical and Experimental Research. 2012;**24**(6):570-579

[32] Boyce JM, Shone GR. Effects of ageing on smell and taste. Postgraduate Medical Journal. 2006;**82**(966):239-241

[33] Morley JE, Silver AJ, Miller DK, Rubenstein LZ. The anorexia of the elderly. Annals of the New York Academy of Sciences. 1989;**575**(1):50-59

[34] Toffanello ED, Inelmen EM, Imoscopi A, Perissinotto E, Coin A, Miotto F, Donini LM, Cucinotta D, Barbagallo M, Manzato E, Sergi G. Taste loss in hospitalized multimorbid elderly subjects. Clinical Interventions in Aging. 2013;**8**:167-174

[35] Doty RL, Shaman P, Applebaum SL, Giberson R, Siksorski L, Rosenberg L. Smell identification ability: Changes with age. Science. 1984;**226**:1441-1443

[36] Gaines AD. Anosmia and hyposmia. In: Allergy and Asthma Proceedings. OceanSide Publications, Inc.; 2010 May;**31**(3):185-189

[37] Murphy C, Schubert CR, Cruickshanks KJ, Klein BE, Klein R, Nondahl DM. Prevalence of olfactory impairment in older adults. JAMA. 2002;**288**(18):2307-2312

[38] Schiffman SS, Zervakis J. Taste and smell perception in the elderly: Effect of medications and disease. Advances in Food and Nutrition Research. 2002;**44**:247-346

[39] Sinding C, Puschmann L, Hummel T. Is the age-related loss in olfactory sensitivity similar for light and heavy molecules? In: Chemical Senses. 2014. p. bju004

[40] Roberts SB, Rosenberg I. Nutrition and aging: Changes in the regulation of energy metabolism with aging. Physiological Reviews. 2006;**86**(2):651-667

[41] Wickremaratchi MM, Llewelyn JG. Effects of ageing on touch. Postgraduate Medical Journal. 2006;**82**(967):301-304

[42] Carpenter MG, Adkin AL, Brawley LR, Frank JS. Postural, physiological and psychological reactions to challenging balance: Does age make a difference? Age and Ageing. 2006;**35**(3):298-303

[43] Villa-Forte A. Effects of aging on the musculoskeletal system. Last Full Review/Revision July 2014; 2015

[44] Basu R, Basu A, Nair KS. Muscle changes in aging. The Journal of Nutrition, Health & Aging. 2001;**6**(5):336-341

[45] Faulkner JA, Larkin LM, Claflin DR, Brooks SV. Age-related changes in the structure and function of skeletal muscles. Clinical and Experimental Pharmacology and Physiology. 2007;**34**(11):1091-1096

[46] McGowen J, Raisz L, Noonan A, Elderkin A. Bone health and osteoporosis: A report of the surgeon general. US Dep. Health Hum. Serv; 2004. pp. 69–87

[47] Morley JE, Baumgartner RN, Roubenoff R, Mayer J, Nair KS. Sarcopenia. Journal of Laboratory and Clinical Medicine. 2001;**137**(4):231-243

[48] Van Kan GA, Rolland YM, Morley JE, Vellas B. Frailty: Toward a clinical definition. Journal of the American Medical Directors Association. 2008;**9**(2):71

[49] Fell J, Williams AD. The effect of aging on skeletal-muscle recovery from exercise: Possible implications for aging athletes. Journal of Aging and Physical Activity. 2008;**16**(1):97

[50] Williams GN, Higgins MJ, Lewek MD. Aging skeletal muscle: Physiologic changes and the effects of training. Physical Therapy. 2002;**82**(1):62-68

[51] Melzer I, Kurz I, Oddsson LI. A retrospective analysis of balance control parameters in elderly fallers and non-fallers. Clinical Biomechanics. 2010;**25**(10):984-988

[52] Bottaro M, Machado SN, Nogueira W, Scales R, Veloso J. Effect of high versus low-velocity resistance training on muscular fitness and functional performance in older men. European Journal of Applied Physiology. 2007;**99**(3):257-264

[53] Wang CY, Olson SL, Protas EJ. Test-retest strength reliability: Hand-held dynamometry in community-dwelling elderly fallers. Archives of Physical Medicine and Rehabilitation. 2002;**83**(6):811-815

[54] Pontifex MB, Hillman CH, Fernhall BO, Thompson KM, Valentini TA. The effect of acute aerobic and resistance exercise on working memory. Medicine & Science in Sports & Exercise. 2009;**41**(4):927-934

[55] Macaluso A, De Vito G. Muscle strength, power and adaptations to resistance training in older people. European Journal of Applied Physiology. 2004;**91**(4):450-472

[56] Puggaard L. Effects of training on functional performance in 65, 75 and 85 year-old women: Experiences deriving from community based studies in Odense, Denmark. Scandinavian Journal of Medicine & Science in Sports. 2003;**13**(1):70-76

[57] Duren DL, Sherwood RJ, Czerwinski SA, Lee M, Choh AC, Siervogel RM, Chumlea WC. Body composition methods: Comparisons and interpretation. Journal of Diabetes Science and Technology. 2008;**2**(6):1139-1146

[58] Barbosa AR, Santarem JM, Jacob FW, Meirelles ES, Marucci JM. Comparison of body fat using anthropometry bioelectrical impedance and DEXA in elderly women. Archivos Latinoamericanos de Nutricion. 2001;**51**(1):49-56

[59] Jiang Y, Zhang Y, Jin M, Gu Z, Pei Y, Meng P. Aged-related changes in body composition and association between body composition with bone mass density by body mass index in Chinese Han men over 50-year-old. PLoS One. 2015;**10**(6):e0130400

[60] Ferraro FR, Muehlenkamp JJ, Paintner A, Wasson K, Hager T, Hoverson F. Aging, body image, and body shape. The Journal of General Psychology. 2008;**135**(4):379-392

[61] Hughes VA, Frontera WR, Wood M, Evans WJ, Dallal GE, Roubenoff R, Singh MAF. Longitudinal muscle strength changes in older adults influence of muscle mass, physical activity, and health. The Journals of Gerontology Series A: Biological Sciences and Medical Sciences. 2001;**56**(5):B209-B217

[62] Baumgartner RN, Koehler KM, Gallagher D, Romero L, Heymsfield SB, Ross RR, Garry PJ, Lindeman RD. Epidemiology of sarcopenia among the elderly in New Mexico. American Journal of Epidemiology. 1998;**147**(8):755-763

[63] Frontera WR, Hughes VA, Lutz KJ, Evans WJ. A cross-sectional study of muscle strength and mass in 45-to 78-yr-old men and women. Journal of Applied Physiology. 1991;**71**(2): 644-650

[64] Rajkamal R, Singh Z, Stalin P, Muthurajesh E. Prevalence and determinants of overweight and obesity among elderly population in an urban area of Puducherry. International Journal of Medical Science and Public Health. 2015;**4**(3):369-372

[65] Shebl AM, Hatata ESZ, Boughdady AM, El-Sayed SM. Prevalence and risk factors of obesity among elderly attending geriatric outpatient clinics in Mansoura City. Journal of Education and Practice. 2015;**6**(30):136-147

[66] Andrade FBD, Caldas Junior ADF, Kitoko PM, Batista JEM, Andrade TBD. Prevalence of overweight and obesity in elderly people from Vitória-ES, Brazil. Ciência & Saúde Coletiva. 2012;**17**(3):749-756

[67] Hunt RH, Xiao SD, Megraud F, Leon-Barua R, Bazzoli F, Van Der Merwe S, Vaz Coelho LG, Fock M, Fedail S, Cohen H, Malfertheiner P. Helicobacter pylori in developing countries. World gastroenterology organisation global guideline. Journal of Gastrointestinal and Liver Diseases. 2011;**20**(3):299-304

[68] Johnson CL, Paulose-Ram R, Ogden CL, Carroll MD, Kruszan-Moran D, Dohrmann SM, Curtin LR. National Health and Nutrition Examination Survey. Analytic Guidelines, 1999-2010. 2013

[69] Ahluwalia N. Aging, nutrition and immune function. Journal of Nutrition, Health & Aging. 2004

[70] Donini LM, Savina C, Gennaro E, De Felice MR, Rosano A, Pandolfo MM, Del Balzo V, Cannella C, Ritz P, Chumlea WC. A systematic review of the literature concerning the relationship between obesity and mortality in the elderly. The Journal of Nutrition, Health & Aging. 2012;**16**(1):89-98

[71] World Health Organization. Global Database on Body Mass Index; 2006

[72] Rhoades JA. Overweight and Obese Elderly and near Elderly in the United States, 2002: Estimates for the Noninstitutionalized Population Age 55 and Older. Medical Expenditure Panel Survey, Agency for Healthcare Research and Quality; 2005

[73] Fakhouri TH, Ogden CL, Carroll MD, Kit BK, Flegal KM. Prevalence of obesity among older adults in the United States, 2007–2010. NCHS Data Brief. 2012;**106**(106):1-8

[74] Villareal DT, Apovian CM, Kushner RF, Klein S. Obesity in older adults: Technical review and position statement of the American Society for Nutrition and NAASO, the Obesity Society. Obesity Research. 2005;**13**(11):1849-1863

[75] Mathus-Vliegen EM, Basdevant A, Finer N, Hainer V, Hauner H, Micic D, Maislos M, Roman G, Schutz Y, Tsigos C, Toplak H. Prevalence, pathophysiology, health consequences and treatment options of obesity in the elderly: A guideline. Obesity Facts. 2012; **5**(3):460-483

[76] Arterburn DE, Crane PK, Sullivan SD. The coming epidemic of obesity in elderly Americans. Journal of the American Geriatrics Society. 2004;**52**(11):1907-1912

[77] Flegal KM, Carroll MD, Ogden CL, Johnson CL. Prevalence and trends in obesity among US adults, 1999–2000. JAMA. 2002;**288**(14):1723-1727

[78] Wong E, Woodward M, Stevenson C, Backholer K, Sarink D, Peeters A. Prevalence of disability in Australian elderly: Impact of trends in obesity and diabetes. Preventive Medicine. 2016;**82**:105-110

[79] Sassi F, Devaux M. OECD Obesity Update 2012. 2014

[80] Olds TS, Tomkinson GR, Ferrar KE, Maher CA. Trends in the prevalence of childhood overweight and obesity in Australia between 1985 and 2008. International Journal of Obesity. 2010;**34**(1):57-66

[81] Bennett SA, Magnus P, Gibson D, Bennett AS. Obesity Trends in Older Australians. Australian Institute of Health and Welfare; 2004

[82] Blokstra A, Vissink P, Venmans LMAJ, Holleman P, Van der Schouw YT, Smit HA, Verschuren WMM. Measuring the Netherlands: A Monitoring Study of Risk Factors in the General Population, 2009–2010. Bilthoven: National Institute for Public Health and the Environment (RIVM); 2011

[83] Putrik P, van Amelsvoort L, De Vries NK, Mujakovic S, Kunst AE, van Oers H, Jansen M, Kant I. Neighborhood environment is associated with overweight and obesity, particularly in older residents: Results from cross-sectional study in Dutch municipality. Journal of Urban Health. 2015;**92**(6):1038-1051

[84] Diouf I, Charles MA, Ducimetière P, Basdevant A, Eschwege E, Heude B. Evolution of obesity prevalence in France: An age-period-cohort analysis. Epidemiology (Cambridge, Mass.). 2010;**21**(3):360

[85] Charles MA, Eschwège E, Basdevant A. Monitoring the obesity epidemic in France: The Obepi surveys 1997–2006. Obesity. 2008;**16**(9):2182-2186

[86] Tanaka H, Kokubo Y. Epidemiology of obesity in Japan. Japan Medical Association Journal. 2005;**48**(1):34-41

[87] Han TS, Tajar A, Lean MEJ. Obesity and weight management in the elderly. British Medical Bulletin. 2011;**97**(1):169-196

[88] Castle A. Obesity in Scotland. SPICe Briefing. Edinburgh: Scottish Parliament Information Centre (SPICe); January 2015

[89] Parkes A, Sweeting H, Wight D. Growing up in Scotland: Overweight, Obesity and Activity-Main Report. 2012

[90] WHO EC. Appropriate body-mass index for Asian populations and its implications for policy and intervention strategies. Lancet (London, England). 2004;**363**(9403):157

[91] Ellulu M, Abed Y, Rahmat A, Ranneh Y, Ali F. Epidemiology of obesity in developing countries: Challenges and prevention. Global Epidemic of Obesity. 2014;**2**(1):2

[92] Ng SW, Zaghloul S, Ali HI, Harrison G, Popkin BM. The prevalence and trends of overweight, obesity and nutrition-related non-communicable diseases in the Arabian gulf states. Obesity Reviews. 2011;**12**(1):1-13

[93] WHO, UNICEF, UNFPA, The World Bank. Trends in Maternal Mortality: 1990 to 2010. World Health Organization, UNICEF, UNFPA, and The World Bank; 2012

[94] Xu W, Zhang H, Paillard-Borg S, Zhu H, Qi X, Rizzuto D. Prevalence of overweight and obesity among Chinese adults: Role of adiposity indicators and age. Obesity Facts. 2016;**9**(1):17-28

[95] Gao Y, Ran XW, Xie XH, Lu HL, Chen T, Ren Y, Long Y, Tian HM. Prevalence of overweight and obesity among Chinese Yi nationality: A cross-sectional study. BMC Public Health. 2011;**11**(1):1

[96] Mehio Sibai A, Nasreddine L, Mokdad AH, Adra N, Tabet M, Hwalla N. Nutrition transition and cardiovascular disease risk factors in Middle East and North Africa countries: Reviewing the evidence. Annals of Nutrition and Metabolism. 2010;**57**(3–4):193-203

[97] Ranasinghe C, Gamage P, Katulanda P, Andraweera N, Thilakarathne S, Tharanga P. Relationship between Body mass index (BMI) and body fat percentage, estimated by bioelectrical impedance, in a group of Sri Lankan adults: A cross sectional study. BMC Public Health. 2013;**13**(1):1

[98] Katulanda P, Jayawardena MAR, Sheriff MHR, Constantine GR, Matthews DR. Prevalence of overweight and obesity in Sri Lankan adults. Obesity Reviews. 2010;**11**(11):751-756

[99] Oladapo OO, Salako L, Sodiq O, Shoyinka K, Adedapo K, Falase AO. Cardiovascular topics. Cardiovascular Journal of Africa. 2010;**21**(1):26-31

[100] Grover S, Sahoo S, Dogra S, Ghormode D. Steroid induced mania in an elderly patient. Journal of Geriatric Mental Health. 2014;**1**(2):115

[101] Gopalan C. Obesity in the Indian urban 'Middle Class'. NFI Bulletin. 1998;**19**:1-4

[102] Visweswara Rao K, Balakrishna N, Shatrugna V. Variations in forms of malnutrition in well-to-do adults and the associated factors. Man in India. 1995;**75**(3):241-249

[103] Gopinath N, Chadha SL, Sood AK, Shekhawat S, Bindra SP, Tandon R. Epidemiological study of hypertension in young (15-24 yr) Delhi urban population. The Indian Journal of Medical Research. 1994;**99**:32-37

[104] Swami HM, Bhatia V, Gupta AK, Bhatia SPS. An epidemiological study of obesity among elderly in Chandigarh. Indian Journal of Community Medicine. 2005;**30**(1):11-13

[105] Swami HM, Bhatia V, Gupta M, Bhatia SPS, Sood A. Population based study of hypertension among the elderly in northern India. Public Health. 2002;**116**(1):45-49

[106] Newman A. Obesity in older adults. The Online Journal of Issues in Nursing. 2009;**14**(1)

[107] Corpas E, Harman SM, Blackman MR. Human growth hormone and human aging. Endocrine Reviews. 1993;**14**(1):20-39

[108] La Berge AF. How the ideology of low fat conquered America. Journal of the History of Medicine and Allied Sciences. 2008;**63**(2):139-177

[109] Vissink P, Venmans LMAJ, Holleman P, van der Schouw YT, Smit HA, Verschuren WMM. Measuring the Netherlands: A monitoring study of risk factors in the general population, 2009–2010. Bilthoven: National Institute for Public Health and the Environment (RIVM); 2011

[110] Thompson PM, Stein JL, Medland SE, Hibar DP, Vasquez AA, Renteria ME, Toro R, Jahanshad N, Schumann G, Franke B, Wright MJ. The ENIGMA consortium: Large-scale collaborative analyses of neuroimaging and genetic data. Brain Imaging and Behavior. 2014;**8**(2):153-182

[111] Herrera BM, Keildson S, Lindgren CM. Genetics and epigenetics of obesity. Maturitas. 2011;**69**(1):41-49

[112] Walley AJ, Blakemore AI, Froguel P. Genetics of obesity and the prediction of risk for health. Human Molecular Genetics. 2006;**15**(Suppl 2):R124-R130

[113] Lyon HN, Hirschhorn JN. Genetics of common forms of obesity: A brief overview. The American Journal of Clinical Nutrition. 2005;**82**(1):215S-217S

[114] Chung WK, Leibel RL. Considerations regarding the genetics of obesity. Obesity. 2008: Dec 1;**16**(S3)

[115] Amarya S, Singh K, Sabharwal M. Health consequences of obesity in the elderly. Journal of Clinical Gerontology and Geriatrics. 2014;**5**(3):63-67

[116] Milanović Z, Pantelić S, Trajković N, Sporiš G, Kostić R, James N. Age-related decrease in physical activity and functional fitness among elderly men and women. Clinical Interventions in Aging. 2013;8:549-556

[117] Sugiura H, Demura S. Possibility of stretch-shortening cycle movement training using a jump rope. The Journal of Strength & Conditioning Research. 2014;28(3):700-705

8

Thymic Rejuvenation: Are we there Yet?

Jamilah Abusarah, Fatemeh Khodayarian, Yun Cui,
Abed El-Hakim El-Kadiry and Moutih Rafei

Abstract

Vaccination is an appealing form of immunotherapy for frail senior patients. However, several studies have shown that in contrast to younger adults, older patients do not effectively respond to vaccines. This phenomenon is greatly attributed to immunosenescence, a hallmark of aging defined by a general decline in immunity caused by thymic involution. Historically, the study of thymic involution brought to attention several factors and components involved in thymopoiesis, as contributors to the phenomena. Depicting the underlying cause(s) of the dramatic changes in the production and properties of the naïve T-cell pool in the event of acute thymic injury or due to inovulation can therefore, help focus the efforts on the best strategy to reverse or overcome these hurdles. Here, we discuss some of the well-studied approaches for rejuvenating the thymus, and introduce interleukin-(IL) 21 as the most recent thymo-stimulatory agent in the field.

Keywords: thymus, thymocytes, thymic epithelial cells, thymic involution, interleukin-21

1. Introduction

With the advances in health sciences and services, the life expectancy of the general population is increasing. The U.S. Census Bureau estimates that by 2050, one quarter of the U.S. population will be over 60 years old [1]. A similar demographic trend is predicted for both developed and developing countries according to the world health organization [2]. A longer life expectancy is accompanied with the increase in chronic diseases [3], susceptibility to infections [4], prevalence of cancer [5], and certain forms of degenerative diseases [6]. All these challenges put a great burden not only on individuals, but on the whole population and health system [7]. Therefore, it is crucial to adopt new strategies aimed at keeping the aging population healthy.

Several of the prominent challenges facing the efforts to achieve healthy aging are being linked to changes in the immune system [6, 8, 9]. More specifically, the natural process of aging is concomitant with immunosenescence; a degeneration of the immune system caused by thymic atrophy or involution [10]. As a result, the production of T-cells through thymopoiesis is compromised, and the output of newly developed naïve T-cells endowed with the capacity of effectively responding to new antigenic challenges decreases dramatically [11]. For example, accumulated extrinsic and intrinsic T-cell receptor (TCR) signaling defects in aging naïve T-cells are found to impede their response to new antigenic challenges [12]. The elucidation of such changes and defects related to thymic aging can therefore help conclude that the elderly's optimal responses to vaccines that may strongly rely on the development of strategies aimed at rejuvenating their weakened thinned-out T-cell repertoire. In addition, immunosenescence compromises the patients' immunocompetency and makes the body more prone to the development of different pathological conditions such as cancer [13]. Although most cancer types can be removed by surgery followed by radiation and/or chemotherapy, these multimodality therapies are primarily effective against localized tumors as opposed to spread metastases [14]. Cancer vaccination represents therefore, an appealing alternative due to its limited toxicity compared to chemo- or radiotherapies and the ability to stimulate the host's own immune system to seek and destroy metastatic cancer cells [15]. Unfortunately, however, vaccines are less effective at older age due to immunosenescence [16]. Thus, there is an urgent need for the development or improvement of immunotherapies to stimulate and rejuvenate the immune response in the elderly population.

The knowledge of the elements involved in the deterioration of thymic function can help identify potential approaches for protecting or rejuvenating the thymus. We will be summarizing in this chapter most of the concepts related to thymus aging and discuss the most promising developments aimed at stimulating thymic function as a mean to rejuvenate elders' immunity. In addition, we will highlight the experimental models along with the outcomes of our work on IL-21 as a thymo-stimulatory agent [17–19]. Optimizing and adopting such concept will strengthen multi-disciplinary collaborations and lead to innovative IL-21-based strategies directed against two key elderly-related health problems: (i) providing superior responsiveness to protective and therapeutic vaccines, and (ii) reducing the incidence and/or relapse of cancer or severe infections in this vulnerable population.

2. Background

2.1. The thymus

Functional immunity relies on the balance between innate immunity as a first responder in the presence of an external insult and the development of a rather specific adaptive immune response [20]. Primary lymphoid organs such as the bone marrow (BM), the fetal liver, and the thymus are the major sites for lymphopoiesis, whereby the common lymphoid progenitors (CLP) proliferate and complete their differentiation into mature effector B and T lymphocytes. The uniqueness of the thymus stems from it being the sole specialized organ where the microenvironment and the cellular content are perfectly orchestrated to support the maturation and development of T-cells [20]. This bilobed organ is located in the thoracic cavity between the heart and the sternum. Histologically, the thymus was believed to be mainly composed of a perivascular space (PVS) and a thymic epithelial space (TES) [21]. The latter is the main site for thymopoiesis and is subdivided into two anatomically and functionally distinct compartments: the cortex and the medulla [22]. These two compartments are connected by a cortico-medullary junction (CMJ), where the entry of lymphoid progenitors and the exit of mature thymocytes take place [23]. Furthermore, each of these two compartments is characterized by the presence of specific thymic epithelial cells (TECs), which guide and support thymocytes at their different differentiation and maturation stages [24]. Interestingly, the cortical (c-) and medullary (m) TECs have distinct expression profile for chemokines and cytokines, transcription factors and costimulatory molecules [25, 26]. As a result, cTECs and mTECs create a unique profile and microenvironment within the cortex and the medulla, respectively, which in turn affect the development and selection of thymocytes [25, 26]. Specifically, within the same compartment, cTECs and mTECs show heterogeneity in their markers and secretary profiles creating distinct microenvironments suitable for specific stages of thymopoiesis [26–28]. For example, cTECs express the thymoproteasome component β5t [29], Cathepsin L [30], in addition to thymus-specific serine protease, which facilitate the generation of major histocompatibility complex (MHC)-associated self-peptides required for positive selection [30, 31]. Moreover, it is being proposed that the crosstalk between thymocytes and different TECs is fundamental not only for supporting thymopoiesis but for maintaining the thymus homeostasis as well [24–26, 32]. Particularly, the interaction of developing thymocytes with certain TEC subsets sustains the regeneration of cTECs and mTECs [32–34].

Thymopoiesis or T-cell development starts with the settling of BM-derived early lymphocyte progenitors (ELP) in the thymus where they proliferate to give rise to early thymic progenitors (ETP) [35, 36]. Upon their interaction with cTECs, rapidly dividing ETPs undergo differentiation to the double-negative (DN) stage while initiating complex gene rearrangements to express a candidate TCR. At that stage, both CD4 and CD8 co-receptors are expressed and the resulting double-positive (DP) thymocyte undergoes positive selection; a process aimed at testing the rearrangement of a functional TCR. If successful, DP thymocytes receive a survival signal and continue their migration to the medulla [37]. Interaction of DP thymocytes with dendritic cells or mTECs is essential to sustain central tolerance as it deletes autoreactive clones leading finally to self-tolerant single-positive (SP) CD4 or CD8 naïve T-cells, which are determined by their restriction to MHCII or MHCI, respectively [38]. Newly developed recent thymic emigrants (RTEs—e.g., naïve CD4 or CD8 T cells) egress to the periphery where they complete their maturation and contribute to establishing a competent peripheral T-cell pool [39–41].

Despite its undisputed role in the development of T-cells, the thymus is commonly portrayed as a temporary organ due to its gradual decrease in size (progressive and irreversible loss of TES). This natural thymic atrophy/involution consequently results in gradual thymopoiesis decay.

2.2. Acute thymic atrophy

Through history, the thymus has been considered as a mysterious organ with no obvious function or purpose until 1961 [42, 43]. In the late 1800 and early 1900, scientists searching for the cause of unexplained sudden death of healthy babies and children labeled the thymus as the villain [44]. The origin of the confusion started as an attempt to understand and find a cure for what is known today as sudden infant death syndrome (SIDS). For instance, several scientists observed that suddenly dying babies had a much larger thymus in comparison to normal subjects. These observations led to the establishment of a medical condition known as status thymicolymphaticus [45–47]. As a result, thousands of infants received prophylactic irradiation to reduce the size of their thymus [45–47]. Interestingly, studies conducted in the mid-1930s on cadavers from ill or malnourished patients revealed that the thymus of these subjects was indeed smaller than those of healthy individuals of the same age [47–49]. These new findings not only acquitted the thymus from any role in SIDS, but also opened the door to better understand the physiology and role of the thymus [50]. Furthermore, subjects that have undergone 'precautious' irradiation in their younger age were later shown to exhibit higher thyroid malignancy and breast cancer risk [51, 52].

Nonchronic thymic atrophy is the first indication for the presence of a given insult(s). There are common morphological characteristics of acute thymic atrophy such as loss of cortical thickness due to sharp decline in cortical thymocytes. Longer exposure to insults leads to thinner, irregular, and lower cortical to medulla ratio, while the CMJ becomes less apparent. Conversely, insult(s) removal is usually sufficient to reverse thymic atrophy and allow the rebound of the cortex and its contents [53–55]. Such insults include a variety of physiological factors such as pregnancy, malnutrition/starvation, stress as well as pathological factors such as infections, corticosteroids, or immunosuppressive therapy [49, 55–58]. The exact mechanism(s) and pathways involved in acute thymic atrophy upon exposure to one or more of these conditions is poorly understood and may vary [55]. For instance, the pathophysiological stress from infections upregulates serum glucocorticoids (GC) secretion by the hypothalamus-pituitary adrenal axis and pro-inflammatory cytokines levels [59, 60]. Thymocytes are highly affected by changes in GC levels, which can promote DP thymocytes apoptosis through caspase 8 and caspase 9 activation resulting consequently in lower naïve T-cell output [61, 62]. On the other hand, medical interventions such as irradiation regimens coupled with chemotherapy induce death of thymocytes, DCs and TECs [63, 64]. These interventions also affect the stromal compartment leading to slower TEC renewal [65]. This explains the delay in immune reconstitution following preparative regimen for BM transplantation (BMT), which leaves the patient immunocompromised [66]. It is therefore essential to elucidate and understand the patho-physiological factors triggering thymic atrophy in order to design strategies aimed at reversing their effect.

2.3. Chronic thymic involution

The progressive age-dependant atrophy of the thymus starts at birth and reaches its peak during puberty before continuing at a stable rate throughout life [53, 67]. The two main factors forming the basis of thymic involution are: (i) defects in the pre-thymic hematopoietic progenitor pool or their migration to the thymus, and (ii) the loss of the stromal compartment [68]. The latter factor is particularly problematic as it implies reduction of cTECs [67], loss of tissue structure, and changes in the microenvironmental niche [69]. Consequently, the body's homeostatic compensatory system helps maintain the existing T-cell pool in the periphery through the expansion of mature T-cells [70, 71], which restricts the ability of aged subjects to benefit from new vaccines [71, 72]. Moreover, aged naïve T-cells are smaller and show defects in antigen recognition, antigen-induced activation and in their ability to proliferate [69, 73, 74]. Such changes in the properties of naïve T-cells and the microenvironment of the thymus can also affect the negative selection process, which in turn, potentiates the emergence of autoreactive or defective T-cells [75]. Besides, the increased longevity of naïve T-cells and the accompanying accumulation of reactive oxygen species lead to reduced TCR diversity and impair the function of effector and memory T cells in the periphery [76–78] translating into weakened immune responses to infections and immunotherapies such as vaccines [79].

Several factors have been proposed to explain and understand the circumstances taking part in the involution of the thymus. One of the earliest factors to be investigated was the change in the level of sex hormones, which peaks during puberty. GCs are believed to negatively affect both TECs and thymocytes mostly by inducing their apoptosis [80–82]. In fact, surgical or chemical castration of male mice was sufficient to restore atrophied thymi back to their normal size and function [83]. However, the decline in androgen levels with age is not accompanied with a concomitant reversal of thymic involution [21], suggesting that additional players are involved in chronic thymic atrophy. Some of these factors include: (i) changes in BM-derived T cell progenitors [84], (ii) alterations in the profile of circulating cytokines and factors such as the leukemia inhibitory factor, interleukin (IL)-6, Oncostatin M, and stem cell factor [73], (iii) a blockade in TCR rearrangement, decreased proliferation and increased apoptosis of ETPs [85, 86], and (iv) a shift towards the myeloid lineage in the elderly [87].

Altogether, the aging of the immune system is an ongoing complex process and is related to numerous clinical challenges. To properly tackle these challenges, it is imperative to adequately understand and elucidate the defects in the aging immune system response. Ultimately, acquired knowledge will guide the efforts for designing counteracting therapies to rejuvenate the immune system.

3. Strategies to stimulate intrathymic T-cell development

T-lymphopoiesis remains functional at older age albeit to a limited extent [88]. Thus, enhancing thymic function in aged hosts remains a promising therapeutic goal. The thymus lacks self-renewing progenitors and relies heavily on sustained seeding with BM-derived ETPs [35]. Unfortunately, ETP numbers decline markedly with age due to increased apoptosis rates as well as reduced proliferative capacities [84, 88]. This in turn negatively impacts the delicate thymic stromal compartment, which depends heavily on cross talk interactions with thymic progenitors for its sustained survival [89–91]. As the magnitude of thymic output correlates closely with the overall number of DN and DP thymocytes [92], pre-conditioning of aged subjects to enhance the development/recovery of these thymic subsets is critical to actively stimulate *de novo* intrathymic naïve T-cell development.

In an attempt to reverse/block this vicious thymic involution cycle, a variety of strategies including cytokines, growth factors, hormonal therapies, in addition to adoptive transfer of precursor T cells or castration have been tested and reviewed in the literature [93–96]. However, few of these interventions stoodout as the most propitious including: (i) sex-steroid ablation (SSA), (ii) keratinocyte growth factor (KGF), (iii) ghrelin (GRL), (iv) IL-7 as well as, and (v) IL-21.

3.1. SSA: to reverse aging-induced changes in the thymus

Steroid hormones elicit their effect in the body by interacting with their specific receptors, where they translocate to the nucleus and directly affect gene transcription [97, 98]. In the thymus, both thymocytes and TECs express receptors for steroid hormones and are affected by changes in their levels [99–101]. For example, testosterone induces DP thymocyte apoptosis through tumor necrosis factor-α upregulation, whereas estrogen binding to receptors expressed by DN thymocytes inhibits their proliferation [100, 102]. Due to the concurrent decline in the size of thymus around puberty, sex steroids are being widely studied as a main factor in thymus involution. For instance, studies designed to evaluate the effect of androgens on T-cell output showed that androgens do indeed have a strong effect on the output of T-cells [94, 101]. Specifically, the reported decline in thymic output is mediated mainly by the sensitivity of TECs to androgens [101–103]. Therefore, adopting a plan to promote thymic activity by antagonizing or preventing the effect of sex hormones on the thymus is perceived as both rational and reasonable [96]. SSA can indeed be achieved either surgically or chemically. Both approaches show positive impact on thymic function, cellularity, as well as architecture, and can significantly enhance thymopoiesis [96, 104]. For instance, castration conducted in different animal models resulted in an increase in thymic output, T-cell responses and helped sustain the size and function of the thymus [105–108]. More specifically, surgical castration in old mice led to rapid reversal of thymic atrophy and restoration of SP and DP thymocyte to comparable levels in young mice [107]. In addition, this approach increased T-cell responsiveness and facilitated the immune recovery of aged mice after chemotherapy and/or BMT [96, 109]. On the other hand, chemical SSA offers a transient and reversible effect by either targeting the upstream signaling events or by directly blocking steroid receptors [96, 110]. Therapeutic agents initially developed for prostate and uterine cancer such as the luteinizing hormone releasing hormone agonist or androgen receptor blocker increased both lymphoid and myeloid progenitors and accelerated thymic recovery after allogeneic BMT [102, 104]. Clinical studies on SSA have further shown increased repertoire diversity in the CD4 and CD8 T-cell populations [111]. Collectively, these preclinical data validated the idea that using SSA to enhance thymic function could lead to beneficial outcomes in both aged and immunocompromised patients [112].

Overall, SSA has a profound positive effect on the thymus. However, the long-term systemic effects of both surgical and chemical SSA are neither yet clear nor are the potential side effects. Therefore, more in depth investigations are required to assess the safety of SSA-based therapy. Moreover, the failure to restore thymic function by the natural decline in sex hormones levels in senile patients provides an evident that thymic involution is a complex process [21, 113]. Therefore, a more comprehensive approach involving different factors and mechanisms should be further investigated.

3.2. KGF: to guard the thymic epithelium

Also known as fibroblast growth factor 7, KGF is a member of the fibroblast growth factor family. It is mainly produced by mesenchymal cells [114, 115] and elects its activity through binding to its receptor fibroblast growth factor R2-IIIb (FgfR2-IIIb or KGFR) [116]. KGF has a notable effect on triggering the proliferation of epithelial cells [116]. Therefore, Palifermin®, a truncated form of KGF is clinically prescribed for patients undergoing stem cell replacement after high-dose chemotherapy and radiation [117]. Specially, Palifermin® is administered to reduce the incidence and duration of mucositis; an inflammation and ulceration of the mucous membranes lining the digestive tract [117].

In the thymus, both TECs and thymocytes produce KGF. However, only TECs express the KGFR, which explains the protective effect of KGF on thymic epithelium [116, 118]. Furthermore, studies conducted on KGFR-deficient mice support a major role for KGF in the thymus. Particularly, these deficient mice, which die at birth due to the absence of functional lungs, present with severely hypoplastic thymus [119]. In the same context, KGFR deficiency is found to be associated with significant defects in thymopoiesis accompanied by a decrease in thymic cellularity, in addition to signs of TEC proliferation blockade [119, 120]. Interestingly, the protective effect of KGF was evaluated in mouse models for allogeneic BMT where KGF pretreatment was found to enhance the immune development post-BMT by improving the function of thymic microenvironment [118]. In the same study, Min et al. reported that KGF pretreatment did improve thymopoiesis and positively affect the functional T-cells pool in the periphery [118].

As KGFR is expressed by several organs targeted by alloreactive T-cells, it was compelling to evaluate the effect of KGF in the setting of acute graft-versus-host disease (GVHD). In fact, current data have shown that KGF administration post-allogeneic BMT can: (i) facilitate alloengraftment [121], (ii) alleviate GVHD [122–124], (iii) protect epithelial cell in the gut mucosa while enhancing its repair [125], (iv) reduce the release of inflammatory cytokine [126], and (v) diminish allogeneic T-cell responses [121, 127]. A subsequent study by Berent-Maoz et al. further demonstrated that KGF not only protects TECs, but could also stimulate thymopoiesis indirectly by triggering them to secrete soluble factors [128]. Conversely, data from two separate phase I/II clinical trials conducted on patients undergoing allogeneic BMT revealed ameliorated mucositis with no significant improvements on the incidence and severity of acute GVHD, T-lymphopoiesis, infections, overall survival, or cancer relapse rates [129, 130]. As such, KGF can improve mucotoxicity following allogeneic BMT without exhibiting beneficial outcome on immune recovery in BMT patients.

3.3. GRL: increasing thymopoiesis appetite

The polypeptide hormone GRL, also named the hunger hormone, is normally released by specialized cells within the stomach into the circulation where it induces hunger and the release of growth hormone by stimulating the hypothalamus and the pituitary gland, respectively [131]. Moreover, GRL is known to play an important role in maintaining energy homeostasis [132, 133]. Interestingly, the GRL receptor (GRLR) is expressed by the pituitary gland, the central nervous system as well as on various immune cells including resting and activated T-cells [134]. Moreover, GRL deficiency in mice is associated with reduced thymopoiesis and increased thymic adiposity [135, 136]. Therefore, a potential role for GRL has been proposed in reversing age-related thymic involution [95]. In fact, scientists believe that GRL represents the next generation of hormonal-based rejuvenation therapy due to its astonishing effect on the aging thymus. Specifically, GRL administration to aged mice (14–22 months) resulted in improved TCR diversity, increased thymic cellularity (including cTECs, mTECs, and ETPs) and RTE output [134, 137]. In addition, Dixit et al. demonstrated that GRL administration inhibits adipogenesis and production of pro-inflammatory cytokines in the thymus; two important characteristics of thymic involution [134, 135, 138]. Despite these promising pleiotropic thymopoietic-stimulating effects, the progressive loss of GRLR expression with aging overshadows the potential use of GRL as a thymo-stimulatory therapy [134].

3.4. IL-7: a toolkit for thymus rejuvenation

Discovered in 1988 as a stimulator for murine B-cell progenitors, IL-7 is a member of the type-I-cytokine-family and signals through its heterodimer IL-7 receptor (IL-7R) [139]. Unlike other cytokines, IL-7 is mainly produced by nonhematopoietic cells [140]. Soon after its discovery, the profound and nonredundant effect of IL-7 on T-lymphopoiesis was underlined as it could: (i) enhance the expansion of naïve peripheral CD4 and CD8 SP T-cells [141], (ii) ameliorate the antiviral/antitumor activity of cytotoxic T-cells [142, 143], and (iii) support the survival/proliferation of CD8 memory T-cells [143–145]. These unique properties made IL-7 a central research topic in the context of viral infections, cancer therapies, and in T-cell reconstitution following BMT [140, 145]. However, the outstanding role of IL-7 as the cornerstone of T-lymphopoiesis in preclinical studies was challenged by contradicting observations made in higher species. For example, data from an autologous hematopoietic stem cell transplantation study in nonhuman primates [146] and from two IL-7 phase I clinical trials conducted on cancer patients failed to provide evidence for significant *de novo* thymopoiesis [147, 148]. This discrepancy with the results obtained from rodent models indicates the need to further elucidate the role of IL-7 in higher species. Nonetheless, IL-7 may still be clinically relevant as a potent adjuvant to stimulate T-cell effector functions in various illnesses.

3.5. IL21: a new thymostimulatory agent

IL-21 is the most recently identified member of the type-I-cytokine-family [149]. Produced mainly by activated CD4 T-cells [150], IL-21 was found to: (i) promote CD4 T-cell differentiation down the Th17 pathway [151], (ii) co-stimulate activated NK and CD8 lymphocytes [152], (iii) desensitize responding cells to the inhibitory effects of regulatory T-cells [150], and (iv) act as a switch for IgG production in B-cells [153]. In addition, similar to other type-I-cytokine-family members, IL-21 signals through its heterodimer IL-21 receptor (IL21-R), which is expressed by different hematopoietic cells such as, natural killers, B and T lymphocytes [154]. Moreover, we have recently showed that *in vitro* peptide-mediated TCR-engagement triggers potent cell surface expression of the IL-21R on DP thymocytes [18]. Although not required for hematopoiesis, BM progenitors expanded in response to IL-21 overexpression *in vivo* [155]. Likewise, IL-21 did not seem to be essential for thymopoiesis due to normal T-cell development in IL-21R$^{-/-}$ mice [149]. Moreover, IL-21 supplementation to positively selected DP thymocytes did not trigger their differentiation to CD8 SP T-cells as did IL-7 [156]. Instead, it led to DP thymocyte expansion and a 3–4-fold increase in the absolute number of *in vitro* differentiated CD8 T-cells when combined with other differentiation-inducing cytokines such as IL-4, IL-7, or IL-13 [157, 158]. These findings prompt further investigations using three pre-clinical settings with impaired thymopoiesis: (i) ensuing pharmacologically-induced thymic atrophy, (ii) in age-related thymic involution, and (iii) for T-cell reconstitution following allogeneic BMT.

So far, no treatments are available to protect against acute thymic atrophy or to accelerate thymic recovery under such circumstances, thereby leaving the immune system compromised. Of note, sepsis caused by bacterial infections can trigger GCs (corticosterone in rodents and cortisol in humans) secretion by the hypothalamus-pituitary adrenal axis. As a result, DP thymocytes undergo apoptosis due to their inability to express the anti-apoptotic molecule Bcl-2 [82]. Such acute thymosuppressive state can be easily replicated in mice via injection of the synthetic corticosteroid dexamethasone (DEX) [159]; hence, the utility of this model in evaluating the capacity of IL-21 in accelerating thymic recovery. One day following intraperitoneal (IP) injection of wild-type C57Bl/6 mice (4–6 months old) with PBS or DEX, IL-21R was found to be expressed on total or fractionated DN as well as CD4/CD8 SP thymocytes in both animal groups [18]. In contrast, DP thymocytes expressed the IL-21R exclusively following DEX injection [18]. To further ascertain these observations, a functional *in vitro* proliferation assay was conducted using sorted DN and DP subsets. Cell counts revealed that DN thymocytes derived from PBS or DEX-treated mice proliferated similarly in a dose-dependent manner in response to IL-21 [18]. In contrast, only positively selected (CD69$^+$) or DEX-derived DP thymocytes expanded in response to IL-21 [18]. To directly assess its effect on thymopoiesis *in vivo*, DEX-treated mice were IP-injected with IL-21 versus equivalent volume of PBS. Thymi derived from the IL-21 group displayed accelerated size and cellularity recovery compared to control DEX/PBS-injected animals. Analysis of the percentages obtained by flow-cytometry revealed that IL-21 treatments enhance the recovery of DP thymocytes. The response to IL-21 administration also culminated in a noticeable remodeling of the thymic architecture [18]. Furthermore, extrapolation of absolute numbers using flow-cytometry percentages revealed a significant increase in the DN and DP populations within the IL-21 group with no observed effects on the TEC compartment. This is not surprising as TECs do not express the IL-21R. To confirm that IL-21-mediated effects are due to proliferation as opposed to survival of thymic progenitors, DN and DP thymocytes were analyzed for their expression of the anti-apoptotic molecules Bcl-2 (expressed only in DN thymocytes) and Bcl-XL (expressed normally in both DN and DP thymocytes) [18]. Interestingly, none of these anti-apoptotic proteins were up-regulated in both populations supporting the notion that IL-21 administration leads to thymocyte expansion as opposed to their enhanced survival. Pertinent to this project, IL-21 administration did not skew the TCR repertoire diversity as T-cells derived from PBS, DEX/PBS-, or DEX/IL-21-treated mice displayed comparable TCRVβ distribution within intrathymic and peripheral CD4/CD8 SP T-cell populations. This point is particularly important as it clearly demonstrates that IL-21 administration under acute thymic atrophy does not lead to nonspecific mono- or oligoclonal T-cell proliferation. Finally, IL-21 signaling is characterized by the preferential activation of the JAK-STAT pathways [160]. Biochemical responsiveness of sorted thymic subsets in response to IL-21 stimulation *in vitro* clearly demonstrated phosphorylation of STAT1, STAT3, and STAT5 in all thymic subsets except for DP thymocytes; unless they were derived from DEX-treated mice. This was expected as nonpositively selected (CD69$^-$) or nonDEX-treated DP thymocytes do not express the IL-21R [18].

In contrast to acute thymic atrophy, chronic age-related involution is characterized by a gradual expansion of the PVS and reduction of the stromal compartment capable of supporting thymopoiesis [74]. To further explore the thymopoietic potential of IL-21 in such model, assessment of IL-21R expression with aging was conducted to discard the possibility that IL-21R expression declines progressively akin to the GRLR situation [134]. Analysis performed on total and fractionated thymocytes (DN, DP, and SPs) revealed that IL-21R expression profiles are comparable between young and aged mice (unpublished data). Next, wild type-aged C57Bl/6 mice (14–18 months old) received three IP injections of IL-21 prior to their analysis on the following day. This treatment led to increased thymic size, weight, and cellularity. Analysis of thymic subsets showed a drastic increase in the proportion of DN thymocytes as it reached 15% in contrast to 3% in PBS control mice. Likewise, a notable increase in the frequency of CD4 and CD8 SP T cells was also observed in the IL-21 group. This outcome was further reflected in the overall absolute number of DN, DP, and SP thymocytes. As one of the predominant deficiencies occurring with chronic thymic atrophy is decreased migration, proliferation, and survival of ETPs, we assessed the effect of IL-21 administration on the scarcity of this central progenitor population in the thymus. Flow-cytometry analysis of ETPs showed a significant increase in their frequencies within the IL-21 group suggesting preferential expansion of ETPs in response to IL-21 administration. As the aim of using IL-21 focuses on rejuvenating T-cell immunity of aged mice, T-cell output was analyzed weekly in PBS- vs. IL-21-treated aged mice over a total period of 3 weeks. Interestingly, aged mice undergoing IL-21 treatment showed distinctively improved T-cell responses [18]. In addition, while IL-21 administration had no impact on the absolute number of all peripheral lymphocytes, the frequency of peripheral GFP$^+$ T-cells increased substantially in comparison with control mice [18]. This can also explain the improved anti-tumoral response observed in IL-21-pre-conditionned aged mice prior to cancer vaccination [18]. The sum of these results serves as the basis to investigate the use of IL-21 as an elderly pre-conditioning therapy to rejuvenate immunity, and thus, improve T-cell responsiveness to vaccination.

The above findings provided the impetus to investigate the use of IL-21 in T-cell reconstitution post-BMT. Although this medical procedure is adopted as a life-saving procedure for specific malignant and non-malignant conditions [161], it remains unfortunately associated with dangerous life-threatening complications. The high morbidity and mortality associated with BMT persist as a major clinical problem associated with increased risks of: (i) relapse or development of secondary malignancies [162, 163], (ii) infection [162, 164, 165], and (iii) reduced responsiveness to vaccination [166]. The primary factors associated with these complications are the significant delay and improper reconstitution of T-cells post-BMT [165, 167] mostly due to the significant damage inflicted to TECs [168–171]. Therefore, the ability of IL-21 to improve *de novo* T-cell reconstitution post-BMT was investigated. For this purpose, T-cell-depleted RAG2p-GFP-derived BM cells (H2-K^b) were transplanted into irradiated LP/J (H2-K$^{b/c}$) recipient animals followed by IL-21 administration. In this experiment, GFP expression driven by the Rag2 promoter allows direct assessment of *de novo* peripheral T-cell reconstitution [172]. Analysis of transplanted mice revealed that IL-21: (i) accelerates lymphocyte reconstitution including T-cells (also observed in NOD scid gamma (NSG) mice receiving human IL-21 following cord-blood transplantation), (ii) slightly improved TECs recovery, (iii) regenerates a naïve peripheral T-cell pool with a diverse TCR repertoire, (iv) enhances regulatory B-cell development, and (v) protects from GHVD while retaining the graft-versus-tumor effect. Of note, IL-21 was originally believed to specifically affect the thymus [154]. In line with a previous study, however, BM analyses conducted on transplanted mice revealed increased counts of $Lin^-Sca1^+cKit^+$ (LSK) cells in IL-21-treated mice [17, 155]. This observation is particularly interesting as HSC/HSC progenitors capable of generating lineages of the hematopoietic system are enriched within the LSKs population [173].

4. Conclusion

So far, the use of IL-21 in the clinic remains limited to cancer immunotherapy (IL-21-based stimulation) or in the setting of autoimmune diseases (IL-21 inhibition). The latter clinical objective is particularly important as it raises major concerns related to the use of IL-21 in patients prone to develop autoimmune ailments. Therefore, additional studies are warranted to specifically address the clinical use of IL-21 in indications such as immunotherapies. Alternatively, all pre-clinical observations related to IL-21 strongly suggest that this cytokine could be exploited either as a monotherapy or in combination with other standards of care. This would ensure, at least in the context of thymopoiesis, improved *de novo* T-cell development in aged subjects as a mean to reverse thymic involution or post-BMT to accelerate the regeneration of naive T cells.

Acknowledgements

The work completed by the group of Dr. Rafei and summarized in this book chapter was supported by the Canadian Cancer Society (Innovation grant #2013-701623; the Louisa Gale Scholar), the Cole Foundation (Transition grant), the Cancer Research Society (Operating grant #18278 and Operating grant #21012) and by a generous donation from the Gagnon family. Jamilah Abusarah is a Vanier scholar. Moutih Rafei holds a Fonds de la Recherche en Santé du Québec Junior I and II Awards.

Author details

Jamilah Abusarah[1], Fatemeh Khodayarian[2], Yun Cui[2], Abed El-Hakim El-Kadiry[2,3] and Moutih Rafei[1,2,4*]

*Address all correspondence to: moutih.rafei.1@umontreal.ca

1 Department of Microbiology and Immunology, McGill University, Montreal, Canada

2 Department of Pharmacology and Physiology, Université de Montréal, Montreal, Canada

3 Department of Biochemistry, The Lebanese University, Beirut, Lebanon

4 Department of Microbiology, Infectious Diseases and Immunology, Université de Montréal, Montreal, Canada

References

[1] National Center for Health, S., Health, United States, in Health, United States, 2007: With Chartbook on Trends in the Health of Americans. 2007, National Center for Health Statistics (US): Hyattsville (MD)

[2] Organization, W.H. Ageing and health. 2015 [cited 2017 09-22]; Available from: http://www.who.int/mediacentre/factsheets/fs404/en/

[3] Denton FT, Spencer BG. Chronic health conditions: Changing prevalence in an aging population and some implications for the delivery of health care services. Canadian Journal on Aging. 2010;29(1):11-21

[4] Effros RB. Role of T lymphocyte replicative senescence in vaccine efficacy. Vaccine. 2007;25(4):599-604

[5] Peto J. Cancer epidemiology in the last century and the next decade. Nature. 2001;411(6835):390-395

[6] Deleidi M, Jaggle M, Rubino G. Immune aging, dysmetabolism, and inflammation in neurological diseases. Frontiers in Neuroscience. 2015;9:172

[7] Dorshkind K, Montecino-Rodriguez E, Signer RA. The ageing immune system: Is it ever too old to become young again? Nature Reviews. Immunology. 2009;9(1):57-62

[8] Pera A et al. Immunosenescence: Implications for response to infection and vaccination in older people. Maturitas. 2015;82(1):50-55

[9] Derhovanessian E et al. Immunity, ageing and cancer. Immunity & Ageing. 2008;5:11

[10] Hakim FT, Gress RE. Immunosenescence: Deficits in adaptive immunity in the elderly. Tissue Antigens. 2007;70(3):179-189

[11] Goronzy JJ et al. Naive T cell maintenance and function in human aging. Journal of Immunology. 2015;194(9):4073-4080

[12] Larbi A et al. Impact of age on T cell signaling: A general defect or specific alterations? Ageing Research Reviews. 2011;10(3):370-378

[13] Fulop T et al. Aging, immunity, and cancer. Discovery Medicine. 2011;11(61):537-550

[14] Urruticoechea A et al. Recent advances in cancer therapy: An overview. Current Pharmaceutical Design. 2010;16(1):3-10

[15] Nabel GJ. Designing tomorrow's vaccines. The New England Journal of Medicine. 2013;368(6):551-560

[16] Gravekamp C. The importance of the age factor in cancer vaccination at older age. Cancer Immunology, Immunotherapy. 2009;58(12):1969-1977

[17] Tormo A et al. Interleukin-21 promotes thymopoiesis recovery following hematopoietic stem cell transplantation. Journal of Hematology & Oncology. 2017;10(1):120

[18] Al-Chami E et al. Interleukin-21 administration to aged mice rejuvenates their peripheral T-cell pool by triggering de novo thymopoiesis. Aging Cell. 2016;**15**(2):349-360

[19] Al-Chami E et al. Therapeutic utility of the newly discovered properties of interleukin-21. Cytokine. 2016;**82**:33-37

[20] Murphy K et al. Janeway's Immunobiology. 7th ed. New York: Garland Science; 2008. xxi, 887 p

[21] Steinmann GG, Klaus B, MÜLler-Hermelink HK. The involution of the ageing human thymic epithelium is independent of puberty. Scandinavian Journal of Immunology. 1985;**22**(5):563-575

[22] Blackburn CC, Manley NR. Developing a new paradigm for thymus organogenesis. Nature Reviews. Immunology. 2004;**4**(4):278-289

[23] Haynes BF et al. The role of the thymus in immune reconstitution in aging, bone marrow transplantation, and HIV-1 infection. Annual Review of Immunology. 2000;**18**:529-560

[24] Pearse G. Normal structure, function and histology of the thymus. Toxicologic Pathology. 2006;**34**(5):504-514

[25] Griffith AV et al. Spatial mapping of thymic stromal microenvironments reveals unique features influencing T lymphoid differentiation. Immunity. 2009;**31**(6):999-1009

[26] Takahama Y et al. Generation of diversity in thymic epithelial cells. Nature Reviews. Immunology. 2017;**17**(5):295-305

[27] Takada K et al. Development and function of cortical thymic epithelial cells. Current Topics in Microbiology and Immunology. 2014;**373**:1-17

[28] Ohigashi I, Kozai M, Takahama Y. Development and developmental potential of cortical thymic epithelial cells. Immunological Reviews. 2016;**271**(1):10-22

[29] Ripen AM et al. Ontogeny of thymic cortical epithelial cells expressing the thymoproteasome subunit beta5t. European Journal of Immunology. 2011;**41**(5):1278-1287

[30] Nakagawa T et al. Cathepsin L: Critical role in Ii degradation and CD4 T cell selection in the thymus. Science. 1998;**280**(5362):450-453

[31] Gommeaux J et al. Thymus-specific serine protease regulates positive selection of a subset of CD4+ thymocytes. European Journal of Immunology. 2009;**39**(4):956-964

[32] Meireles C et al. Thymic crosstalk restrains the pool of cortical thymic epithelial cells with progenitor properties. European Journal of Immunology. 2017;**47**(6):958-969

[33] van Ewijk W et al. Stepwise development of thymic microenvironments in vivo is regulated by thymocyte subsets. Development. 2000;**127**(8):1583-1591

[34] Alves NL et al. Thymic epithelial cells: The multi-tasking framework of the T cell "cradle". Trends in Immunology. 2009;**30**(10):468-474

[35] Schwarz BA, Bhandoola A. Trafficking from the bone marrow to the thymus: A prerequisite for thymopoiesis. Immunological Reviews. 2006;**209**:47-57

[36] Lind EF et al. Mapping precursor movement through the postnatal thymus reveals specific microenvironments supporting defined stages of early lymphoid development. The Journal of Experimental Medicine. 2001;**194**(2):127-134

[37] Takada K et al. Development and function of cortical Thymic epithelial cells. In: Boehm T, Takahama Y, editors. Thymic Development and Selection of T Lymphocytes. Berlin, Heidelberg: Springer Berlin Heidelberg; 2014. pp. 1-17

[38] Anderson G et al. Mechanisms of thymus medulla development and function. In: Boehm T, Takahama Y, editors. Thymic Development and Selection of T Lymphocytes. Berlin, Heidelberg: Springer Berlin Heidelberg; 2014. pp. 19-47

[39] Miyasaka M et al. Characterization of lymphatic and venous emigrants from the thymus. Thymus. 1990;**16**(1):29-43

[40] Petrie HT. Cell migration and the control of post-natal T-cell lymphopoiesis in the thymus. Nature Reviews. Immunology. 2003;**3**(11):859-866

[41] Toro I, Olah I. Penetration of thymocytes into the blood circulation. Journal of Ultrastructure Research. 1967;**17**(5):439-451

[42] Miller JF. The discovery of thymus function and of thymus-derived lymphocytes. Immunological Reviews. 2002;**185**:7-14

[43] Lavini C. The thymus from antiquity to the present day: The history of a mysterious gland. In: Lavini C et al, editors. Thymus Gland Pathology: Clinical, Diagnostic, and Therapeutic Features. Milano: Springer Milan; 2008. pp. 1-12

[44] Solis-Cohen S. The therapeutic uses of the thymus gland. Journal of the American Medical Association. 1900;**XXXV**(7):421-424

[45] Rosenow EC 3rd, Hurley BT. Disorders of the thymus. A review. Archives of Internal Medicine. 1984;**144**(4):763–770

[46] Wilson DS. Status thymicolymphaticus; presentation and discussion of a case. Current Researches in Anesthesia & Analgesia. 1950;**29**(6):356-358

[47] Jacobs MT, Frush DP, Donnelly LF. The right place at the wrong time: Historical perspective of the relation of the thymus gland and pediatric radiology. Radiology. 1999; **210**(1):11-16

[48] RM S. Poverty's remains. The Sciences (NY Acad Sci). 1990;**31**(5):8-10

[49] Chandra RK. Nutritional deficiency and susceptibility to infection. Bulletin of the World Health Organization. 1979;**57**(2):167-177

[50] Ritterman JB. To Err is Human: Can American Medicine Learn from Past Mistakes? The Permanente Journal. 2017;**21**:16-181

[51] Duffy BJ Jr, Fitzgerald PJ. Thyroid cancer in childhood and adolescence; a report on 28 cases. Cancer. 1950;**3**(6):1018-1032

[52] Hildreth NG, Shore RE, Dvoretsky PM. The risk of breast cancer after irradiation of the thymus in infancy. The New England Journal of Medicine. 1989;**321**(19):1281-1284

[53] Elmore SA. Enhanced histopathology of the thymus. Toxicologic Pathology. 2006;**34**(5): 656-665

[54] Pearse G. Histopathology of the thymus. Toxicologic Pathology. 2006;**34**(5):515-547

[55] Gruver AL, Sempowski GD. Cytokines, leptin, and stress-induced thymic atrophy. Journal of Leukocyte Biology. 2008;**84**(4):915-923

[56] Choyke PL et al. Thymic atrophy and regrowth in response to chemotherapy: CT evaluation. AJR. American Journal of Roentgenology. 1987;**149**(2):269-272

[57] Clarke AG, Kendall MD. The thymus in pregnancy: The interplay of neural, endocrine and immune influences. Immunology Today. 1994;**15**(11):545-551

[58] Lynch HE et al. Thymic involution and immune reconstitution. Trends in Immunology. 2009;**30**(7):366-373

[59] de Meis J et al. Thymus atrophy and double-positive escape are common features in infectious diseases. Journal of Parasitology Research. 2012;**2012**:574020

[60] Billard M, Gruver A, Sempowski G. Acute stress-induced thymic atrophy is mediated by intrathymic inflammatory and wound healing responses (113.25). The Journal of Immunology. 2011;**186**(1 Supplement):113.25-113.25

[61] Tuckermann JP et al. Molecular mechanisms of glucocorticoids in the control of inflammation and lymphocyte apoptosis. Critical Reviews in Clinical Laboratory Sciences. 2005;**42**(1):71-104

[62] Distelhorst CW. Recent insights into the mechanism of glucocorticosteroid-induced apoptosis. Cell Death and Differentiation. 2002;**9**(1):6-19

[63] Perry GA, Jackson JD, Talmadge JE. Effects of a multidrug chemotherapy regimen on the thymus. Thymus. 1994;**23**(1):39-51

[64] Hakim FT et al. Constraints on CD4 recovery postchemotherapy in adults: Thymic insufficiency and apoptotic decline of expanded peripheral CD4 cells. Blood. 1997;**90**(9): 3789-3798

[65] Randle-Barrett ES, Boyd RL. Thymic microenvironment and lymphoid responses to sublethal irradiation. Developmental Immunology. 1995;**4**(2):101-116

[66] Daley JP et al. Retarded recovery of functional T cell frequencies in T cell-depleted bone marrow transplant recipients. Blood. 1987;**70**(4):960-964

[67] Hale LP. Histologic and molecular assessment of human thymus. Annals of Diagnostic Pathology. 2004;**8**(1):50-60

[68] Boehm T, Swann JB. Thymus involution and regeneration: Two sides of the same coin? Nature Reviews. Immunology. 2013;**13**(11):831-838

[69] Salam N et al. T cell ageing: Effects of age on development, survival & function. The Indian Journal of Medical Research. 2013;**138**(5):595-608

[70] Tanchot C, Rocha B. The peripheral T cell repertoire: Independent homeostatic regulation of virgin and activated CD8+ T cell pools. European Journal of Immunology. 1995; **25**(8):2127-2136

[71] Taub DD, Longo DL. Insights into thymic aging and regeneration. Immunological Reviews. 2005;**205**:72-93

[72] Gravekamp C, Chandra D. Aging and cancer vaccines. Critical Reviews in Oncogenesis. 2013;**18**(6):585-595

[73] Sempowski GD et al. Leukemia inhibitory factor, oncostatin M, IL-6, and stem cell factor mRNA expression in human thymus increases with age and is associated with thymic atrophy. Journal of Immunology. 2000;**164**(4):2180-2187

[74] Valiathan R, Ashman M, Asthana D. Effects of ageing on the immune system: Infants to elderly. Scandinavian Journal of Immunology. 2016;**83**(4):255-266

[75] Stacy S et al. Immunological memory and late onset autoimmunity. Mechanisms of Ageing and Development. 2002;**123**(8):975-985

[76] Jones SC et al. Impact of post-thymic cellular longevity on the development of age-associated CD4+ T cell defects. Journal of Immunology. 2008;**180**(7):4465-4475

[77] Eaton SM et al. Age-related defects in CD4 T cell cognate helper function lead to reductions in humoral responses. The Journal of Experimental Medicine. 2004;**200**(12):1613-1622

[78] Kay MM. Immunological aspects of aging: Early changes in thymic activity. Mechanisms of Ageing and Development. 1984;**28**(2–3):193-218

[79] Haynes L, Swain SL. Why aging T cells fail: Implications for vaccination. Immunity. 2006;**24**(6):663-666

[80] Ansar Ahmed S, Penhale WJ, Talal N. Sex hormones, immune responses, and autoimmune diseases. Mechanisms of sex hormone action. The American Journal of Pathology. 1985;**121**(3):531-551

[81] Ansar Ahmed S, Dauphinee MJ, Talal N. Effects of short-term administration of sex hormones on normal and autoimmune mice. Journal of Immunology. 1985;**134**(1):204-210

[82] Herold MJ, McPherson KG, Reichardt HM. Glucocorticoids in T cell apoptosis and function. Cellular and Molecular Life Sciences. 2006;**63**(1):60-72

[83] Fitzpatrick FT et al. Reappearance of thymus of ageing rats after orchidectomy. The Journal of Endocrinology. 1985;**106**(3):R17-R19

[84] Min H, Montecino-Rodriguez E, Dorshkind K. Reduction in the developmental potential of intrathymic T cell progenitors with age. Journal of Immunology. 2004;**173**(1):245-250

[85] Sharp A, Kukulansky T, Globerson A. In vitro analysis of age-related changes in the developmental potential of bone marrow thymocyte progenitors. European Journal of Immunology. 1990;**20**(12):2541-2546

[86] Eren R et al. Age-related changes in the capacity of bone marrow cells to differentiate in thymic organ cultures. Cellular Immunology. 1988;**112**(2):449-455

[87] Rossi DJ et al. Cell intrinsic alterations underlie hematopoietic stem cell aging. Proceedings of the National Academy of Sciences of the United States of America. 2005;**102**(26): 9194-9199

[88] Linton PJ, Dorshkind K. Age-related changes in lymphocyte development and function. Nature Immunology. 2004;**5**(2):133-139

[89] Li L et al. Cellular mechanism of thymic involution. Scandinavian Journal of Immunology. 2003;**57**(5):410-422

[90] Takahama Y. Journey through the thymus: Stromal guides for T-cell development and selection. Nature Reviews. Immunology. 2006;**6**(2):127-135

[91] Aw D, Silva AB, Palmer DB. Is thymocyte development functional in the aged? Aging (Albany NY). 2009;**1**(2):146-153

[92] Hale JS et al. Thymic output in aged mice. Proceedings of the National Academy of Sciences of the United States of America. 2006;**103**(22):8447-8452

[93] Henson SM, Pido-Lopez J, Aspinall R. Reversal of thymic atrophy. Experimental Gerontology. 2004;**39**(4):673-678

[94] Ventevogel MS, Sempowski GD. Thymic rejuvenation and aging. Current Opinion in Immunology. 2013;**25**(4):516-522

[95] Taub DD, Murphy WJ, Longo DL. Rejuvenation of the aging thymus: Growth hormone-mediated and ghrelin-mediated signaling pathways. Current Opinion in Pharmacology. 2010;**10**(4):408-424

[96] Velardi E, Dudakov JA, van den Brink MR. Sex steroid ablation: An immunoregenerative strategy for immunocompromised patients. Bone Marrow Transplantation. 2015;**50**(Suppl 2):S77-S81

[97] Evans RM. The steroid and thyroid hormone receptor superfamily. Science. 1988; **240**(4854):889-895

[98] Marcinkowska E, Wiedlocha A. Steroid signal transduction activated at the cell membrane: From plants to animals. Acta Biochimica Polonica. 2002;**49**(3):735-745

[99] Luster MI et al. Estrogen immunosuppression is regulated through estrogenic responses in the thymus. Journal of Immunology. 1984;**133**(1):110-116

[100] Zoller AL, Kersh GJ. Estrogen induces thymic atrophy by eliminating early thymic progenitors and inhibiting proliferation of beta-selected thymocytes. Journal of Immunology. 2006;**176**(12):7371-7378

[101] Olsen NJ et al. Androgen receptors in thymic epithelium modulate thymus size and thymocyte development. Endocrinology. 2001;**142**(3):1278-1283

[102] Lai KP et al. Targeting thymic epithelia AR enhances T-cell reconstitution and bone marrow transplant grafting efficacy. Molecular Endocrinology. 2013;**27**(1):25-37

[103] Olsen NJ, Kovacs WJ. Effects of androgens on T and B lymphocyte development. Immunologic Research. 2001;**23**(2–3):281-288

[104] Kompella UB et al. Luteinizing hormone-releasing hormone agonist and transferrin functionalizations enhance nanoparticle delivery in a novel bovine ex vivo eye model. Molecular Vision. 2006;**12**:1185-1198

[105] Goodall A. The post-natal changes in the thymus of guinea-pigs, and the effect of castration on thymus structure. The Journal of Physiology. 1905;**32**(2):191-198

[106] Henderson J. On the relationship of the thymus to the sexual organs: I. The influence of castration on the thymus. The Journal of Physiology. 1904;**31**(3–4):222-229

[107] Heng TS et al. Effects of castration on thymocyte development in two different models of thymic involution. Journal of Immunology. 2005;**175**(5):2982-2993

[108] Heng TS et al. Impact of sex steroid ablation on viral, tumour and vaccine responses in aged mice. PLoS One. 2012;**7**(8):e42677

[109] Goldberg GL et al. Enhanced immune reconstitution by sex steroid ablation following allogeneic hemopoietic stem cell transplantation. Journal of Immunology. 2007;**178**(11): 7473-7484

[110] Greenstein BD et al. Regeneration of the thymus in old male rats treated with a stable analogue of LHRH. The Journal of Endocrinology. 1987;**112**(3):345-350

[111] Sutherland JS et al. Activation of thymic regeneration in mice and humans following androgen blockade. Journal of Immunology. 2005;**175**(4):2741-2753

[112] van Poppel H, Nilsson S. Testosterone surge: Rationale for gonadotropin-releasing hormone blockers? Urology. 2008;**71**(6):1001-1006

[113] Griffith AV et al. Persistent degenerative changes in thymic organ function revealed by an inducible model of organ regrowth. Aging Cell. 2012;**11**(1):169-177

[114] Rubin JS et al. Keratinocyte growth factor as a cytokine that mediates mesenchymal-epithelial interaction. EXS. 1995;**74**:191-214

[115] Rubin JS et al. Purification and characterization of a newly identified growth factor specific for epithelial cells. Proceedings of the National Academy of Sciences of the United States of America. 1989;**86**(3):802-806

[116] Finch PW, Rubin JS. Keratinocyte growth factor expression and activity in cancer: Implications for use in patients with solid tumors. Journal of the National Cancer Institute. 2006;**98**(12):812-824

[117] Spielberger R et al. Palifermin for oral mucositis after intensive therapy for hematologic cancers. The New England Journal of Medicine. 2004;**351**(25):2590-2598

[118] Min D et al. Protection from thymic epithelial cell injury by keratinocyte growth factor: A new approach to improve thymic and peripheral T-cell reconstitution after bone marrow transplantation. Blood. 2002;**99**(12):4592-4600

[119] Revest JM et al. Development of the thymus requires signaling through the fibroblast growth factor receptor R2-IIIb. Journal of Immunology. 2001;**167**(4):1954-1961

[120] Zhang X et al. Receptor specificity of the fibroblast growth factor family. The complete mammalian FGF family. Journal of Biological Chemistry. 2006;**281**(23):15694-15700

[121] Bruinsma M et al. Keratinocyte growth factor improves allogeneic bone marrow engraftment through a CD4+Foxp3+ regulatory T cell-dependent mechanism. Journal of Immunology. 2009;**182**(12):7364-7369

[122] Rossi S et al. Keratinocyte growth factor preserves normal thymopoiesis and thymic microenvironment during experimental graft-versus-host disease. Blood. 2002;**100**(2): 682-691

[123] Panoskaltsis-Mortari A et al. Keratinocyte growth factor administered before conditioning ameliorates graft-versus-host disease after allogeneic bone marrow transplantation in mice. Blood. 1998;**92**(10):3960-3967

[124] Krijanovski OI et al. Keratinocyte growth factor separates graft-versus-leukemia effects from graft-versus-host disease. Blood. 1999;**94**(2):825-831

[125] Vanclee A et al. Keratinocyte growth factor ameliorates acute graft-versus-host disease in a novel nonmyeloablative haploidentical transplantation model. Bone Marrow Transplantation. 2005;**36**(10):907-915

[126] Hill GR, Ferrara JL. The primacy of the gastrointestinal tract as a target organ of acute graft-versus-host disease: Rationale for the use of cytokine shields in allogeneic bone marrow transplantation. Blood. 2000;**95**(9):2754-2759

[127] Panoskaltsis-Mortari A et al. Keratinocyte growth factor facilitates alloengraftment and ameliorates graft-versus-host disease in mice by a mechanism independent of repair of conditioning-induced tissue injury. Blood. 2000;**96**(13):4350-4356

[128] Berent-Maoz B et al. Fibroblast growth factor-7 partially reverses murine thymocyte progenitor aging by repression of Ink4a. Blood. 2012;**119**(24):5715-5721

[129] Filicko J, Lazarus HM, Flomenberg N. Mucosal injury in patients undergoing hematopoietic progenitor cell transplantation: New approaches to prophylaxis and treatment. Bone Marrow Transplantation. 2003;**31**(1):1-10

[130] Freytes CO et al. Phase I/II randomized trial evaluating the safety and clinical effects of repifermin administered to reduce mucositis in patients undergoing autologous hematopoietic stem cell transplantation. Clinical Cancer Research. 2004;**10**(24):8318-8324

[131] Inui A et al. Ghrelin, appetite, and gastric motility: The emerging role of the stomach as an endocrine organ. The FASEB Journal. 2004;**18**(3):439-456

[132] Cheng KC et al. The role of ghrelin in energy homeostasis and its potential clinical relevance (review). International Journal of Molecular Medicine. 2010;**26**(6):771-778

[133] De Vriese C, Delporte C. Influence of ghrelin on food intake and energy homeostasis. Current Opinion in Clinical Nutrition and Metabolic Care. 2007;**10**(5):615-619

[134] Dixit VD et al. Ghrelin promotes thymopoiesis during aging. The Journal of Clinical Investigation. 2007;**117**(10):2778-2790

[135] Youm YH et al. Deficient ghrelin receptor-mediated signaling compromises thymic stromal cell microenvironment by accelerating thymic adiposity. The Journal of Biological Chemistry. 2009;**284**(11):7068-7077

[136] Sun Y et al. Ghrelin stimulation of growth hormone release and appetite is mediated through the growth hormone secretagogue receptor. Proceedings of the National Academy of Sciences of the United States of America. 2004;**101**(13):4679-4684

[137] Dixit VD, Taub DD. Ghrelin and immunity: A young player in an old field. Experimental Gerontology. 2005;**40**(11):900-910

[138] Dixit VD et al. Ghrelin inhibits leptin- and activation-induced proinflammatory cytokine expression by human monocytes and T cells. The Journal of Clinical Investigation. 2004;**114**(1):57-66

[139] Namen AE et al. Stimulation of B-cell progenitors by cloned murine interleukin-7. Nature. 1988;**333**(6173):571-573

[140] Fry TJ, Mackall CL. Interleukin-7: From bench to clinic. Blood. 2002;**99**(11):3892-3904

[141] Seddon B, Zamoyska R. TCR and IL-7 receptor signals can operate independently or synergize to promote lymphopenia-induced expansion of naive T cells. Journal of Immunology. 2002;**169**(7):3752-3759

[142] Wiryana P et al. Augmentation of cell-mediated immunotherapy against herpes simplex virus by interleukins: Comparison of in vivo effects of IL-2 and IL-7 on adoptively transferred T cells. Vaccine. 1997;**15**(5):561-563

[143] Lynch DH, Namen AE, Miller RE. In vivo evaluation of the effects of interleukins 2, 4 and 7 on enhancing the immunotherapeutic efficacy of anti-tumor cytotoxic T lymphocytes. European Journal of Immunology. 1991;**21**(12):2977-2985

[144] Khaled AR, Durum SK. Lymphocide: Cytokines and the control of lymphoid homeostasis. Nature Reviews. Immunology. 2002;**2**(11):817-830

[145] Mackall CL, Fry TJ, Gress RE. Harnessing the biology of IL-7 for therapeutic application. Nature Reviews. Immunology. 2011;**11**(5):330-342

[146] Lu H et al. Interleukin-7 improves reconstitution of antiviral CD4 T cells. Clinical Immunology. 2005;**114**(1):30-41

[147] Rosenberg SA et al. IL-7 administration to humans leads to expansion of CD8+ and CD4+ cells but a relative decrease of CD4+ T-regulatory cells. Journal of Immunotherapy. 2006;**29**(3):313-319

[148] Sportes C et al. Administration of rhIL-7 in humans increases in vivo TCR repertoire diversity by preferential expansion of naive T cell subsets. The Journal of Experimental Medicine. 2008;**205**(7):1701-1714

[149] Spolski R, Leonard WJ. Interleukin-21: A double-edged sword with therapeutic potential. Nature Reviews. Drug Discovery. 2014;**13**(5):379-395

[150] Spolski R, Leonard WJ. Interleukin-21: Basic biology and implications for cancer and autoimmunity. Annual Review of Immunology. 2008;**26**:57-79

[151] Zhou L et al. IL-6 programs T(H)-17 cell differentiation by promoting sequential engagement of the IL-21 and IL-23 pathways. Nature Immunology. 2007;**8**(9):967-974

[152] Li Y, Bleakley M, Yee C. IL-21 influences the frequency, phenotype, and affinity of the antigen-specific CD8 T cell response. Journal of Immunology. 2005;**175**(4):2261-2269

[153] Ozaki K et al. A critical role for IL-21 in regulating immunoglobulin production. Science. 2002;**298**(5598):1630-1634

[154] Parrish-Novak J et al. Interleukin 21 and its receptor are involved in NK cell expansion and regulation of lymphocyte function. Nature. 2000;**408**(6808):57-63

[155] Ozaki K et al. Overexpression of interleukin 21 induces expansion of hematopoietic progenitor cells. International Journal of Hematology. 2006;**84**(3):224-230

[156] Zeng R et al. Synergy of IL-21 and IL-15 in regulating CD8+ T cell expansion and function. The Journal of Experimental Medicine. 2005;**201**(1):139-148

[157] Rafei M et al. Differential effects of gammac cytokines on postselection differentiation of CD8 thymocytes. Blood. 2013;**121**(1):107-117

[158] Rafei M et al. Development of a novel method for in vitro analysis of γc-cytokine effects on CD8 T cells positive selection (111.15). The Journal of Immunology. 2012;**188**(1 Supplement): 111.15-111.15

[159] Boersma W, Betel I, van der Westen G. Thymic regeneration after dexamethasone treatment as a model for subpopulation development. European Journal of Immunology. 1979; **9**(1):45-52

[160] Leonard WJ, Wan C-K. IL-21 Signaling in Immunity. F1000Research, 2016;**5**:p. F1000 Faculty Rev-224

[161] Sureda A et al. Indications for allo- and auto-SCT for haematological diseases, solid tumours and immune disorders: Current practice in Europe, 2015. Bone Marrow Transplantation. 2015;**50**(8):1037-1056

[162] Auletta JJ, Lazarus HM. Immune restoration following hematopoietic stem cell transplantation: An evolving target. Bone Marrow Transplantation. 2005;**35**(9):835-857

[163] Drobyski WR. Evolving strategies to address adverse transplant outcomes associated with T cell depletion. Journal of Hematotherapy & Stem Cell Research. 2000;**9**(3):327-337

[164] Baddley JW et al. Invasive mold infections in allogeneic bone marrow transplant recipients. Clinical Infectious Diseases. 2001;**32**(9):1319-1324

[165] Marr KA. Delayed opportunistic infections in hematopoietic stem cell transplantation patients: A surmountable challenge. Hematology. American Society of Hematology. Education Program. 2012;**2012**:265-270

[166] Avigan D, Pirofski LA, Lazarus HM. Vaccination against infectious disease following hematopoietic stem cell transplantation. Biology of Blood and Marrow Transplantation. 2001;**7**(3):171-183

[167] Takatsuka H et al. Complications after bone marrow transplantation are manifestations of systemic inflammatory response syndrome. Bone Marrow Transplantation. 2000; **26**(4):419-426

[168] Williams KM, Gress RE. Immune reconstitution and implications for immunotherapy following haematopoietic stem cell transplantation. Best Practice & Research. Clinical Haematology. 2008;**21**(3):579-596

[169] Chung B et al. Radiosensitivity of thymic interleukin-7 production and thymopoiesis after bone marrow transplantation. Blood. 2001;**98**(5):1601-1606

[170] Weinberg K et al. Factors affecting thymic function after allogeneic hematopoietic stem cell transplantation. Blood. 2001;**97**(5):1458-1466

[171] Banfi A et al. Bone marrow stromal damage after chemo/radiotherapy: Occurrence, consequences and possibilities of treatment. Leukemia & Lymphoma. 2001;**42**(5):863-870

[172] Monroe RJ et al. RAG2:GFP knockin mice reveal novel aspects of RAG2 expression in primary and peripheral lymphoid tissues. Immunity. 1999;**11**(2):201-212

[173] Okada S et al. Enrichment and characterization of murine hematopoietic stem cells that express c-kit molecule. Blood. 1991;**78**(7):1706-1712

9

Characteristics of Hearing in Elderly People

Maria Boboshko, Ekaterina Zhilinskaya and
Natalia Maltseva

Abstract

The authors define the term presbycusis and discuss the prevalence of hearing loss in elderly people, its etiology, and methods of diagnostics (anamnesis, evaluation of the peripheral and central parts of the hearing system). The authors emphasize that central auditory processing disorder (CAPD) significantly impairs speech perception in elderly people and makes difficult the rehabilitation of patients with presbycusis. The possibility of improving speech intelligibility by using auditory training is considered. Improved functioning of the central auditory pathways in hearing aid (HA) users with moderate to moderately severe chronic sensorineural hearing loss (SNHL) and symptoms of CAPD was shown after the auditory training with the use of two approaches ("bottom-up" and "top-down"). The algorithm of the auditory training was designed based on distinction between nonverbal and verbal stimuli of varying complexity, as well as tasks to improve memory (e.g., memorizing poetry). The benefits of the auditory training in the rehabilitation of HA users with low speech intelligibility were demonstrated. Improvement of speech intelligibility in elderly patients with SNHL proves that plasticity of the auditory regions of the brain remains possible throughout the life. Options of the presbycusis prophylaxis are summarized.

Keywords: presbycusis, central auditory processing disorder (CAPD), diagnosis, hearing aids, rehabilitation

1. Introduction

Presbycusis is a range of hearing disorders caused by an aging process (from Greek presbus "aged" and akousis "hearing"). It is one of the most common conditions affecting older and elderly adults. Zwaardemaker was the first who has used the term "presbycusis" in 1893.

Different authors sometimes interpret this term differently. Some researchers meant (imply under this term) age-related hearing disorders caused by involutional changes only in the cochlea, and others meant that changes involve all parts of the auditory system [1, 2]. Presbycusis is considered to be one of the forms of progressive SNHL, which is associated with age-related involutional changes of different parts of the hearing system and is presented by symmetric pure tone audiogram with flat loss toward high-frequency range (less steep than 20 dB/oct) [3]. Numerous studies are dedicated to anatomical and functional risk factors of the presbycusis [4–9]. The significance of the presbycusis problem is determined by its social importance, lack of data about its etiology, and need for clinical practice to accurately determine an impaired area of auditory system and to identify the presbycusis genesis.

2. Prevalence

Presbycusis is a rather common disorder. According to the World Health Organization (WHO), more than 5% of global population (about 328 millions of adults) suffers from any degree of hearing loss, while among people older than 65 years of age, the prevalence of hearing loss exceeds 30% [10].

Its prevalence increases every year that may be due to the general trend of increased life duration—much more adults reach aged (from 60 to 74 years old according to the WHO classification) and senile (75 years old and more) periods. The world population is rapidly aging. At the period between 2000 and 2050, the proportion of the world's population over 60 years will double from about 11 to 22%. The absolute number of people aged 60 years and over is expected to increase from 605 million to 2 billion over the same period. The number of people aged 80 years or older will have almost quadrupled between 2000 and 2050 to 395 million [11]. Approximately one in three people in the United States between the age of 65 and 74 has hearing loss, and nearly half of those older than 75 have difficulties in hearing. Having trouble hearing can make it hard to understand and follow a doctor's advice, respond to warnings, and hear phones, doorbells, and smoke alarms. Hearing loss can also make it hard to enjoy talking with family and friends, leading to feelings of isolation.

3. Etiology

There are many causes of age-related hearing loss. Most commonly, it not only arises from changes in the inner ear as we age but can also result from changes in the middle ear, or from multiple changes that occur along the nerve pathways directed toward the brain from the inner ear. Associated medical conditions and some medications may also exert an influence. Many factors can contribute to hearing loss as you get older. It can be difficult to distinguish age-related hearing loss and hearing impairment caused by other reasons, for example, noise-induced hearing loss. Noise-induced hearing loss is caused by long-term exposure to sounds that are either too loud or last too long. This kind of noise exposure can damage the sensory hair cells of the inner ear and is responsible for hearing loss. Once these hair cells are damaged, they do not grow back, and the ability to hear is diminished.

Conditions that are more common in older people, such as high blood pressure or diabetes, can contribute to hearing loss. Medications that are toxic to the sensory cells in our ears (e.g., some chemotherapy drugs) can also cause hearing loss. Aged and senile persons have a lot of biological and social risk factors of hearing disorder development. According to some authors [3], age-related hearing loss results from biological aging process of tissue elements in the auditory system and prolonged noise exposure. SNHL is considered to be a polyetiological process with partly unidentified factors of pathogenesis. There are more than 100 causes of SNHL: infections, intoxications, acoustic trauma, genetic factors, unfounded use of aminoglycoside antibiotics, irrational treatment of acute and chronic middle ear disorders, autoimmune diseases, and so on.

Genetic determinacy of the presbycusis cannot be excluded, and diseases acquired throughout the lifetime, hemorheological changes, and other factors can trigger or exacerbate age-related hearing loss. It is difficult to define that whether or not presbycusis depends on genetic factors because other factors potentially contributing to a hearing loss development are closely associated with an aging process. Nevertheless, some epidemiological studies argue in favor of genetic influence on age-related hearing loss development, especially in the case of metabolic type of the presbycusis, according to Schuknecht [12], which is caused by the atrophy of the stria vascularis [13, 5]. Genetic factor in the presbycusis origin is acknowledged by many authors [3, 14, 15]. This fact is confirmed in our study as well. Hearing heredity is revealed to be presented more often in patients with presbycusis. Identification of genes, underlying this pathology, could be extremely helpful for many people in our aging society.

Numerous genes are responsible for functioning of the auditory system, and some of them can contribute to the presbycusis development and determine a degree and time of onset of age-related hearing loss. However, neither of them is known to be the gene responsible for the presbycusis [4, 5]. The gene of age-related hearing loss was identified in mice. This gene encodes cadherin 23 (Cdh23) and is supposed to predispose an early onset of age-related hearing loss in mice [16]. A mutation of a similar gene in human Cdh23 can incline a susceptibility to the presbycusis [17]. However, genes of monogenic deafness detected in mice are doubtfully to be the same in human.

The last gene that was considered to be a cause of the presbycusis development in human was revealed in wide genome study of age-related hearing loss, which was conducted in the House Ear Institute, Gonda Research Center for Cell and Molecular Biology, USA. Specialists from Los Angeles collaborated with Translational Genomics Research Institute and University of Antwerp (Belgium). Friedman et al. [18] studied 3434 twins aged between 53 and 67 years old—patients of eight medical centers from six European countries. After hearing assessment using routine methods, 846 pairs with one normal hearing and one hearing impaired brother or sister have been selected. Family genomes were marked by numerous genetic markers, and the comparative analysis was performed. Scientists looked for spots with different nucleotides in the same genes. And a number of such genes were revealed. After applying an excluding method, only one potential gene was left in result. It was the gene GRM7 (metabotropic glutamate receptor type 7), which takes a part in a glutamate metabolism—it encodes one of the receptors of this amino acid. Glutamate (or glutamic acid) is one of the most important excitatory neurotransmitters of the mammal's neural system. It is involved in the functioning of different brain areas and provides neurotransmission. Studies performed on mice and humans showed that gene GRM7 is highly active in the hair cells and the spiral ganglion cells of the inner ear. The glutamate is very toxic in high concentration. Its overexciting results in neuron disruption. The excess amount of the glutamate is suspected to cause a hearing loss in twins as the study authors considered. Genetic analysis showed that after getting "protein casts" with certain variations in a gene GRM7 improperly operating glutamate receptor was obtained. It can result in the amino acid storage in the synaptic fissure and damage of the outer and the inner hair cells in the cochlea [18].

Of the genetic point of view, presbycusis is the complex pathology. In the case of monogenic disease, a simple mutation is enough to cause a clinical onset/presentation. This type of disease is easy to determine. Meanwhile, in the case of complex genetic disorder, the interaction between genetic and environmental factors is obligatory, and the only factor is not enough for disease manifestation. In the case of genetic predisposition, a degree of hearing loss and a duration of hearing impairment depend on the summary of ototoxic factors, environmental noise during lifetime, as well as acquired diseases, changes of the blood quilts, and other factors contributing to hearing loss progression [19]. These studies are considered to define various factors that influence on the presbycusis development and to determine a degree of hearing disorder in aged and senile periods. They are still significant and must result in developing standards for prognosticating and preventing this pathology.

Thus, all abovementioned endo- and exogenous factors that are presented throughout the lifetime are considered to contribute to hearing disorder development in aged and senile periods. Nevertheless, hearing impairment does not occur in everyone and is affected by harmful factors.

The role of the atherosclerosis in the age-related hearing loss development has been studied since the middle of the last century. Does the severity of the atherosclerosis and the cochlear dysfunction correlate? Some authors confirm the presence of this correlation between these pathologies [20, 21]. A close interrelation between hearing loss and high serum cholesterol levels is shown in several studies, and the dependence of hearing function on some other atherogenic lipid levels in the blood is found. Inverse correlation of high significance between high-density lipoproteins (HDL) level of the peripheral blood and hearing acuity at the frequency of 4 kHz was revealed [22]. Morphological and functional damages of the cochlea and their correlations with hyperlipidemia, atherosclerosis, and endothelial dysfunction in mice are described in studies of Guo et al. [23].

Increased blood viscosity is known to influence a SNHL development. Hildesheimer et al. examined a group of 33 patients with SNHL with unknown cause; a high-blood viscosity was revealed in many of them, which was interpreted by the authors as a possible etiologic factor of SNHL [24]. Other authors also suggest that rheological properties of the blood and characteristics of the red blood cells can be considered to be a SNHL development risk factor in all patients [25].

In the majority of countries, women are registered to have longer lifespan than men that is explained by the biological distinguishing features of the female organism and differences of the atherosclerosis development process in people of different sex [26]. This mismatch has to be taken into account in the study of presbycusis problem. Efimova performed a complex clinical and audiological examination of women of different ages: 28 elderly women with presbycusis (the main group) and 28 elderly women with normal hearing (the control group). The mean age of menopause onset was less in patients of the main group than in the control one by 3.2 ± 1.0 years, which argues in favor of the earlier aging of a whole organism including the auditory system in patients with presbycusis. The comparison of biochemical and clinical blood profiles of the main and control groups did not reveal any significant differences. The essential role of hyperlipidemia in the hearing loss progression was revealed by analysis of correlation between the lipid profile and hearing thresholds in the patients of the main group: the worse the lipid profile, the worse the hearing thresholds have been revealed [27].

Some authors mention that variable professions are not statistically associated with presbycusis [19]. However, Lopotko et al. noted that intellectuals in aged and senile periods have better hearing than people of the same age with diminished intellectual activity [3].

4. Diagnostics and clinical presentation of the presbycusis

In the middle of the last century, Schuknecht described four forms of the presbycusis: (1) sensory (caused by gradual degeneration of sensorineural elements of the inner ear); (2) neural (determined by the cell reduction in the spiral ganglion, auditory nerve fibers, and central auditory pathways); (3) metabolic (associated with atrophic changes in the stria vascularis); and (4) cochlear conductive or mechanical (associated with the process of the basal membrane thickening and loss of its elasticity). According to the author, all these forms manifest in increased tonal thresholds, and the neural one also manifests in the impaired speech intelligibility [12]. CAPD is shown to join the peripheral disorders with the aging process, so they also contribute to the presbycusis [28]. One of the keys of solving presbycusis problem is to define the proportion of peripheral and central disorders. Currently, potential role of disorders at all levels of the auditory system is taken into account, and it is realized as an integrated functional system and taken into consideration while understanding the age-related involutional hearing loss pathogenesis [29].

4.1. Asking about complaints and anamnesis

To diagnose an age-related hearing loss and to determine all risk factors of rapid hearing loss progression complete examination is necessary to begin with history taking (anamnesis), complex audiologic examination using instrumental methods in order to identify a level of a disorder, and finally, biochemical blood tests and general practitioner and neurologist consultations. All these examinations should be performed in the morning in kindly calm and comfortable conditions. The total duration of the audiological examination should not exceed 60 minutes to avoid the fatigue of a patient and loss of his attention.

While collecting a medical history, the absence of any reasons of hearing loss except of the age is noted. These patients do not have any serious somatic illnesses, middle ear pathology, professional noisy environment, or other determined reasons of the impaired hearing. Genetic factors and hearing loss duration should be taken into account while analyzing an anamnesis. Patients with presbycusis commonly cannot determine exactly the onset time of hearing loss due to its gradual progression. The early periods of hearing impairment often remain unnoticed for a patient; meanwhile, in this period, we expect the maximal effectiveness of a therapy. That is why annual prophylactic audiologic examinations of people older than 60 years of age seem to be rational.

4.2. Evaluation of the peripheral part of the hearing system

The first step of audiological examination is the peripheral part of the auditory system functioning evaluation. Subjective examination (pure tone audiometry for auditory threshold assessment, speech audiometry, and psychoacoustic tests for recruitment identification) and objective examination (tympanometry and acoustic reflex testing) must be listed as the main methods.

Symmetric binaural pure tone audiogram with flat loss toward high frequencies is typical for patients with presbycusis. Finding out the patient's age, we are able to suggest a degree of hearing loss properly for "normal" age-related hearing loss. Commonly, hearing in women with physiologic presbycusis gradually impairs and reaches the borderline with the mild hearing loss toward 60 years old [3, 27]. The mild hearing loss was detected in 67.9% of women with presbycusis from 60 to 74 years old. The loudness recruitment phenomenon is usually presented in the case of peripheral forms of SNHL. It is the sign of damaged neuroepithelial structures of the cochlea, especially the outer hair cells. Recruitment results in exaggeration of sound perception. Even though there is only a small increase in the noise level, sound may seem to be much louder, can be distorted, and cause a severe discomfort. The measurement of an uncomfortable loudness level is one of the simplest and most informative methods to detect recruitment [30, 31].

Speech audiometry is an issue of high significance among subjective methods of aged people examination. In cases of peripheral SNHL, especially with steeply sloping audiograms or the recruitment presence, the intelligibility usually does not exceed 70–80%. If monaural intelligibility in patient with mild or moderate hearing loss is less than 50%, CAPD can be suspected. It is due to the fact that pathology of central auditory pathways is responsible for the conversion, encoding, processing, and recognizing the speech signals. CAPD leads to the appearance of additional distortions caused by impaired binaural interaction, threshold and loudness adaptation, temporal analysis, and so on. Significantly reduced intelligibility with comparatively good tonal thresholds is defined as of tonal and speech hearing dissociation (phonemic regression); age-related hearing loss often manifests this way [27, 28, 31, 32].

Impedancemetry has to be included into the list of obligatory objective methods using patient's examination. Tympanometry evaluates the middle ear condition. Age-related alterations can be observed in both the sound conductive and receptive parts of the auditory system. Sometimes the external auditory canal narrows in the isthmus area and collapses, and the epithelial migration decreases. The eardrum in aged people thickens and dims. Lipid deposits appear around the handle of the malleus and the fibrous tympanic ring. In some cases, the eardrum does not thicken but on the contrary atrophies. Age-related changes of the middle ear matter a lot and manifest in ankylosis of the joints of auditory ossicles with the development of adhesions among the eardrum, auditory ossicles and promontorium, ossification of the circular ligament, and so on [3, 33]. However, as far as in the middle of the last century, an age-related hearing loss was already considered to be the primary consequence of degenerative alterations in sound perceptive part of the ear. The main disorders are suggested to take place in the cochlear membranes, which become rigid, thicken, and lose their form as aging progresses [29].

Changes of the spiral organ neuroepithelial elements play a leading role in the age-related hearing loss development. But according to some authors, isolated hair cell damage cannot be the only reason of selective high frequencies affected impairment in older age [34]. Involutional and dystrophic changes in the cochlea can be primary or secondary, and it is associated with blood vessel dysfunctions [35]. The reduced number of bipolar cells of the spiral ganglion can be named the steadiest morphologic manifestation of the cochlear aging in humans and animals. Changes of the auditory nerve also play a certain role in the presbycusis development [36].

4.3. The evaluation of central auditory pathways

CAPD occurs very often in elderly or senile persons, reaching up to 80% and contributing to the age-related hearing loss [28]. Stach et al. revealed CAPD symptoms in 70% of adults older than 60 years of age, and its occurrence increases with aging: adults of 50–54 years old had CAPD in 17% of cases; meanwhile, adults older than 80 years old had CAPD in 95% of cases [37]. According to Golovanova et al., 31% of elderly patients with normal hearing thresholds complained of hearing impairment, which was explained by the authors as impaired speech intelligibility caused by central auditory pathway dysfunction [38]. Australian investigators, Golding et al., also confirm the increase of CAPD occurrence associated with aging and note the prevalence of men with this pathology [39]. The difficulties of the occurrence of CAPD assessment are associated either with similarity of its symptoms with other pathologies (cognitive disorders, attention deficit, memory impairments, etc.) or with the absence of any standards of this disorder diagnostics.

Audiologic methods of evaluation of the central auditory pathway functioning are divided into behavioral (subjective) and objective. Subjective methods are subdivided into verbal and nonverbal methods. Advantages of speech tests are associated with their social significance, the ability to use them both for identifying a level of hearing pathology and for hearing aid fitting. The following speech tests are advised to use by the American work group on CAPD: (1) monaural low redundant; (2) dichotic; and (3) tests of binaural interaction [40]. The first group of tests is believed to be sensitive to auditory cortical disorders, the second is sensitive to dysfunctions of interhemisherical connections, the third is sensitive to the dysfunctions of higher auditory centers or, according to some authors, to brain stem damages [41].

Monaural low redundant speech tests evaluate the ability of the auditory system for auditory closure. There are tests with speech signals passed through filters with different cutoff frequencies, signals with distorted temporal characteristics, and tests with speech in background noise. In the tests mentioned above, the auditory closure (the ability to understand a whole word or phrase when a part of them is missing) or the ability to recognize signals in background noise are assessed [28, 32]. While testing with speech in background noise, a speech signal is presented simultaneously with a masker (different types of noise or speech signals). For Russian language, Prof. Lopotko [30] created the Russian speech audiometric express test, during which polysyllable words are presented in the background of different noises (white noise, noise of transport, etc.). In the last year, the matrix sentence test has become rather popular, aimed to evaluate phrases intelligibility in background noise, and approbated for many European languages including Russian (Russian matrix sentence test—RuMatrix) [42]. In the presence of CAPD, intelligibility of distorted speech or speech in background noise is very poor [28].

In the dichotic tests, different speech signals, for example, monosyllable words, are presented through headphones to each ear simultaneously. In these tests, binaural integration (when a patient is instructed to repeat all signals presented to both ears) and binaural separation (when a patient is instructed to repeat signals presented only to one ear) are assessed. Numerous studies proved that in conditions of competition between right and left auditory channels, an ear that is contralateral to a dominant in the processing of presented signal hemisphere dominates. The majority of people are right-handed, and the speech center is located mainly in the left hemisphere, so the right auditory channel is dominant. This phenomenon is called "the right ear effect." However, the right ear dominance occurs only in 80% of right-handed, while the speech center is located in the left hemisphere in 95% of right-handed people. The dominance of ipsilateral auditory pathways in some people may be the cause of this fact. A large number of dichotic test modifications were suggested as follows: dichotic digit test [43], dichotic sentence identification [44], and so on. Currently, dichotic tests are among the most popular methods to examine interhemispherical asymmetry in healthy people of different ages and in patients with central neural disorders [28, 30, 32].

In tests of binaural interaction, information is presented to each ear not simultaneously but consecutively: one part of a word/phrase is presented to one ear and the other part is presented to another. The ability of a listener to integrate signals and repeat correctly the whole income information is evaluated [41]. An example of the group tests is the audiometry with binaural alternating speech [45]. For English language, the following examples are CVC Fusion Test, during which consonants are presented to one ear, and vowels are presented to another; Spondee Binaural Fusion Test; and so on. [28].

Results of nonverbal CAPD tests are less influenced by linguistic knowledge of a patient, which is their advantage, but to perform many of them special not commercially manufactured equipment is often required [46]. One of the crucial methods of temporal processing evaluation is the Random Gap Detection Test (RGDT). It is sensitive to cortical pathologies, especially of the left hemisphere. During this test, signals (pure tones and broadband noise) with inserted pauses are presented through headphones at a comfortable loudness level [28, 47]. In the last year, indications to use subjective test diagnosing CAPD are expanded. Impaired speech intelligibility because of CAPD is proved to be one of the predictors of Alzheimer's disease and dementia. To detect at-risk groups, some authors suggest a number of behavioral tests with high sensitivity to subclinical cognitive deficit comparing to screening cognitive tests [48–50].

Electrophysiologic (objective) audiological tests include auditory evoked potentials (AEPs), which are divided into several types by localization of generators and time of onset: cochlear potentials (are registered during cochleography), short latency (brainstem) auditory evoked potentials, middle latency AEP, long latency (cortical) AEP, cognitive potentials, and mismatch negativity. At the moment, the unique criteria to include any type of AEP in the test battery for revealing CAPD do not exist.

Concluding the aforementioned, audiological methods for CAPD diagnosing can be divided into the following ways: speech tests (monaural low redundant, dichotic, and binaural interaction); tests assessing temporal processing; and electrophysiologic tests. Tests to perform should be chosen individually based on patient's complaints and anamnesis. Both verbal and nonverbal tests should be included. The mentioned division of the tests does not mean that tests from all groups must be used. The minimally necessary number of tests is recommended. The use of electrophysiologic tests is determined by the lack of possibility to use behavioral tests or the lack of their accuracy [40, 51]. Thus, the audiologic examination of a patient with presbycusis includes the following steps: (1) collection of complaints, anamnesis, and ENT examination; (2) pure tonal threshold audiometry in silence; (3) impedancemetry; and (4) CAPD tests.

A constant increase in number of elderly and senile people, greater demands on the quality of life in contemporary society, along with extended possibilities of audiological examination dictates a necessity to seek new approaches to the problem of age-related hearing loss. Identification of a pathology level in the auditory system with presbycusis matters a lot while choosing a further tactics of treatment and hearing aid fitting.

5. Rehabilitation of patients with presbycusis

Hearing aid fitting is the only possibility to compensate hearing loss in elderly people in the majority of cases. With the technical progress, hearing aids (HAs) become more complex devices satisfying users' needs, but often HAs do not meet high expectations placed upon it. There are data that only from 6 to 40% of patients with hearing loss use a HA [52, 53]. A number of patients completely satisfied by HA fitting results are about 20%; in elderly people, this percent is even lower, which is associated with several distinguishing features of this group [31, 54, 55]. Memory disorders, impaired ability to capture new information, cognitive disorders, impaired vision, degraded fine motor skills, and the presence of co-morbidities along with specific alterations of auditory perception are among these features [56]. Meanwhile, the refuse of patients with hearing loss to use HA is known to disturb socialization significantly, to lead to social isolation, to intensify cognitive disorders, to reduce the safety of vital activity, and to cause the essential deterioration of quality of life [57]. To evaluate the effectiveness of HA, the speech audiometry in free field is commonly used in adults along with questionnaires [58]. Together with medical parameters, social criteria (ability to practice their profession, to communicate in family without any difficulties, to lead an active social life, etc.) are evaluated. Despite high prevalence of hearing loss, few studies dedicated to the problem of HA effectiveness exist up to the moment [59].

Low effectiveness of HA fitting in elderly and senile patients was shown in our study by results of speech audiometry in 26 (21%) of 125 patients (percent of polysyllabic words intelligibility in quiet with HA was less than 70%). The analysis of results of an audiological examination allowed to conclude that the main factor reducing the effectiveness of HA use in elderly patients was the presence and a degree of CAPD. Studies of other authors confirm this fact [28, 60]. With alterations of the retrocochlear structures, which are often associated with presbycusis, a person's ability to process and differentiate temporal and spectral properties of acoustic signals is violated, especially in conditions of perceiving speech in background noise [60].

Modern HAs are known to solve the problems of peripheral hearing loss but often not the ones of impaired speech intelligibility. Besides, HAs providing enough loudness of speech signal do not always improve signal-to-noise ratio [61], which disturb good intelligibility. Up-to-date technologies, for example, systems of noise reduction and differentiation between speech and noise, directional microphones, and the presence of various listening programs in one HA, allow a user to increase speech intelligibility with HA [62]. According to our study to increase the effectiveness of HA use by elderly patients, a complex of measures is needed including special audiological examination, therapy aimed at correction of CAPD, and HA fitting with consideration of individual features of a patient's auditory system.

Revealing CAPD before HA fitting allows an audiologist to prescribe adequate treatment, to warn a patient and his relatives about possible difficulties with HA use, to avoid excessive expectations from HA use, and to plan rehabilitation after HA fitting. To diagnose CAPD, all tests mentioned above are not necessary to perform, although all of them are performed with the use of standard equipment and do not require a lot of time. A percent of monosyllabic words intelligibility in quiet at a comfortable loudness level could serve as an express criterion to prognosticate an effectiveness of HA. Our study showed that with this percent being less than 60%, the risk of poor results from HA fitting significantly increases. A long adaptation to HA, involving not only an audiologist but also a speech therapist and a psychologist, is often required. The aim of such work is the successful use of a HA, so that in older hearing impaired patients social contacts expand, communication skills improve, and self-esteem and overall quality of life increase [59, 60].

At the moment the designed pharmacological treatment of impaired speech intelligibility associated with CAPD does not exist, this problem is being actively studied [27, 63, 64]. Despite the absence of significant success in creation of drugs for restoring speech intelligibility, improving speech signal processing in central auditory pathways is possible, thanks to the auditory training that helps to correct CAPD.

The auditory training is the complex of acoustic settings and tasks created to activate the auditory and related systems and to cause positive changes of neuronal activity and related auditory behavior. Two types of the auditory training are distinguished: (1) "bottom-up" approach (from the periphery to central parts, due to incoming sound signal) includes the improved audibility and sound quality through the use of hearing aids, FM systems and optimization of room acoustics, as well as sessions with a speech therapist to correct temporal and frequency processing, sensitivity to changes of loudness, and so on [65] and (2) "top-down" approach (from central parts to periphery involving higher functions of central nervous system) combines linguistic, cognitive, and metacognitive strategies of learning and includes special complexes to train the auditory attention, memory, linguistic and cognitive functions, musical education, and learning foreign languages.

Generally, these two approaches complement each other and must be applied together to reach maximum positive results, to improve speech intelligibility, and to compensate a residuary deficit [65]. Concrete rehabilitation plan must be worked out individually depending on deficit profile of a patient, his lifestyle, social and communicative needs, presence of comorbidities,and so on. The concept of the auditory training as acoustic stimulation has been known a few centuries. At the end of 1990, first confirmations of the influence of auditory deprivation on the auditory system and proofs of plasticity inherent to the brain appeared, so the principles of the auditory training regained its development [65].

Results of last studies definitively proved that plasticity was inherent to the brain, that is, the ability of the cortex and lower levels to reorganize, and these modifications were manifested in behavioral changes [66, 67]. Although the plasticity of the brain is maximum in childhood, the ability to reorganize in the response to education persists in the mature CNS as well [68]. The auditory training leads to the reorganization of the cortex and brainstem and the increase in effectiveness of the synaptic transmission and in density of the neural tissue [66, 67, 69, 70]. Even rather peripheral processes such as determination of signal pitch can be altered during the training [71]. Cortical changes stimulated by the auditory training invade rather broad areas and remain for a long time [65]. They include four types of cortical reorganization: (1) expansion of maps, that is, areas responsible for a trained function; (2) a compensatory transmission of performing a trained function into another cortical area; (3) cross modal reorganization with involvement of cortical areas receiving an input signal from other sensory modalities; and (4) adaptation of homologous regions, that is, activation in areas in homologous regions of the contralateral hemisphere [72].

Studies on animal models proved that auditory stimulation induces alterations of inherent neural substrate. For example, tonotopic reorganization of the auditory cortex was revealed in monkeys after intensive frequency discrimination tasks. The cortical representation, the sharpness of tuning, and the latency of the response were greater for the behaviorally relevant frequencies of trained monkeys when compared to the same frequencies of control monkeys [65]. Experiences with rats showed that training-induced improvements occurred in the auditory cortex even if a damage (an impact of noise in the experiences) was done in childhood. This proves the possibility of improvement, or maybe restoration, of auditory function in adult rats even after a long time after the initial damage to the auditory cortex [73]. Another study on rats showed that the age-related deficit in distinguishing sound characteristics could also be restored by the intensive auditory training, and not only functional but also structural changes in the auditory cortex resulted from the training [74]. The human auditory system is assumed to undergo similar changes in conditions of sound stimulation.

Before studying patients with hearing loss, the auditory training was approbated in patients with normal hearing. Positive results of the training in persons with normal functioning of the auditory system (both peripheral and central) were shown: the improved results of behavioral and electrophysiological tests were observed after the auditory training to distinguish sound stimuli consonant-vowel [75, 76]. Significant improvement of speech intelligibility was observed in young persons with normal hearing after the auditory training with multiple tasks (speech in noise and accelerated speech) for 8 weeks. The improved results of behavioral tests were confirmed by the increased sharpness of frequency tuning, especially fundamental frequency and the second harmonic [77]. Thus, the auditory training causes the changes in neural activity and improves the neural impulses, which provide coding speech signals [78]. Positive changes of mismatch negativity and increased amplitudes of P_1, N_1, and P_2 were revealed after the training. N_1-P_2 potential is considered to reflect early cortical processes associated with stimulus decoding and speech detection. Mismatch negativity reflects later processes including distinguishing of speech stimuli changes. The activity of the superior temporal gyrus and planum polare of the right hemisphere on fMRI had decreased in patients after the auditory training, which reflected the enhanced effectiveness of functioning of these areas and improved ability of auditory perception [79]. Some authors consider these improvements to occur only for the trained sound stimulus, and others consider to spread on other stimuli [80]. Neurons of the auditory cortex, which are selectively tuned to some frequencies or amplitudes, were found to be able to change their selectivity after the behavioral auditory training [81].

It can be said that we form our brain as we form our muscles. These data open up new possibilities for rehabilitation, particularly the possibility to train patients' own central resources. Although the compensation of the peripheral deficit (the increased intensity of input signal) dominates in rehabilitation of elderly patients, the role of deficit-specific, intensive auditory training should not be underestimated.

In case of concurrent attention, deficits or intellectual disorder cognitive trainings are also used [65]. Compensatory training belongs to "top-down" approach designed to minimize the impact of auditory processing deficit that persists after the modification of acoustic environment and the auditory training. Compensatory training includes providing information on strategies of communication aimed at strengthening the use of central cognitive resources (linguistic strategies, memory, ability to problem solving, exercises on vocabulary expansion, development of active listening, and training of concentration). General recommendations on lifestyle such as preservation of intellectual activity, maintaining physical activity, minimizing chronic stress, and healthy nutrition are helpful to reduce a risk of development of cognitive deficit [28]. The effectiveness of the auditory training is explained by the fact that neuroplasticity is not completely lost with the aging process, though gradually decreases [60]. The central auditory system in elderly persons preserves its ability for training-induced alterations, which entails the possibility to improve speech intelligibility, especially in noisy environment [65].

In the laboratory of hearing and speech (Saint-Petersburg, Russia), a program of the auditory training with the use of two approaches "bottom-up" and "top-down" was evaluated. The aim of the study was to design an optimal algorithm of the auditory training for adults with SNHL and poor speech intelligibility in noise. Twenty-nine patients, HA users with moderate to moderately severe SNHL and symptoms of CAPD, including poor speech intelligibility in noise, underwent this auditory training: 12 young patients (from 19 to 22 years old) and 17 elderly and senile patients (from 60 to 83 years old). An examination before the training included the pure tonal audiometry, tests evaluating central auditory pathway functioning, and speech audiometry in free field by means of the Russian Matrix sentence test (RUMatrix). The auditory training was conducted individually by a speech therapist and included a distinction between nonverbal and verbal stimuli of varying complexity, as well as tasks to improve memory (e.g., memorizing poetry).

Nonverbal training included the following tasks: (1) to distinguish stimuli by pitch with sets of 18 musical sounds of different pitches. Increase of the stimulation complexity—from the set "1 instrument—1 pause" to the set "3 instruments—2 pauses"; (2) to detect silent pause between two sound signals—three variants (tonal signal, noise signal, and vowel); and (3) to evaluate rhythmic pattern of three signals (long or short).

Verbal training included the following tasks: (1) to distinguish a rhythmical pattern of 15 sequences of three syllables/phonemes (vowel "A," syllables "MA," and "PA") of different duration or intensity; (2) to perceive acoustically similar words and syllables with a choice of the correct word from 6 to 12 homonyms ("dom-tom" and "gora-kora"); (3) to distinguish syllables with a choice from two syllables ("ba-va" and "ga-da"), in more complex variants—from four to eight syllables; and (4) to perceive speech in background speech noise with identifying all vowels presented (eight variants in the set) or words (20 in the set), in the complex variant—to identify the predetermined signal by a speaker's voice (vowels or words spoken by male or female voice) in background speech of another speaker.

Classes lasted for 60 minutes and were carried out twice a week. The course of the auditory training took 8–10 weeks. A percent of correct answers and time of reaction were compared in the beginning and at the end of the training when analyzing the results. After the training, the significantly improved ($p < 0.01$) perception of verbal and nonverbal signals was revealed both in young and elderly HA users (a percent of correct answers increased by $24.4 \pm 5.2\%$ and $15.3 \pm 6.4\%$ accordingly; decrease of time of reaction in the range from 0.4 to 1.6 seconds). Besides, RuMatrix in quiet and noise, performed with hearing aids in free field before and after the training, was used to assess the effectiveness of the training. Signals were presented from a loudspeaker located at an angle of 0° relatively to a patient's head (frontally) on 1 m distance. The effectiveness of the training was evaluated by calculating the difference between first and last results. Significantly improved speech intelligibility ($p < 0.05$) both in quiet and in noise was revealed after the training. According to the results of the RuMatrix in quiet, the intensity, at which 50% sentence intelligibility level was achieved, was 44.5 ± 11.4 dB SPL before the training and 43.5 ± 12.5 dB SPL after the training. The difference of the results is significant ($p < 0.05$). According to the results of the RuMatrix in noise, signal-to-noise ratio, at which 50% sentence intelligibility level was achieved, was 1.5 ± 5.5 dB SNR before the training and -0.33 ± 5.5 dB SNR after the training. The difference between the results is also significant ($p < 0.05$).

Based on the study, improved functioning of the central auditory pathway was shown after the auditory training, so it is appropriate to include it in the rehabilitation of HA users with low speech intelligibility in noise. The following algorithm of the auditory training was designed: (1) the distinction between nonverbal signals with changes in their duration, frequency, and intensity; (2) recognition of speech stimuli of varying complexity, including speech in background noise; and (3) tasks to improve memory. An important aspect of training was a gradual complication of tasks in the process of each session and from lesson to lesson [82].

Improvement of speech intelligibility in elderly patients with SNHL proves that plasticity of the auditory regions of the brain remains possible throughout the life. Stimulation-induced plastic changes in the central auditory pathways were proved by other researchers too [28]. According to some researchers, the decreased latency time and decreased variability between peaks of auditory evoked potentials were revealed in elderly after the course of the auditory training and accompanied by improved speech intelligibility in noise and short-term memory [28]. As shown by our study, improvement of neuronal functioning can be proven by the results of behavioral tests, which were also noted by a number of foreign authors [77].

Neuronal changes depend on the activity of training and amount of stimulation, and the sooner the stimulation begins after the detection of impaired intelligibility, the best results can be expected, however, to start training is never too late [65].

One of the basic principles of the auditory training must be concordance between the used material and age and linguistic skills of a patient. If the materials and tasks exceed the cognitive and linguistic skills of a patient, he/she will have no interest in the training, and there will be no progress. In contrast, material for adult training should not be childish and too simplistic. Motivation is also one of decisive factors in the training success. To increase the motivation, patients should understand the principles and the theory of action of the auditory training.

The use of a various tasks, the variation of a stimulus in the auditory training helps to maintain a patient's attention, increases motivation and makes the training more efficient. The complexity of tasks during the training can vary automatically: as soon as a patient reaches the predetermined level, the task becomes more difficult. Careful monitoring of a patient's progress is important. For each patient, an individual profile of functional deficit, which reflects the processing of information in the central auditory pathways, cognitive and language skills, should be developed, and an emphasis on training deficit skills should be done while planning the rehabilitation.

6. Possibilities of the presbycusis prophylaxis

At the moment, the presbycusis is irreversible; therefore, the prevention of age-related hearing loss must be paid attention to. First of all, it is necessary to educate the population about harmful factors affecting hearing throughout the life, such as ototoxic drugs, noise exposure, vibrations, and others. Audiological care in case of SNHL should be aimed at the enhancement of nonspecific resistance of excitable structures of the auditory analyzer to general pathological damaging factors—tissue hypoxia, oxidative stress, and extinction of the action of endogenous neurotrophic factors [30, 83].

Due to the fact that with age-related hearing loss, it is impossible to obtain gains in tonal hearing, and special emphasis is done on means of improving the auditory attention (the functions of the central auditory pathways), which allows to compensate for the lack of auditory acuity and enhance the efficacy of the hearing aid. If CAPD causing poor speech intelligibility is detected, the auditory training is appropriate.

7. Conclusion

Constantly growing number of aged and senile people, increasing demands to the quality of life in modern conditions, as well as enhancing of audiological examination opportunities requires the necessity of searching the new approaches to the problem of age-related hearing impairment.

Presbycusis does not develop in all people. Genetic mechanisms are considered to be the crucial cause of age-related hearing loss development. Different diseases acquired throughout the lifetime and other factors can contribute to hearing loss progression in the case of hereditary predisposition to presbycusis.

Assessment of pathology level in the auditory system in patients with presbycusis is essential during the choice of further treatment and hearing rehabilitation. Therefore, it is necessary to use various audiologic methods during elderly people examination, including tests to evaluate the central auditory pathways. Elderly patients often suffer from impaired speech intelligibility, especially in background noise. This is one of the central auditory processing disorder symptoms. Currently, there are no data about significant achievements in development of drugs, improving speech intelligibility. According to research on brain neuroplasticity, specially designed auditory training programs have been shown to be able to refine speech signals' processing in central auditory pathways even in aged people. Auditory training designed with consideration of the individual features of auditory deficit should be included into rehabilitation programs of aged people with speech intelligibility disorders.

Conflict of interest

There are no conflicts of interests.

Author details

Maria Boboshko*, Ekaterina Zhilinskaya and Natalia Maltseva

*Address all correspondence to: boboshkom@gmail.com

Laboratory of Hearing and Speech of Academician I.P. Pavlov First St. Petersburg State Medical University, St. Petersburg, Russia

References

[1] Glorig A, Davis H. Age, noise and hearing loss. The Annals of Otology, Rhinology, and Laryngology. 1961;**70**:556-571. DOI: 10.1177/000348946107000219

[2] Hinchliffe R. The anatomical locus of presbyacusis. The Journal of Speech and Hearing Disorders. 1962;**27**(4):301-310. DOI: 10.1044/jshd.2704.301

[3] Lopotko A, Plouzhnikov M, Atamouradov M. Presbyacusis. Ashkhabad: Ylym; 1986. p. 300 [In Russian]

[4] Jennings C, Jones N. Presbyacusis. The Journal of Laryngology and Otology. 2001;**115**:171-178. DOI: 10.1258/0022215011906984

[5] Willott JF, Chisolm TH, Lister JJ. Modulation of presbycusis: Current status and future directions. Audiology & Neuro-Otology. 2001;**6**:231-249. DOI: 10.1159/000046129

[6] Seidman M, Ahmad N, Bai U. Molecular mechanisms of age-related hearing loss. Ageing Research Reviews. 2002;**1**:331-343. DOI: 10.1016/S1568-1637(02)00004-1

[7] Gratton M, Vazquez A. Age-related hearing loss: Current research. Current Opinion in Otolaryngology & Head and Neck Surgery. 2003;**11**(5):367-371. DOI: 10.1097/00020840-200310000-00010

[8] Ohlemiller K. Age-related hearing loss: The status of Schuknecht's typology. Current Opinion in Otolaryngology & Head and Neck Surgery. 2004;**12**(5):439-443. DOI: 10.1097/01.moo.0000134450.99615.22

[9] Pickles O. Mutation in mitochondrial DNA as a cause of presbyacusis. Audiology & Neuro-Otology. 2004;**9**(1):23-33. DOI: 10.1159/000074184

[10] World Health Organization. Deafness and hearing loss. Fact sheet N 300. [Internet]. 2015. Available from: http://www.who.int/mediacentre/factsheets/fs300/en/ [Accessed: 2018.01.20]

[11] World Health Organization. Facts about ageing. [Internet]. 2014. Available from: http://www.who.int/ageing/about/facts/en/ [Accessed: 2018.01.20]

[12] Schuknecht H. Further observations on the pathology of presbycusis. Archives of Otolaryngology. 1964;**80**:369. DOI: 10.1001/archotol.1964.00750040381003

[13] Gates G, Couropmitree N, Myers R. Genetic associations in age-related hearing thresholds. Archives of Otolaryngology – Head & Neck Surgery. 1999;**125**(6):654-659. DOI: 10.1001/archotol.125.6.654

[14] Rodriguez-Paris J, Ballay J, Inserra M, Stidham K, Colen T, Roberson J, Gardner P, Schrijver I. Genetic analysis of presbycusis by arrayed primer extension. Annals of Clinical and Laboratory Science. 2008;**38**(4):352-360. DOI: 10.1016/j.otohns.2007.06.277

[15] Raynor L, Pankow J, Miller M, et al. Familial aggregation of age-related hearing loss in an epidemiological study of older adults. American Journal of Audiology. 2009;**18**(2):114-118. DOI: 10.1044/1059-0889(2009/08-0035)

[16] Noben-Trauth K, Zheng Q, Johnson K. Association of cadherin 23 with polygenic inheritance and genetic modification of sensorineural hearing loss. Nature Genetics. 2003;**35**(1):21-23. DOI: 10.1038/ng1226

[17] Siemens J, Lillo C, Dumont R, et al. Cadherin 23 is a component of the tip link in hair-cell stereocilia. Nature. 2004;**428**(6986):950-955. DOI: 10.1038/nature02483

[18] Friedman R, Van Laer L, Huentelman M, et al. GRM7 variants confer susceptibility to age-related hearing impairment. Human Molecular Genetics. 2009;**18**(4):785-796. DOI: 10.1093/hmg/ddn402

[19] Sousa C, Larsson E, Ching T. Risk factors for presbycusis in a socio-economic mid-dle-class sample. Brazilian Journal of Otorhinolaryngology. 2009;**75**(4):530-536. DOI: 10.1590/s1808-86942009000400011

[20] Syka J, Ouda L, Nachtigal P, et al. Atorvastatin slows down the deterioration of inner ear function with age in mice. Neuroscience Letters. 2007;**411**(2):112-116. DOI: 10.1016/j. neulet.2006.10.032

[21] Park S, Schwartz J, Wright R, Spiro A, Vokonas P, Hu H. Atherosclerosis-related genes, low-level lead exposure and age-related hearing loss: The normative aging study. Epidemiology. 2009;**20**(6):S211. DOI: 10.1097/01.ede.0000362708.72273.23

[22] Erdem T, Ozturan O, Miman M, Ozturk C, Karatas E. Exploration of the early audi-tory effects of hyperlipoproteinemia and diabetes mellitus using otoacoustic emis-sions. European Archives of Oto-Rhino-Laryngology. 2003;**260**(2):62-66. DOI: 10.1007/ s00405-002-0519-1

[23] Guo Y, Zhang C, Du X, Nair U, Yoo T. Morphological and functional alterations of the cochlea in apolipoprotein E gene deficient mice. Hearing Research. 2005;**208**(1-2):54-67. DOI: 10.1016/j.heares.2005.05.010

[24] Hildesheimer M, Bloch F, Muchnik C, Rubinstein M. Blood viscosity and sensorineural hearing loss. Archives of Otolaryngology – Head & Neck Surgery. 1990;**116**(7):820-823. DOI: 10.1001/archotol.1990.01870070068012

[25] Gatehouse S, Lowe G. Whole blood viscosity and red cell filterability as factors in sen-sorineural hearing impairment in the elderly. Acta Oto-Laryngologica. 1991;**111**(476):37-43. DOI: 10.3109/00016489109127254

[26] Ohhira S, Miyahara H, Fujita N, et al. Influence of hyperlipidemia and smoking on age-related changes in caloric response and pure-tone hearing. Acta Oto-Laryngologica. 1998;**118**(1):40-45. DOI: 10.1080/00016489850183737

[27] Boboshko M, Efimova M. Aspects of topical diagnostics of hearing disorders by presbya-cusis. Russian Otorhinolaryngology. 2011;**52**(3):23-26 [In Russian]

[28] Musiek F, Chermak G. Handbook of Central Auditory Processing Disorder. Vol. 1. Auditory Neuroscience and Diagnosis. 2nd ed. San Diego: Plural Publishing; 2014. p. 745

[29] Fetoni A, Picciotti P, Paludetti G, Troiani D. Pathogenesis of presbycusis in animal models: A review. Experimental Gerontology. 2011;**46**(6):413-425. DOI: 10.1016/j.exger. 2010.12.003

[30] Lopotko A. Practical Guidance on Audiology. St. Petersburg: Dialog; 2008. p. 273 [In Russian]

[31] Tavartkiladze G. Handbook on Clinical Audiology. Moskow: Meditsina; 2013. p. 676 [In Russian]

[32] Boboshko M. Speech Audiometry. St. Petersburg: SPbGMU; 2012. p. 64 [In Russian]

[33] Gaihede M, Koefoed-Nielsen B. Mechanics of the middle ear system: Age-related changes in viscoelastic properties. Audiology and Neurotology. 2000;**5**(2):53-58. DOI: 10.1159/000013867

[34] Fu B, Le Prell C, Simmons D, et al. Age-related synaptic loss of the medial olivoco-chlear efferent innervation. Molecular Neurodegeneration. 2010;**5**(1):53. DOI: 10.1186/1750-1326-5-53

[35] Nakashima T, Naganawa S, Sone M, et al. Disorders of cochlear blood flow. Brain Research Reviews. 2003;**43**(10):17-28. DOI: 10.1016/s0165-0173(03)00189-9

[36] Bao J, Ohlemiller K. Age-related loss of spiral ganglion neurons. Hearing Research. 2010;**264**(1-2):93-97. DOI: 10.1016/j.heares.2009.10.009

[37] Stach B, Spretnjak M, Jerger J. The prevalence of central presbyacusis in a clinical popu-lation. Journal of the American Academy of Audiology. 1990;**1**:109-115

[38] Golovanova L, Boboshko M, Takhtaeva N, Zhilinskaya E. Hearing disorders in patients of older age groups. Advances in Gerontology. 2014;**27**(2):376-381 [In Russian]

[39] Golding M, Carter N, Mitchell P, Hood L. Prevalence of central auditory processing (CAP) abnormality in an older Australian population: The Blue Mountains hearing study. Journal of the American Academy of Audiology. 2004;**15**(9):633-642. DOI: 10.3766/jaaa.15.9.4

[40] Diagnosis, Treatment and Management of Children and Adults with Central Auditory Processing Disorder. Clinical Practice Guidelines. American Academy of Audiology. [Internet]. 2010. Available from: http://audiology-web.s3.amazonaws.com/migrated/CAPD%20Guidelines%208-2010.pdf_539952af956c79.73897613.pdf [Accessed: 2018.01.20]

[41] Bellis T. Assessment and Management of Central Auditory Processing Disorders in the Educational Setting: From Science to Practice. 2nd ed. Thomson: Delmar Learning; 2003. p. 533

[42] Kollmeier B, Warzybok A, Hochmuth S, Zokoll M, Uslar V, Brand T, Wagener K. The multi-lingual matrix test: Principles, applications, and comparison across languages – A review. International Journal of Audiology. 2015;**54**(2):3-16. DOI: 10.3109/14992027.2015.1020971

[43] Musiek F. Assessment of central auditory dysfunction: The dichotic digit test revisited. Ear and Hearing. 1983;**4**(2):79-83. DOI: 10.1097/00003446-198303000-00002

[44] Fifer R, Jerger J, Berlin C, Tobey E, Campbell J. Development of a dichotic sentence identification test for hearing impaired adults. Ear and Hearing. 1983;**4**:300-305. DOI: 10.1097/00003446-198311000-00007

[45] Ryndina A, Berdnikova I, Tsvyleva I. Alternating signal speech audiometry in the diag-nosis of central lesions of the acoustic analyzer. Vestnik Otorinolaringologii. 1998;**6**:13-14 [In Russian]

[46] Boboshko M, Garbaruk E, Maltceva N. Diagnostic of Central Auditory Disorders. St-Petersburg: PSPbGMU; 2013. p. 48 [In Russian]

[47] Random Gap Detection Test [Internet]. 2000. Available from: https://auditecincorporated.wordpress.com/2015/09/28/random-gap-detection-test-rgdt/ [Accessed: 2018-01-20]

[48] Gates G, Anderson M, McCurry S, Feeney M, Larson E. Central auditory dysfunction as a harbinger of Alzheimer's dementia. Archives of Otolaryngology–Head & Neck Surgery. 2011;**137**(4):390-395. DOI: 10.1001/archoto.2011.28

[49] Lin F, Metter E, O'Brien R, Resnick S, Zonderman A, Ferrucci L. Hearing loss and incident dementia. Archives of Neurology. 2011;**68**(2):214-220. DOI: 10.1001/archneurol.2010.362

[50] Schneider B. How age affects auditory-cognitive interactions in speech comprehension. Audiology Research. 2011;**1**(1S). DOI: 10.4081/audiores.2011.e10

[51] Central Auditory Processing Disorders. Technical Report. American Speech Language Hearing Association. [Internet]. 2005. Available from: https://www.asha.org/policy/TR2005-00043/ [Accessed: 2018-01-20]

[52] Davis A. Population study of the ability to benefit from amplification and the provision of a hearing aid in 55-74-year-old first-time hearing aid users. International Journal of Audiology. 2003;**42**(2):39-52. DOI: 10.3109/14992020309074643

[53] Popelka M, Cruickshanks K, Wiley T, Tweed T, Klein B, Klein R. Low prevalence of hearing aid use among older adults with hearing loss: The epidemiology of hearing loss study. Journal of the American Geriatrics Society. 1998;**46**(9):1075-1078. DOI: 10.1111/j.1532-5415.1998.tb06643.x

[54] Golovanova L, Boboshko M, Takhtaeva N, Zhilinskaya E. Rehabilitation in elderly people with hearing loss. Advances in Gerontology. 2014;**27**(4):758-762. [In Russian] Available from: http://www.gersociety.ru/netcat_files/userfiles/10/AG_2014-27-04.pdf [Accessed: 2018-01-20]

[55] Boboshko M, Golovanova L, Zhilinskaia E, Ogorodnikova E. The effectiveness of hearing aids in elderly people. Advances in Gerontology. 2017;**30**(1):114-120 [In Russian]

[56] Desjardins J, Doherty K. Do experienced hearing aid users know how to use their hearing aids correctly? American Journal of Audiology. 2009;**18**(1):69-76. DOI: 10.1044/1059-0889(2009/08-0022)

[57] Kelly R, Atcherson S. Quality of life for individuals with hearing impairment who have not consulted for services and their significant others: Same- and different-sex couples. Journal of Communication Disorders. 2011;**44**(3):336-344. DOI: 10.1016/j.jcomdis.2011.01.004

[58] Boboshko M, Zhilinskaia E, Golovanova L, Legostaeva T, Di Berardino F, Cesarani A. The use of speech audiometry in the practice of the geriatric center. Advances in Gerontology. 2017;**7**(2):166-169. DOI: 10.1134/S2079057017020023

[59] Pacala J, Yueh B. Hearing deficits in the older patient: "I Didn't notice anything". Journal of the American Medical Association. 2012;**307**(11):1185-1194. DOI: 10.1001/jama.2012.305

[60] De Miranda E, Gil D, Iório M. Formal auditory training in elderly hearing aid users. Revista Brasileira de Oto-Rino-Laringologia. 2008;**74**(6):919-925. DOI: 10.1016/s1808-8694(15)30154-3

[61] Burk M, Humes L. Effects of long-term training on aided speech-recognition performance in noise in older adults. Journal of Speech, Language, and Hearing Research. 2008;**51**(3):759-771. DOI: 10.1044/1092-4388(2008/054)

[62] Mueller H, Ricketts T, Bentler R. Modern Hearing Aids. San Diego: Plural Publishing; 2014. p. 462

[63] Gopal K, Bishop C, Carney L. Auditory measures in clinically depressed individuals. II. Auditory evoked potentials and behavioral speech tests. International Journal of Audiology. 2004;**43**(9):499-505. DOI: 10.1080/14992020400050064

[64] Gleich O, Hamann I, Klump G, Kittel M, Strutz J. Boosting GABA improves impaired auditory temporal resolution in the gerbil. Neuroreport. 2003;**14**(14):1877-1880. DOI: 10.1097/00001756-200310060-00024

[65] Chermak G, Musiek F. Handbook of Central Auditory Processing Disorder. Vol. 2. Comprehensive Intervention. 2nd ed. San Diego: Plural Publishing; 2014. p. 792

[66] Song J, Skoe E, Wong P, Kraus N. Plasticity in the adult human auditory brainstem following short-term linguistic training. Cognitive Neuroscience. 2008;**20**(10):1892-1902. DOI: 10.1162/jocn.2008.20131

[67] Snyder R, Bonham B, Sinex D. Acute changes in frequency responses of inferior colliculus central nucleus (ICC) neurons following progressively enlarged restricted spiral ganglion lesions. Hearing Research. 2008;**246**(1-2):59-78. DOI: 10.1016/j.heares.2008.09.010

[68] Ohl F, Scheich H. Learning-induced plasticity ion animal and human auditory cortex. Current Opinion in Neurobiology. 2005;**15**(4):470-477. DOI: 10.1016/j.conb.2005.07.002

[69] De Boer J, Thornton A. Neural correlates of perceptual learning in the auditory brainstem: Efferent activity predicts and reflects improvement at a speech-in-noise discrimination task. The Journal of Neuroscience. 2008;**28**(19):4929-4937. DOI: 10.1523/jneurosci.0902-08.2008

[70] Johnson K, Nicol T, Zecker S, Kraus N. Developmental plasticity in the human auditory brainstem. The Journal of Neuroscience. 2008;**28**(15):4000-4007. DOI: 10.1523/jneurosci.0012-08.2008

[71] Carcagno S, Plack C. Subcortical plasticity following perceptual learning in a pitch discrimination task. Journal of the Association for Research in Otolaryngology. 2011;**12**(1):89-100. DOI: 10.1007/s10162-010-0236-1

[72] Grafman J, Christen Y. Neuronal Plasticity: Building a Bridge from the Laboratory to the Clinic. New York: Spriner-Verlag; 1999. p. 187. DOI: 10.1007/978-3-642-59897-5

[73] Pan Y, Zhang J, Zhou R, Sun X. Developmentally degraded directional selectivity of the auditory cortex can be restored by auditory discrimination training in adults. Behavioural Brain Research. 2011;**225**(2):596-602. DOI: 10.1016/j.bbr.2011.08.033

[74] de Villers-Sidani E, Alzghoul L, Zhou X, Simpson K, Lin R, Merzenich M. Recovery of functional and structural age-related changes in the rat primary auditory cortex with

operant training. Proceedings of the National Academy of Sciences of the United States of America. 2010;**107**(31):13900-13905. DOI: 10.1073/pnas.1007885107

[75]   Kraus N, McGee T, Carrell T, King C, Tremblay K, Nicol T. Central auditory system plasticity associated with speech discrimination training. Journal of Cognitive Neuroscience. 1995;**7**(1):25-32. DOI: 10.1162/jocn.1995.7.1.25

[76]   Tremblay K, Kraus N, Carrell T, McGee T. Central auditory system plasticity: Generalization to novel stimuli following listening training. The Journal of the Acoustical Society of America. 1997;**102**(12):3762-3773. DOI: 10.1121/1.420139

[77]   Song J, Skoe E, Banai K, Kraus N. Training to improve hearing speech in noise: Biological mechanisms. Cerebral Cortex. 2012;**22**(5):1180-1190. DOI: 10.1093/cercor/bhr196

[78]   Tremblay K, Kraus N, McGee T. The time course of auditory perceptual learning: Neurophysiological changes during speech-sound training. Neuroreport. 1998;**9**(16): 3556-3560. DOI: 10.1097/00001756-199811160-00003

[79]   Jäncke L, Gaab N, Wüstenberg T, Scheich H, Heinze H. Short-term functional plasticity in the human auditory cortex: An fMRI study. Brain Research. 2001;**12**(3):479-485. DOI: 10.1016/s0926-6410(01)00092-1

[80]   Delhommeau K, Micheyl C, Jouvent R. Generalization of frequency discrimination learning across frequencies and ears: Implications for underlying neural mechanisms in humans. Journal of the Association for Research in Otolaryngology. 2005;**6**(2):171-179. DOI: 10.1007/s10162-005-5055-4

[81]   Weinberger N. Auditory associative memory and representational plasticity in the primary auditory cortex. Hearing Research. 2007;**229**(1-2):54-68. DOI: 10.1016/j.heares. 2007.01.004

[82]   Kaplun D, Gnezdilov D, Efimenko G, Pochechuev A, Ogorodnikova E, Boboshko M. Development and evaluation of the program for auditory training in the correction of central auditory processing disorders. In: Proceedings of the 2017 IEEE II International Conference on Control in Technical Systems (CTS); 25-27 October 2017; St.Petersburg, p. 106-109. DOI: 10.1109/CTSYS.2017.8109501

[83]   Bielefeld E, Tanaka C, Chen G, Henderson D. Age-related hearing loss: Is it a preventable condition? Hearing Research. 2010;**264**(1-2):98-107. DOI: /10.1016/j.heares.2009.09.001

10

The Basics of Biogerontology

Mark Rinnerthaler and Klaus Richter

Abstract

Aging is an enormously complicated process. Despite a great many of theories (among them "Program Theories", "Combined Theories", "Damage Theories", "Inflamm-Aging", "Garb-Aging" and the "Rising Deleteriome"), so far there is none which is able to explain this phenomenon satisfactorily and completely. A different approach to address the complexity of aging is to characterize the major "Hallmarks of Aging". These are genomic instability, telomere attrition, epigenetic alterations, loss of proteostasis, deregulated nutrient sensing, mitochondrial dysfunction, cellular senescence, stem cell exhaustion and an altered intercellular communication. From research on these hallmarks, new avenues were opened on how to interfere with the aging process. Some of these possible therapeutic interventions are described here too.

Keywords: aging, aging theories, hallmarks of aging, senescence, healthy aging, anti-aging interventions

1. Introduction

Aging has ever been a puzzling phenomenon for mankind. It is already an important topic in ancient Greek mythology: Eos goddess of the dawn did fall in love with Tithonus son of Laomedon king of Troy. Eos asked Zeus to grant Tithonus immortality, she did forget to ask for eternal youth too, however. Therefore Tithonus was living happily, but the process of aging continued inexorably. Over time, there was not much more left of him than a croaking voice and finally, he was transformed into a cicada.

The question of then still remains today: Is aging really unavoidable? Not necessarily, as some organisms do not seem to age. Most prominent of them is the tiny fresh water polyp *Hydra*. It does already have a simple nervous system and does not display any signs of aging.

This remarkable feature of *Hydra* is due to the fact that its stem cells have an unlimited capacity for self-renewal. In this respect, the transcription factor FoxO plays a crucial role [1]. In contrast to Hydra, all vertebrates are aging although at a very different rate. The lifespan of the mouse is between 2 and 4 years, whereas the lifespan of the Greenland shark is beyond 400 years [2]. If we look at mammals, the lifespan can vary up to 100-fold: The Etruscan shrew has a lifespan up to 2 years, whereas for the bowhead whale a lifespan beyond 200 years has been estimated [3]. In general, large animals are living longer than small ones. A dog lives considerably longer than a mouse and an Elephant lives much longer than a dog. There is, however, a great variety in lifespans: as already mentioned, the lifespan of the mouse is in the range of 2–4 years, whereas the related naked mole rat which is roughly the same size lives up to 30 years [4]. Some organisms are aging very fast and some are aging quite slowly. Nevertheless for all of them is true: Aging is characterized by a reduction of fitness, an increase of age-related diseases and a massive increase of the risk of dying. Considering humans, the risk of dying of an 80-year-old is 300 times higher than for a 20-year-old person [5]. With this chapter, we want to give a short overview on major topics of current aging research. Furthermore, we want to point out possibilities that are arising from this research field which will probably help to increase the healthy lifespan quite considerably.

2. Theories of aging

In the quest to explain aging, many theories have been developed. In 1990, Zhores Medvedev collected all these different theories and their number exceeded 300 [6]. In the meantime, a number of new ones have been presented. Considering only this fact, one can easily imagine that aging is a very complex process. Accordingly, aging is far away from being understood completely. In a recent publication, the different theories are divided into "Program Theories", "Combined Theories" and "Damage Theories" [7]. The program theories are based on the assumption that aging is genetically programed. Among these theories is the theory of replicative senescence [8]. Already in 1965, Hayflick has observed that cells in cell culture divide about 40–50 times after which they enter a permanent cell cycle arrest from which they cannot escape any more. This phenomenon has been explained by the shortening of telomeres taking place at each cell division. If telomeres are becoming too short, the shelterin complex is lost and the cell recognizes this as a DNA double-strand break triggering a permanent DNA damage response [9]. Furthermore, it turned out that cellular senescence can be triggered by a variety of different stress factors, among them oxidative stress or overexpression of cellular oncogenes. Cellular senescence is a potent anti-tumor mechanism preventing damaged cells from dividing any further. Senescent cells undergo dramatic phenotypic changes and start secreting many proteins (among them cytokines and chemokines), this is known as the senescence-associated secretory phenotype (SASP). These proteins attract immune cells like macrophages, neutrophils and natural killer cells, which are supposed to remove the senescent cells. Nevertheless, senescent cells are accumulating with increasing age and triggering pathological changes in the particular organ. In a mouse model, it has been demonstrated that pathological changes in lung [10], kidney, heart and adipose tissue [11] can be prevented if senescent cells are cleared from the organism. There is convincing evidence that senescent cells play a major role in reducing the function of old organs and the emergence of age-associated pathologies [9, 12].

The formation of senescent cells might also be seen as kind of antagonistic pleiotropy. This "program" aging theory claims that during evolution mutations are taking place which provide an advantage for early stages of life but are detrimental late in life [13]: Damaged cells becoming senescent prevent tumor formation early in life but they produce a number of adverse effects late in life. The "disposable soma theory" [14] also a "program" theory claims that resources for an organism are limited and they have to be allocated between maintenance of the organism and reproduction. Furthermore does the "neuroendocrine theory of aging" [15] belong to the "program theories". It states that aging is regulated by hormones similar to puberty and menopause. As a matter of fact, animals that reach sexual maturity in a short period of time have also a short lifespan. The mouse reaches sexual maturity within 6–8 weeks and has a lifespan of 2–4 years, whereas for the Greenland shark it takes some 150 years to reach sexual maturity but then its lifespan exceeds 400 years [2]. Interesting in this respect is that in parabiosis experiments, it was demonstrated that blood from young mice has a rejuvenating effect on old mice [16]. Recent research furthermore points to the fact that changes in the regulation of gene expression during aging are predominantly affecting genes which are responsible for growth and development [17]. The age an organism is able to live up to is without any doubt depending on its genome. Even under identical environmental conditions, a human will be living much much longer than a mouse. But up to now, there has been no gene identified that would actively regulate the aging process.

On the other end of the spectrum of aging theories are the damage theories. Among them the most prominent is the free radical theory of aging [18, 19]. According to it, reactive oxygen species (ROS) a byproduct of oxidative phosphorylation in mitochondria, damage DNA, lipids and proteins. They will be briefly discussed as follows:

1. DNA damage: It is of utmost importance that DNA damage will be repaired efficiently. If not this causes a rapidly accelerated aging process as can be observed in patients with a progeria syndrome (Werner Syndrome). Therefore we have a number of DNA repair systems (direct reversal pathway, mismatch repair, base excision repair, nucleotide excision repair, homologous recombination and non-homologous end joining) which repair DNA damage very efficiently [20]. Altogether there are more than 100 DNA repair enzymes known [21] which take care that DNA damage is not a major cause for aging until their activity diminishes during aging. Most probably contributing to the aging process are DNA double-strand breaks [22].

2. Lipid peroxidation: ROS predominantly attack unsaturated fatty acids in the membranes of a cell. By this lipid peroxidation fatty acids literally become chopped down producing chemically very active aldehydes [23]. These aldehydes react with DNA and proteins resulting in irreversible modifications. Proteins modified this way often loose their function and form aggregates which are not degradable by the cell which is in particular problematic in the brain. It has been demonstrated that lipid peroxidation triggers neurodegeneration [24].

3. Protein oxidation: Proteins are also attacked by ROS. In particular, sulfur-containing amino acids are being oxidized. The first stage of oxidation can be reversed enzymatically but later stages not any more [25]. Oxidatively damaged proteins too have the tendency to denature and to form aggregates which the cell is not able to degrade. Such aggregates may

cause death of the cell eventually as is the case in Alzheimer patients. ROS are damaging cells in many locations in particular if they are produced excessively. On the other hand, ROS are important signaling molecules, therefore their complete removal by antioxidants is definitely counterproductive. In recent years, a modification of the free radical theory of aging gained attention: It claims that not ROS are driving the aging process but the disturbed redox homeostasis is a major culprit [26, 27].

Also a damage theory is the theory of "Inflamm-Aging" which claims that aging is caused by ongoing low level sterile inflammatory processes [28]. In fact all degenerative diseases in aging have an inflammatory component as there are: Alzheimer, Parkinson, arteriosclerosis, arthritis, multiple sclerosis, osteoporosis and diabetes type II [29]. Responsible for many inflammatory reactions are debris of dead cells and un-degradable protein aggregates which have not been removed completely. This was the basis to coin the term "Garb-Aging" (from garbage and aging) as an addition to inflamm-aging [30]. None of the so far mentioned theories, however, is able to explain all facets of the aging process. Therefore a new perspective was presented recently: "Aging: progressive decline in fitness due to the rising deleteriome" [31]. According to this theory neither the synthesis of biomolecules nor the repair systems in a cell are working absolute flawlessly. Furthermore there are chemical reactions between many biomolecule. The resulting compounds cannot be removed completely. That means that unwanted reaction products as well as non-repaired damage (= deleteriome) increases with time and causes the aging process.

3. Hallmarks of aging

A completely different approach than to explain aging by theories is to describe it by its major characteristic features: "The Hallmarks of Aging" [32]:

3.1. Genomic instability

DNA is permanently exposed to a great variety of damage caused by ROS, lipid peroxidation products, environmental mutagens, hydrolytic reactions, UV irradiation and many more.

Besides chemical modifications to DNA, there can be single- and double-strand breaks, depurination as well as cross links between bases. Addition, deletion or substitution of bases is causing mutations. All together, these changes can also lead to epigenetic alterations causing changes in gene expression. To repair this damage efficiently is of utmost importance as can be seen in progeria or premature aging syndromes. In these diseases, defects in DNA repair systems are causing a dramatically accelerated aging process [33].

Usually, DNA damage is repaired very efficiently, however, the activity of the repair systems declines during aging [34].

3.2. Telomere attrition

Telomeres are protective caps on the ends of chromosomes preventing degradation or fusion of chromosome ends. At every cell division, telomeres are getting shorter and if they reach a critical length the cells, are not able to divide anymore. This telomere attrition eventually leads to replicative senescence. The degree of shortening is proportionate to risks of a number of aging diseases [35]. In particular, short telomeres lead to bone marrow failure causing anemia and immune senescence and to enterocolitis in the intestinal epithelium. Furthermore, short telomeres are causing premature onset of emphysema and pulmonary fibrosis in the lung, fibrosis in the liver and also osteoporosis [36]. In addition, short telomeres have an impact on gene expression through telomere position effects on nearby genes [37]. Through the expression of telomerase in mice, the normal aging process could be delayed [38]. In humans, 11 mutations inactivating a single gene are known which directly affect telomere maintenance and they lead to age-related diseases and accelerated aging [35]. Also a telomere biology disorder is the Hoyeraal-Hreidarsson (HH) syndrome which is caused by mutations in genes with telomeric functions. It is characterized by very short telomeres and affected individuals die in childhood mostly due to bone marrow failure [39]. Interestingly, it has been shown that in wild animals, telomeres shorten more slowly in slow-aging than in fast-aging ones [40].

3.3. Epigenetic alterations

Epigenetic changes are comprising alterations in histone marks, DNA methylation, nucleosome positioning and non-coding RNAs [41]. Histone modifications and methylation patterns of CpG islands have a tremendous influence on gene expression. For a set of 353 CpG islands, a clear correlation with age could be demonstrated. Of these, 193 CpGs get hypermethylated and 160 get hypomethylated during aging [42]. According to its reliable changes in methylation status, this set has been termed the epigenetic clock [27, 42, 43]. With this epigenetic clock, it is possible to predict the biological age and an age-related functional decline. Furthermore, it has been demonstrated that lifestyle factors like diet, exercise and education have an influence on this epigenetic clock [44]. In addition to DNA, the histones are subject to modifications (acetylation, methylation, phosphorylation and more). There are also a number of methylation marks that are changing with age. But the present picture is less clear than with DNA methylation [41]. A lot of attention has been focused on sirtuins. Sirtuins are class III histone deacetylases, which need NAD^+ as a cofactor and remove acetyl groups from previously modified lysines in the histone N-terminal tails. By removing the acetyl groups, lysines regain their positive charge and bind more tightly to DNA. The result is a more compact chromatin structure and down-regulation of gene expression. The removal of histone acetyl groups by sirtuins results in an extension of lifespan [45]. In total, seven sirtuins are known, of which SIRT1, SIRT6 and SIRT7 are localized in the nucleus. SIRT2 is predominantly found in the cytoplasm and is only localized to chromatin during the G/M phase of the cell cycle. SIRT3, SIRT4 and SIRT5 are the three mitochondrial deacetlyases. Sirtuins do not only deacetylate histones but regulate the activity of a number of other proteins too. This way they play a central role in regulatory networks important for aging and longevity [46]. Mutant mice where single sirtuin genes have been deleted show a number of different pathologies connected to metabolism, cancer and inflammation [47].

3.4. Loss of proteostasis

Proteins not only have to be synthesized but they have to be removed and degraded eventually. Among many others, there are two major ways to remove damaged proteins: either to degrade them by the proteasome or via autophagy [48, 49]. In addition, the cell has chaperones. These proteins help to fold proteins correctly or enable the renaturation of already denatured proteins. If refolding is impossible, chaperons are also able to target misfolded proteins to the proteasome. Therefore proteostasis, the maintenance of an intact proteome, includes not only synthesis and degradation of proteins but also folding and conformational maintenance. The disturbance of proteostasis is considered to be a major cause of aging [50, 51]. Not only the amount of chaperones is decreasing [52], but also the proteasomal activity and autophagy are declining during aging. This decline causes an accumulation of denatured proteins which have the tendency to form aggregates that cannot be removed by the cell anymore. These aggregates are detrimental to the cell and can even cause death of the cell (e.g. nerve cells in Alzheimer and Parkinson patients) [53]. Furthermore, it has been demonstrated that long-living animals have less denatured proteins than short-living ones [54]. In addition, the activity of the proteasome is remarkably higher in the long-living naked mole rat than in the short-lived mouse [55]. Particularly interesting in this respect is that experimental interventions which reduce the aging process are stimulating autophagy like caloric restriction, rapamycin, metformin, resveratrol and spermidine [56].

3.5. Deregulated nutrient sensing

Nutrient sensing is of utmost importance for every cell. The major nutrient sensing pathways that are also longevity pathways are [57]:

- IGF-1 and insulin signaling pathway

- mTOR pathway

- AMP-activated protein kinase (AMPK) pathway

- NAD^+ dependent sirtuins

IGF-1 is like insulin a growth factor for many cells and acts via the insulin and IGF-1 signaling (IIS) pathway. The down-regulation of this pathway leads to a prolonged lifespan [58]. IGF-1 but also EGF and high amino acid levels are activating the mTOR pathway which stimulates protein synthesis and growth in general but down-regulates autophagy [59]. AMPK is the sensor and regulator for energy metabolism and homeostasis of the cell. AMPK activity can extend the lifespan of yeast, *C. elegans* and drosophila and the healthspan of mice [60].

NAD-dependent sirtuins are a family of deacylases which not only deacetylate histones but modify a large number of non-histone proteins too. They show impressive activities to prevent diseases and some aspects of aging [61].

During aging, the synthesis of these sensor proteins is reduced however [62].

The different signal transduction pathways that are sensing the availability of nutrients are deregulated during aging by metabolic diseases [63].

3.6. Mitochondrial dysfunction

As mitochondria are not only the power plants of the cell but also important signaling centers they play a central role in the aging process. For energy production in form of ATP, they reduce oxygen to water. If accidentially oxygen gets only one electron, it leads to the production of ROS instead of water. This has inspired Harman already in 1956 to present his "Free Radical Theory of Aging," which he has repeatedly improved [18]. Furthermore, it has been demonstrated that ROS are not only causing damage but also are important signaling molecules, which are able to regulate many pathways. For example, ROS can induce autophagy (mitophagy) [64].

The events of biogenesis, fusion, fission and mitophagy are collected under the term mito-chondrial dynamics [65]. Function as well as quality of mitochondria is regulated by mito-chondrial dynamics. Nutrients in excess cause fragmentation (fission) of mitochondria and a low level of nutrients leads to fusion and elongation [66]. Mitochondrial dynamics is also influenced by external signals like hormones, nutrients and physical exercise. A number of pathways are involved like mTOR, AMP-activated kinase and sirtuins [67]. In particular, sir-tuins play an important role as they do not regulate a few target enzymes but regulate func-tional clusters (e.g. TCA cycle, fatty acid metabolism, electron transport chain and others). This way they are involved in the regulation of ROS-mediated signaling pathways as well as in the detoxification of damaging ROS. Furthermore they regulate metabolic plasticity. SIRT3, for example, promotes switching to fatty acid oxidation upon caloric restriction [68]. The modulation of metabolic changes plays a crucial role in senescence too. In addition, defect mitochondria are stimulating inflammatory reactions which are triggering inflamm-aging [69]. Altogether, mitochondrial dysfunction leads to a number of age-related diseases includ-ing metabolic, cardiovascular and neurodegenerative pathologies, sarcopenia and fibrosis in different organs [65].

All these facts demonstrate that the quality of mitochondria has a tremendous impact on the aging process [70, 71].

3.7. Cellular senescence

Cellular senescence is characterized by an irreversible arrest of the cell cycle. This means that cellular senescence can only affect cells that are able to divide like stem cells, progenitor cells or cells that are not yet terminally differentiated. This phenomenon has been discovered with cells in cell culture. It turned out that they cannot divide without limits but stop growing after about 40–50 cell divisions [72].

The irreversible cell cycle arrest can be induced by erosion of telomeres, substantial DNA dam-age, oxidative stress, overexpression of oncogenes, mitochondrial dysfunction and proteotox-icity [73]. Cells in the state of senescence change their morphology, they are getting larger and there are massive changes in the organization of chromatin [74]. Furthermore, they start to secret a large number of proteins. The sum of all these proteins is called the senescence-asso-ciated secretory phenotype (SASP). Among these proteins are pro-inflammatory cytokines, chemokines, growth factors and matrix metalloproteases (MMPs). The pro-inflammatory cytokines are causing local sterile inflammations which contribute substantially to "inflamm-aging". They attract cells of the immune system which are killing senescent cells. The over-proportional increase of senescent cells during aging is probably due to a decline in immune function [75]. An important additional feature of senescent cells is the active suppression of apoptosis [76]. At the level of gene expression, permanent cell cycle arrest is mediated by the protein p16[Ink4a] which is an inhibitor of the cyclin dependent kinases 4 and 6 (CDK4 and CDK6).

In healthy young cells, p16[Ink4a] expression is low or undetectable but increases dramatically in senescent cells [9]. This way it is evident that an essential function of senescence (maybe the most important one for the organism) is to pull the emergency brake to prevent uncontrolled cell division which otherwise could cause tumor formation. Senescent cells have also an important additional function in wound healing. After a wound has been inflicted many cells are produced in excess to close the wound. During the subsequent remodeling process, the surplus of cells is entering senescence and will be removed by the immune system. For years it has been discussed by researchers if cellular senescence has any influence on the aging process itself. During the past few years, scientists came to the conclusion that cellular senescence is one of the major causes of aging [77]. In genetically modified mice, it was already possible to delete senescent cells (p16[Ink4a] positive cells). These animals showed less age-related pathologies, an improved healthspan and a prolonged median lifespan [9, 11]. Therefore, there are already a number of different interventions under investigation how senescent cells can be removed from the human body [78, 79]. To succeed in this respect could dramatically improve human healthspan. Senescent cells are detrimental to the function of organs they are residing in and this way they have a tremendous impact on age-dependent degenerative diseases [12, 78].

3.8. Stem cell exhaustion

Stem cells are of utmost importance for tissue homeostasis and regeneration and stem cell exhaustion is among the most significant hallmarks of aging. Stem cell exhaustion is leading to a reduced regenerative capacity during the aging process. Premature stem cell exhaustion is also seen in age-related diseases [80]. Stem cells are usually very small remaining in a state of quiescence. This state is characterized by low metabolism and the presence of few mitochondria. From dormancy, they can be activated to replace lost stem cells or to produce transit amplifying cells which will provide many cells for repair or regeneration of their particular tissue. During this differentiation process, they are going through a developmental program which is tuning them precisely to their new function [81].

There are tissues with a very high turnover of cells like bone marrow, intestine and the epidermis of the skin. There are also tissues where stem cells get activated rarely like muscle and brain. Essential for survival and quiescence of stem cells is their immediate environment which is defined as the stem cell niche. The stem cell niche comprises proteins of the extracellular matrix and surrounding cells which secrete a number of growth regulating proteins (Wnts, BMPs, EGF and Notch). It is essentially regulating the state of quiescence [82, 83]. Different drivers of aging (telomere attrition, cellular senescence, DNA damage, epigenetic alterations, nutrient sensing and disturbed proteostasis) have their impact on stem cells too and are responsible for stem cell aging [84]. As stem cells usually stay in the state of quiescence and divide rarely, many pro-aging impacts affect the stem cells via their niche. Muscle stem cells, so called satellite cells, rarely divide, but proliferate massively upon demand. They produce myoblasts which are the precursor cells necessary for the regeneration process of the muscle. If old satellite cells are transplanted into young muscle tissue their regenerative capacity increases which demonstrates the influence of the young niche [85, 86]. The opposite is true for transforming growth factor beta (TGF-beta1). This factor is produced by the niche and reduces the proliferative potential of satellite cells. During aging under certain circumstances the niche increases the production of fibroblast growth factor 2 (FGF2). This triggers the stem cells to leave quiescence and start to divide which eventually leads to a reduction of satellite cells available for the regeneration of muscle tissue [87]. In a similar way, the prolonged signaling of the growth hormone (GH)/insulin/insulin-like growth factors (IGF) axis is considered to cause a depletion of stem cells [88]. There are also areas in the adult brain where stem cells are residing: in the dentate gyrus of the hippocampus in the hypothalamus and in the subventricular zone of the lateral ventricles [89]. Like in other tissues, there are age-related changes in the stem cell niche and the number of neural stem cells is declining during aging. Not only the numbers of stem cells are decreasing during aging but also the proliferation of the developing precursor cells will be damped via an elevated concentration of TGF-beta1. This way the production of new neurons is reduced while the generation of oligodendroglia remains at about the same level [90]. Furthermore, sterile micro-inflammation in the hypothalamus can cause a reduction of neural stem cells which in turn leads to a reduction of cognitive functions [91]. In addition to the number of stem cells and the contribution of the stem cell niche, the regenerative capacity will be influenced by systemic factors. Via parabiosis experiments (connecting an old mouse to a young one), it was possible to correct malfunction of old satellite cells in muscle tissue. These satellite cells could be reactivated again. In a similar way, it was possible to improve the function of stem cells and neurogenesis in old brains. The proteins responsible for this activity could be identified as growth differentiation factor 11 (GDF11) and oxytocin [92]. There are numerous factors that regulate the biological function of stem cells. Presently, it seems that the most important ones are metabolism and epigenetic changes [80]. As excessive nutrient sensing leads to premature depletion of adult neural stem cells [89] and chronic activation of mTOR leads to loss of stem cells in the airway epithelium of the mouse [93].

3.9. Altered intercellular communication

The regenerative capacity of stem cells is independently influenced by intrinsic and extrinsic determinants [92]. An intrinsic determinant is the maintenance of autophagy. A failure of autophagy in old satellite cells leads to senescence eventually [94]. Among the extrinsic factors, growth hormone/insulin/IGF-1 (somatotrophic axis) is a center piece for the regulation of growth in the mammalian organism. Mouse mutants with defects in the biosynthesis of the growth hormone (Ames dwarf mice, Snell dwarf mice or GHRKO-mice (GH receptor deletion)) are considerably smaller than wild type mice but have an approximately 50% longer lifespan [95]. In humans, the amount of growth hormone and IGF-1 in the circulation is changing during aging. The highest level is reached during the second decade where growth is most prominent. Afterwards the concentration is going down continuously until it reaches a low plateau during the sixth decade. Humans with genetic polymorphisms resulting in a reduced activity of IGF-1 show a significantly increased lifespan. An elevated concentration of IGF-1 is correlated to a higher risk for some tumors [96]. There is also an altered communication between muscle stem cells and the environment. Growth hormone is important for the maintenance of muscle mass [97]. IGF-1 is modulating the differentiation of muscle progenitor cells (myoblasts) and influencing satellite cells [98]. An increased aging of muscle stem cells is caused by an elevated concentration of Wnt-proteins (e.g. Wnt3A) [99]. As an antagonist of Wnt/β-catenin signaling acts the protein klotho. Unfortunately, the amount of klotho in the circulation is decreasing during aging. In the mouse, the silencing of the klotho gene triggered a rapid aging process [100]. Klotho is essential for the homeostasis of mineral metabolism (in particular phosphate) but it also modulates the signaling pathways of IGF-1 and Wnt. The deletion of the klotho gene in mice reduces their lifespan to 2–3 months which is only about 10% of their regular lifespan [101]. A remarkable activity has also been demonstrated for GDF11 which improves regeneration in old organisms and serum levels of GDF11 are significantly lower in old individuals [102]. An increased regenerative activity has been shown for bone [103], brain [104], skeletal muscle [105] and heart [106].

Furthermore, a number of chemokines (CCL2, CCL11, CCL12 and CCL19) have been identified via parabiosis experiments and they have been correlated with impaired neurogenesis in old individuals [107]. Other potential pro-aging factors that increase during lifetime are TGF-beta1, IL-6 and TNF-alpha [107]. Beta2microglobulin too is a systemic pro-aging factor triggering age-related cognitive impairment [108].

Another pro-aging factor is the plasminogen activator inhibitor 1 (PAI-1) which is secreted by senescent cells. It induces the accumulation of p16^{Ink4a} leading to cellular senescence [109]. An anti-aging factor is kallistatin which inhibits oxidative stress and inflammation. It is also able to down-regulate the miRNA synthesis of miR21 and miR-34a, thereby reducing vascular senescence and aging [110]. The protein tissue inhibitor of metalloproteinase 2 (TIMP 2) was isolated from human umbilical cord. It is an anti-aging protein which revitalizes the hippocampus, increases synaptic plasticity and improves cognitive function [111]. The intercellular communication is also altered by numerous pro-inflammatory cytokines which are released by senescent cells. These cytokines are causing inflammatory processes [112]. Furthermore, inflammasomes in the cells of the innate immune system can be activated by DAMPs (damage-associated molecular patterns) [113]. DAMPS are comprised of debris of necrotic cells, amyloide fibers, HMGB1, heat shock proteins, crystals of cholesterol and uric acid. Activated inflammasomes are causing the release of interleukins IL-1beta and IL-18 [114]. These interleukins trigger inflammatory reactions in the surrounding tissue which are causing age-related diseases [115], among them Alzheimer's disease [116].

Exosomes provide an additional possibility for intercellular communication. They are small lipid vesicles which are secreted by the cell and they carry proteins and functional RNAs [117]. They can contact nearby cells or they can be distributed via the circulation across the whole organism. They help the cell to get rid of toxic protein waste [118] or to contribute to intercellular communication [119]. In the latter case, predominantly miRNAs play an important function [120]. During aging, the amount of exosomes in the blood stay more or less constant. Their content, however, becomes more pro-inflammatory [121]. Recently, it has been shown that they also play a role in senescence and aging [122].

4. Possible therapeutic interventions

4.1. Physical exercise

The most simple and probably the most efficient way to attenuate aging is to perform physical exercise. A sedentary lifestyle with minimal physical activity on the contrary is detrimental for health comparable to smoking [123]. It is quite obvious that physical exercise is the best way to keep skeletal muscles in a healthy condition [124] and to prevent sarcopenia and frailty in old age [125]. Physical exercise does not only improve physiological parameters like maximum oxygen consumption and reduced levels of cholesterol and triglycerides in the blood, but it also improves physical and psychical conditions in old age [126]. Although a number of physiological parameters can be improved considerably by physical training, the protective function for the cardiovascular system are about twice as high as can be explained by these parameters only. Therefore there are still many open questions concerning the molecular mechanisms which are activated by physical training [127]. Very well documented is, however, the positive effect on the brain and in particular on cognitive functions and the stimulation of neuronal growth in the hippocampus, an area critically important for memory processes [128]. Physical exercise increases hippocampal volume, functional connectivity and improved connectivity between the default mode network and the prefrontal cortex [129]. In this context, it should also be mentioned that physical exercise leads to a significant improvement of memory functions in Alzheimer patients [130].

4.2. Caloric restriction/dietary restriction

Already in 1935 it has been demonstrated on rats that reducing the amount of food intake can extend the lifespan by 30% [131]. This experiment has been repeated many times and it turned out that animals are not only living longer but they also show less age-related deficits. During the past years, it has been demonstrated that the amount of calories is less important than the amount of proteins. Therefore the term caloric restriction has been replaced in most cases by the term dietary restriction. In addition to the amount of food, the timing of food uptake is important. Animals getting their food evenly distributed during the day did not show positive effects but animals fed only once a day did show the positive effects. Also did fasting every second day result in an increase of lifespan by 30% [132]. Altogether a great many experiments have been performed concerning this topic and results are sometimes contradictory. Some authors are pointing out explicitly that it is necessary to test many different combinations of carbohydrates and proteins in a single experiment. It has been demonstrated that a relation of 1:10 (proteins:carbohydrates) results in the longest lifespan in mice. Remarkable in this respect is the fact that the traditional diet of the population of Okinawa consists of protein to carbohydrates in a relation of 9:85 and it is well documented that the people of Okinawa have the highest life expectancy worldwide [133]. It has to be mentioned that not only permanent dietary restriction is effective but intermittent fasting too. In rats and mice as well as in humans, there are profound health benefits. Results of intermittent fasting (2 days per week or every other day) decreased insulin levels, increased resistance to stress of heart and brain, reduced inflammation, enhanced autophagy, mitochondrial health and DNA repair [134]. Concerning DNA repair, the following experiment is really remarkable: mice lacking the DNA excision repair gene Ercc1 are aging very fast with a lifespan of 4–6 months. If they are subjected to a dietary restriction of 30%, this treatment triples their lifespan [33]. The single cell senses the availability of nutrition via nutrient sensing pathways which are GH/insulin/IGF-1, mTOR, sirtuins and AMPK and via these pathways the metabolic influence on the aging process is regulated [57].

4.2.1. The somatotrophic axis (GH/insulin/IGF-1)

Attenuating the signaling of the somatotrophic axis results in an increased lifespan. This has been demonstrated in animal models, in genetic polymorphisms or functional mutations in the IGF1R gene in humans [96]. Pharmaceutical interventions to block the signaling of this pathway are being tested but there are no drugs available yet to be used in humans [96].

4.2.2. mTOR

mTOR is a serine/threonine kinase which is "the grand conductor of metabolism and aging" and is either part of the multiprotein complex mTORC1 or mTORC2 [135]. Growth factors, insulin, IGF-1, amino acids and glucose are activating mTOR which in turn stimulates growth and inhibits autophagy.

Rapamycin binds to FKBP12 in this way inhibiting mTOR. Blockage of mTOR increases the lifespan in different organisms among them mice. But unfortunately there are numerous side effects which prohibit the use on a daily basis for healthy individuals [135].

4.2.3. Sirtuins

Sirtuins interact with IGF-1, mTOR and AMPK signaling pathways and regulate many other proteins involved in energy metabolism, DNA repair, cell survival, inflammation and tissue regeneration. SIRT1, for example, besides deacetylating histones H1, H3 and H4 modifies more than 50 other proteins [61]. Sirtuin-activating compounds (STACs) have gained much attention since their discovery 2003 and more than 14,000 STACs have been identified since then [61]. Essentially there are two different classes: sirtuin activators and compounds that raise NAD$^+$ levels. Using rodents numerous studies have shown that STACs promote health during aging involving protection against cardiovascular disease, diabetes type 2, neurodegeneration and even cancer [61].

4.2.4. AMP-activated protein kinase (AMPK)

AMP-activated protein kinase is a heterotrimeric protein and a key enzyme in cellular energy sensing. The alpha subunit kinase domain contains a conserved threonine which is phosphorylated by upstream kinases activating AMPK. The beta subunit binds the alpha and gamma subunits and has an additional domain to sense glycogen. The gamma domain has four sites that can bind AMP, ADP and ATP which provides AMPK with the ability to sense AMP:ATP and ADP:ATP ratios [136, 137]. These features make AMPK the centerpiece of "an energy-sensing pathway with multiple inputs and outputs" [136].

AMPK turns on glucose uptake, fatty acid oxidation, autophagy and mitochondrial biogenesis and it inhibits mTOR and the synthesis of lipids and proteins. It is therefore a central regulator of metabolic pathways including their effects on age-related diseases. It is also involved in the process of inflamm-aging via the regulation of the NLRP3 inflammasome during aging [138]. The capacity of AMPK signaling declines with aging which has a negative effect on the maintenance of cellular homeostasis [60]. Considering these facts, it is obvious that there is extensive research going on how to restore or boost AMPK activity by metformin [139] or by other nutraceutical compounds in particular polyphenols like resveratrol [140].

4.3. Pharmacological substances

4.3.1. Metformin

Metformin is in use to treat diabetes type 2 since a long time already. The inhibitory effect on the synthesis of glucose in the liver is due to the activation of AMPK [141, 142]. In addition metformin inhibits mTOR and complex I of the mitochondrial electron transfer chain resulting in a reduced production of ROS. In addition metformin stimulates autophagy, dampens inflammatory processes and senescence and increases the lifespan in animal models [58, 143, 144]. There are reports claiming that metformin does not only improves the healthspan and lifespan but also reduces the risk of some cancers and shows positive effects with congestive heart failure, chronic liver disease, chronic kidney disease and multiple sclerosis (summarized in [145]). This had led some researchers to call metformin "the aspirin of the twenty-first century" [145].

4.3.2. Rapamycin

This substance has been isolated from the microorganism *Streptomyces hygroscopicus* which has been found on the island of Rapa Nui, hence the name rapamycin. It is widely used as an immunosuppressant to prevent rejection after organ transplantation. The protein complex inhibited by this substance has been termed "Target of rapamycin" or TOR and it has been demonstrated that it leads to a significant increase in lifespan when applied to mice and most other "aging" model organisms [146].

4.3.3. Resveratrol

Polyphenols are comprising a large group of plant secondary metabolites. They are classified into phenolic acids, lignans, flavonoids and stilbenes [147]. The most prominent member of stilbenes is resveratrol which is synthesized by many plants in particular in wine. Resveratrol activates SIRT1 which mediates the effect of caloric restriction [148]. It could be demonstrated that resveratrol increases the lifespan of some organisms, in mice only if they are fed a high-fat diet [149]. In addition, resveratrol causes a number of positive effects in the cardiovascular system, cancer, diabetes type 2 inflammation and neurodegeneration [150]. As resveratrol is also stimulating autophagy and together with its neuroprotective effects, there are indications that resveratrol might also be applicable to treat Alzheimer's disease [151]. It has to be mentioned that resveratrol not only activates SIRT1 but also AMPK which explains many of its anti-oxidant and anti-inflammatory activities [152]. Furthermore resveratrol activates a number of stimulus-responsive transcription factors and inhibits cAMP-degrading phospho-diesterases which helps to understand its many effects [153–155].

4.3.4. Spermidine

Like rapamycin and resveratrol, the polyamine spermidine also stimulates autophagy although via a different molecular mechanism. Similar to resveratrol, the stimulation of autophagy is achieved by a change in the acetylation status of several proteins, but this occurs in a SIRT1-independent manner (most probably due to an inhibition of acetylases) [156]. For spermidine too, it has been demonstrated that it is increasing the lifespan of mice and all "aging" model organisms [157]. Surprisingly, the amount of this substance that is present in all cells dramatically decreases with aging [158]. In addition spermidine has neuroprotective capacities [159] and reduces the risk for cardiovascular diseases [160].

Spermidine also stimulates the synthesis of anti-inflammatory cytokines and has a positive influence on lipid metabolism [161].

4.3.5. Vitamin D

Muscle and bone are forming a physiological unit whereby both partners are regulating each other via endocrine signals [162]. Vitamin D has an essential function within this regulatory network. A sufficient supply of vitamin D prevents loss of muscle mass (sarcopenia) and age-dependent deposition of fat in muscles [163, 164]. In addition vitamin D shows a positive effect on cognitive function in old age [165]. Mice lacking the vitamin D receptor do age prematurely and the animal model for Alzheimer's disease show better memory performance and a reduction of some markers for Alzheimer's pathology after vitamin D supplementation. Humans with Alzheimer's disease show very low blood levels of vitamin D. Altogether vitamin D is a neuroprotective substance [166].

4.3.6. Soluble proteins/growth factors

Treating age-related ailments with soluble proteins is particularly attractive because it can be performed via simple infusions. Among the best candidates, GDF11 and oxytocin have demonstrated a rejuvenating effect in old mice [92]. In a study comparing very old healthy individuals (beyond the age of 100) with 70–80-year-old persons, a set of proteins have been identified whose levels were elevated in the serum of the 100+ probands. This study correlates "successful aging" with these four proteins: Chemerin, Fetuin-A, FGF19 and FGF21 [167]. In particular, FGF21 is a "systemic enhancer of longevity" [168]. It is involved in the coordination of glucose and lipid metabolism and maintains tissue homeostasis under stress conditions. FGF21 can enhance autophagy and mice overexpressing it live up to 40% longer [168]. Another good candidate to provide a healthy lifespan is adiponectin. Adiponectin is expressed in and secreted from small adipocytes. It increases insulin sensitivity, shows anti-artherosclerotic effects and improves metabolism in skeletal muscle, liver and adipose tissue. Adiponectin activates AMPK and SIRT1 and this way it acts like an exercise mimicking factor [169]. Finally, it has to be mentioned that it also turns on catalase and superoxide dismutase reducing oxidative stress in metabolically active organs (summarized in [169]). A further "pro-youthful" factor is follistatin-like 1 (FSTL1) which together with GDF11 supports heart regeneration, as it increases the survival of cardiomyocytes [170]. Another good candidate is the soluble isoform of Klotho which increases the lifespan of mice and shows a neuroprotective function making it a good candidate for the treatment of Alzheimer's and multiple sclerosis [171].

4.3.7. Acetylcholinesterase inhibitors

Alzheimer's disease (AD) is the most devastating aging disease. For 2013, it was estimated that more than 44 million people were affected worldwide and this number is expected to be beyond 135 million by the year 2050. Although there is presently no cure, there are a few drugs available that make life easier for AD patients. Most prominent are acetylcholinesterase inhibitors which show modest effects on improving cognitive function. The degeneration of cholinergic neurons which is seen in AD as well as Parkinson's disease dementia (PDD) leads to a reduction of acetylcholine levels. Furthermore, cholinergic pathways are not only important for the brain but also for skeletal muscle and the autonomous nervous system [172]. The increase of acetylcholine levels via inhibition of acetylcholinesterase improves cognitive function and has also beneficial effects on some of the comorbidities that usually affect AD and PD patients [173].

4.4. Selective elimination of senescent cells

If senescent cells are not removed by the immune system they are causing organ dysfunction and are a major cause of age-related diseases [174]. The removal of senescent cells in mice has improved their health conditions considerably. The elimination of senescent cells via drugs (senolysis) [175] or to trigger apoptosis (senoptosis) is also a realistic possibility in humans. From the observation that senescent cells do not respond to their own pro-apoptotic SASP, it was concluded that they have senescent-cell anti-apoptotic pathways (SCAPs). Six such SCAPs have been identified and these SCAPs were then screened for targets sensitive to senolytic drugs [176]. A number of senolytic drugs synthetic ones as well as of plant origin have been identified in the meantime. Prominent among them is quercetin which demonstrates promising activities [166]. It has to be mentioned that not every senolytic drug is effective on each senescent cell type and often is the combination of two or three drugs much more effective. An advantage over other medications is that senolytic drugs need not be taken continuously to exert their effect but just administered intermittently [176]. The use of senolytic drugs increase hope for the treatment of diseases for which there are hardly any other therapeutic options like idiopathic pulmonary fibrosis (IPF) a devastating lung disease [177]. Another elegant approach to trigger apoptosis in senescent cells has recently been demonstrated using a synthetic peptide. This cell penetrating peptide (CPP) was deduced from the sequence of the transcription factor FOXO4 and it excludes p53 from the nucleus. Instead of residing in the nucleus p53 is docking on to mitochondria to trigger apoptosis [178]. An additional possibility is to attack senescent cells with specific antibodies or by modified T cells [9].

4.5. Transplantation of stem cells

Stem cells are of utmost importance for regeneration and function of all organs. Transplanting stem cells into target tissues opens the possibility to repair major defects. Here we are at the brink of breathtaking possibilities for regenerative medicine. In particular, multipotent mesenchymal stem cells offer a wide spectrum of applications however these cells are loosing a lot of their regenerative capacity during aging [179]. Substantial progress has been made by the discovery that only four transcription factors (OCT3/4, SOX2, KLF4 and MYC) can induce reprogramming to pluripotency. Somatic cells can be transformed into young embryonic stem cells (induced pluripotent stem cells = iPSCs) [180]. From human fibroblasts such iPSCs could be generated and after specific differentiation processes used in different tissues [181]. In clinical trials, specific cells have been differentiated from iPSCs to treat Alzheimer disease, Parkinson disease, spinal cord injuries, diabetes or congestive heart failure [182]. Such a strategy for rejuvenation of old organs via stem cell therapy offers possibilities almost without limits for the future [183]. There is, however, a number of points that critically affects the success of stem cell transplantation. No matter how the replacement cells have been generated either as induced pluripotent stem cells (iPSCs) and subsequent differentiation steps or by direct transdifferentiation of somatic cells the condition of the stem cell niche is of utmost importance for regenerative success [183]. Also protein factors of the circulation effect transplanted cells massively [184]. Furthermore inflammatory processes which are often increased during aging effect stem cells dramatically as has been demonstrated for satellite cell function [185]. This demands the inhibition of inflammatory signaling as absolutely necessary.

5. Conclusion

Since the turn of the century there has been enormous progress in aging research in many fields. In this book chapter, we made a selection of aging theories and pathways that in our opinion are of great importance. To name them all would by far go beyond the scope of this article. It also has to be stated that of all the organelles in the cell we did just name mitochondria and their role in the aging process. But there is rising knowledge that all organelles have their specific share to aging. In the focus of this article were especially pathways and mechanisms on the cellular level. We did neglect that basically each organ and tissue has its private aging mechanisms [186, 187]. Therefore we believe that aging research will move on from cells toward tissues/organs and whole organisms. The possibilities that epigenetics will provide to increase health span look breathtaking, however, they cannot be really estimated to their full extend today yet. Much more realistic seems the application of stem cells which will provide regenerative medicine with fabulous opportunities. A very positive effect for an increased healthspan for almost all people will be possible if we will be able to boost autophagy without side effects. A similar effect on health span and the prevention of age-related diseases can be expected if it will be possible to eliminate senescent cells. Taken together there are really good chances that in the near future it will be possible to help many humans to live a healthy aging.

Author details

Mark Rinnerthaler and Klaus Richter*

*Address all correspondence to: klaus.richter@sbg.ac.at

Department of Biosciences, University of Salzburg, Salzburg, Austria

References

[1] Boehm AM, Khalturin K, Anton-Erxleben F, Hemmrich G, Klostermeier UC, Lopez-Quintero JA, et al. FoxO is a critical regulator of stem cell maintenance in immortal Hydra. Proceedings of the National Academy of Sciences of USA. 2012;**109**(48):19697-19702

[2] Nielsen J, Hedeholm RB, Heinemeier J, Bushnell PG, Christiansen JS, Olsen J, et al. Eye lens radiocarbon reveals centuries of longevity in the Greenland shark (*Somniosus microcephalus*). Science. 2016;**353**(6300):702-704

[3] George JC, Bockstoce JR. Two historical weapon fragments as an aid to estimating the longevity and movements of bowhead whales. Polar Biology. 2008;**31**(6):751-754

[4] Buffenstein R. Negligible senescence in the longest living rodent, the naked mole-rat: Insights from a successfully aging species. Journal of Comparative Physiology B. 2008;**178**(4):439-445

[5] Lipsky MS. Biological theories of aging. DM Disease-a-Month. 2015;**61**(11):460-466

[6] Medvedev ZA. An attempt at a rational classification of theories of aging. Biological Reviews. 1990;**65**(3):375-398

[7] da Costa JP, Vitorino R, Silva GM, Vogel C, Duarte AC, Rocha-Santos T. A synopsis on aging-theories, mechanisms and future prospects. Ageing Research Reviews. 2016;**29**:90-112

[8] Hayflick L. The limited in vitro lifetime of human diploid cell strains. Experimental Cell Research. 1965;**37**:614-636

[9] Childs BG, Durik M, Baker DJ, van Deursen JM. Cellular senescence in aging and age-related disease: From mechanisms to therapy. Nature Medicine 2015;**21**(12):1424-1435

[10] Hashimoto M, Asai A, Kawagishi H, Mikawa R, Iwashita Y, Kanayama K, et al. Elimination of p19(ARF)-expressing cells enhances pulmonary function in mice. JCI Insight. 2016;**1**(12):e87732

[11] Baker DJ, Childs BG, Durik M, Wijers ME, Sieben CJ, Zhong J, et al. Naturally occurring p16(Ink4a)-positive cells shorten healthy lifespan. Nature. 2016;**530**(7589):184

[12] He SH, Sharpless NE. Senescence in health and disease. Cell. 2017;**169**(6):1000-1011

[13] Williams GC. Pleiotropy, natural-selection, and the evolution of senescence. Evolution. 1957;**11**(4):398-411

[14] Kirkwood TBL, Austad SN. Why do we age? Nature. 2000;**408**(6809):233-238

[15] Finch CE. The menopause and aging, a comparative perspective. Journal of Steroid Biochemistry. 2014;**142**:132-141

[16] Katsimpardi L, Litterman NK, Schein PA, Miller CM, Loffredo FS, Wojtkiewicz GR, et al. Vascular and neurogenic rejuvenation of the aging mouse brain by young systemic factors. Science. 2014;**344**(6184):630-634

[17] de Magalhaes JP. Programmatic features of aging originating in development: Aging mechanisms beyond molecular damage? The FASEB Journal. 2012;**26**(12):4821-4826

[18] Harman D. The aging process. Proceedings of the National Academy of Sciences, India, Section B: Biological Sciences. 1981;**78**(11):7124-7128

[19] Harman D. Aging – A theory based on free-radical and radiation-chemistry. Journal of Gerontology. 1956;**11**(3):298-300

[20] Hoeijmakers JHJ. DNA damage, aging, and cancer. (p. 1475). New England Journal of Medicine. 2009;**361**(19):1914

[21] Cadet J, Davies KJA. Oxidative DNA damage & repair: An introduction. Free Radical Biology & Medicine. 2017;**107**:2-12

[22] White RR, Vijg J. Do DNA double-strand breaks drive aging? Molecular Cell. 2016;**63**(5): 729-738

[23] Negre-Salvayre A, Auge N, Ayala V, Basaga H, Boada J, Brenke R, et al. Pathological aspects of lipid peroxidation. Free Radical Research. 2010;**44**(10):1125-1171

[24] Sultana R, Perluigi M, Butterfield DA. Lipid peroxidation triggers neurodegeneration: A redox proteomics view into the Alzheimer disease brain. Free Radical Biology and Medicine. 2013;**62**:157-169

[25] Go YM, Chandler JD, Jones DP. The cysteine proteome. Free Radical Biology and Medicine. 2015;**84**:227-245

[26] Ursini F, Maiorino M, Forman HJ. Redox homeostasis: The golden mean of healthy living. Redox Biology. 2016;**8**:205-215

[27] Jones DP, Sies H. The redox code. Antioxidants and Redox Signaling. 2015;**23**(9):734-746

[28] Franceschi C, Bonafe M, Valensin S, Olivieri F, De Luca M, Ottaviani E, et al. Inflamm-aging – An evolutionary perspective on immunosenescence. Annals of the New York Academy of Sciences. 2000;**908**:244-254

[29] Xia SJ, Zhang XY, Zheng SB, Khanabdali R, Kalionis B, Wu JZ, et al. An update on Inflamm-aging: Mechanisms, prevention, and treatment. Journal of Immunology Research. 2016; 8426874

[30] Franceschi C, Garagnani P, Vitale G, Capri M, Salvioli S. Inflammaging and 'Garb-aging' Trends in Endocrinology and Metabolism. 2017;**28**(3):199-212

[31] Gladyshev VN. Aging: Progressive decline in fitness due to the rising deleteriome adjusted by genetic, environmental, and stochastic processes. Aging Cell. 2016;**15**(4):594-602

[32] Lopez-Otin C, Blasco MA, Partridge L, Serrano M, Kroemer G. The hallmarks of aging. Cell. 2013;**153**(6):1194-1217

[33] Vermeij WP, Dolle MET, Reiling E, Jaarsma D, Payan-Gomez C, Bombardieri CR, et al. Restricted diet delays accelerated ageing and genomic stress in DNA-repair-deficient mice. Nature. 2016;**537**(7620):427

[34] Kubben N, Misteli T. Shared molecular and cellular mechanisms of premature ageing and ageing-associated diseases. Nature Reviews Molecular Cell Biology. 2017;**18**(10):595-609

[35] Blackburn EH, Epel ES, Lin J. Human telomere biology: A contributory and interactive factor in aging, disease risks, and protection. Science. 2015;**350**(6265):1193-1198

[36] Armanios M, Blackburn EH. The telomere syndromes. Nature Reviews. Genetics. 2012;**13**(10):693-704

[37] Martinez P, Blasco MA. Telomere-driven diseases and telomere-targeting therapies. The Journal of Cell Biology. 2017;**216**(4):875-887

[38] de Jesus BB, Vera E, Schneeberger K, Tejera AM, Ayuso E, Bosch F, et al. Telomerase gene therapy in adult and old mice delays aging and increases longevity without increasing cancer. EMBO Molecular Medicine. 2012;**4**(8):691-704

[39] Glousker G, Touzot F, Revy P, Tzfati Y, Savage SA. Unraveling the pathogenesis of Hoyeraal-Hreidarsson syndrome, a complex telomere biology disorder. British Journal of Haematology. 2015;**170**(4):457-471

[40] Dantzer B, Fletcher QE. Telomeres shorten more slowly in slow-aging wild animals than in fast-aging ones. Experimental Gerontology. 2015;**71**:38-47

[41] Booth LN, Brunet A. The aging Epigenome. Molecular Cell. 2016;**62**(5):728-744

[42] Horvath S. DNA methylation age of human tissues and cell types. Genome Biology. 2013;**14**(10):R115

[43] Zampieri M, Ciccarone F, Calabrese R, Franceschi C, Burkle A, Caiafa P. Reconfiguration of DNA methylation in aging. Mechanisms of Ageing and Development. 2015;**151**:60-70

[44] Quach A, Levine ME, Tanaka T, Lu AT, Chen BH, Ferrucci L, et al. Epigenetic clock analysis of diet, exercise, education, and lifestyle factors. Aging-Us. 2017;**9**(2):419-446

[45] Jing H, Lin HN. Sirtuins in epigenetic regulation. Chemical Reviews. 2015;**115**(6):2350-2375

[46] Imai S, Guarente L. It takes two to tango: NAD(+) and sirtuins in aging/longevity control. NPJ Aging and Mechanisms of Disease. 2016;**2**:16017

[47] Buler M, Andersson U, Hakkola J. Who watches the watchmen? Regulation of the expression and activity of sirtuins. The FASEB Journal. 2016;**30**(12):3942-3960

[48] Hohn A, Weber D, Jung T, Ott C, Hugo M, Kochlik B, et al. Happily (n)ever after: Aging in the context of oxidative stress, proteostasis loss and cellular senescence. Redox Biology. 2017;**11**:482-501

[49] Kaushik S, Cuervo AM. Proteostasis and aging. Nature Medicine. 2015;**21**(12):1406-1415

[50] Klaips CL, Jayaraj GG, Hartl FU. Pathways of cellular proteostasis in aging and disease. The Journal of Cell Biology. 2017;**217**(1):51-63

[51] Labbadia J, Morimoto RI. The biology of Proteostasis in aging and disease. Annual Review of Biochemistry. 2015;**84**:435-464

[52] Hipp MS, Park SH, Hartl FU. Proteostasis impairment in protein-misfolding and -aggregation diseases. Trends in Cell Biology. 2014;**24**(9):506-514

[53] Chiti F, Dobson CM. Protein misfolding, amyloid formation, and human disease: A summary of progress over the last decade. Annual Review of Biochemistry. 2017;**86**:27-68

[54] Treaster SB, Ridgway ID, Richardson CA, Gaspar MB, Chaudhuri AR, Austad SN. Superior proteome stability in the longest lived animal. Age. 2014;**36**(3):1009-1017

[55] Rodriguez KA, Edrey YH, Osmulski P, Gaczynska M, Buffenstein R. Altered composition of liver proteasome assemblies contributes to enhanced proteasome activity in the exceptionally long-lived naked mole-rat. PLoS One. 2012;**7**(5):e35890

[56] Madeo F, Zimmermann A, Maiuri MC, Kroemer G. Essential role for autophagy in life span extension. The Journal of Clinical Investigation. 2015;**125**(1):85-93

[57] Finkel T. The metabolic regulation of aging. Nature Medicine. 2015;**21**(12):1416-1423

[58] Barzilai N, Crandall JP, Kritchevsky SB, Espeland MA. Metformin as a tool to target aging. Cell Metabolism. 2016;**23**(6):1060-1065

[59] Saxton RA, Sabatini DM. mTOR Signaling in growth, metabolism, and disease. Cell. 2017;**168**(6):960-976

[60] Salminen A, Kaarniranta K, Kauppinen A. Age-related changes in AMPK activation: Role for AMPK phosphatases and inhibitory phosphorylation by upstream signaling pathways. Ageing Research Reviews. 2016;**28**:15-26

[61] Bonkowski MS, Sinclair DA. Slowing ageing by design: The rise of NAD(+) and sirtuin-activating compounds. Nature Reviews Molecular Cell Biology. 2016;**17**(11):679-690

[62] Lopez-Otin C, Galluzzi L, Freije JMP, Madeo F, Kroemer G. Metabolic control of longevity. Cell. 2016;**166**(4):802-821

[63] Efeyan A, Comb WC, Sabatini DM. Nutrient-sensing mechanisms and pathways. Nature. 2015;**517**(7534):302-310

[64] Scherz-Shouval R, Elazar Z. ROS, mitochondria and the regulation of autophagy. Trends in Cell Biology. 2007;**17**(9):422-427

[65] Sebastian D, Palacin M, Zorzano A. Mitochondrial dynamics: Coupling mitochondrial fitness with healthy aging. Trends in Molecular Medicine. 2017;**23**(3):201-215

[66] Liesa M, Shirihai OS. Mitochondrial dynamics in the regulation of nutrient utilization and energy expenditure. Cell Metabolism. 2013;**17**(4):491-506

[67] Ruetenik A, Barrientos A. Dietary restriction, mitochondrial function and aging: From yeast to humans. Biochimica et Biophysica Acta-Bioenergetics. 2015;**1847**(11):1434-1447

[68] van de Ven RAH, Santos D, Haigis MC. Mitochondrial sirtuins and molecular mechanisms of aging. Trends in Molecular Medicine. 2017;**23**(4):320-331

[69] Sun N, Youle RJ, Finkel T. The mitochondrial basis of aging. Molecular Cell. 2016;**61**(5): 654-666

[70] Knuppertz L, Osiewacz HD. Orchestrating the network of molecular pathways affecting aging: Role of nonselective autophagy and mitophagy. Mechanisms of Ageing and Development. 2016;**153**:30-40

[71] Wang Y, Hekimi S. Mitochondrial dysfunction and longevity in animals: Untangling the knot. Science. 2015;**350**(6265):1204-1207

[72] Hayflick L, Moorhead PS. The serial cultivation of human diploid cell strains. Experimental Cell Research 1961;**25**:585-621

[73] Sharpless NE, Sherr CJ. Forging a signature of in vivo senescence. Nature Reviews. Cancer 2015;15(7):397-408

[74] Criscione SW, Teo YV, Neretti N. The chromatin landscape of cellular senescence. Trends in Genetics. 2016;**32**(11):751-761

[75] Munoz-Espin D, Serrano M. Cellular senescence: From physiology to pathology. Nature Reviews Molecular Cell Biology. 2014;**15**(7):482

[76] Childs BG, Baker DJ, Kirkland JL, Campisi J, van Deursen JM. Senescence and apoptosis: Dueling or complementary cell fates? EMBO Reports. 2014;**15**(11):1139-1153

[77] Bhatia-Dey N, Kanherkar RR, Stair SE, Makarev EO, Csoka AB. Cellular senescence as the causal nexus of aging. Frontiers in Genetics. 2016;**7**:13

[78] Childs BG, Gluscevic M, Baker DJ, Laberge RM, Marquess D, Dananberg J, et al. Senescent cells: An emerging target for diseases of ageing. Nature Reviews Drug Discovery. 2017;**16**(10):718-735

[79] de Keizer PLJ. The fountain of youth by targeting senescent cells? Trends in Molecular Medicine. 2017;**23**(1):6-17

[80] Ren RT, Ocampo A, Liu GH, Belmonte JCI. Regulation of stem cell aging by metabolism and epigenetics. Cell Metabolism. 2017;**26**(3):460-474

[81] Lepperdinger G. Developmental programs are kept alive during adulthood by stem cells: The aging aspect. Experimental Gerontology. 2013;**48**(7):644-646

[82] Cheung TH, Rando TA. Molecular regulation of stem cell quiescence. Nature Reviews Molecular Cell Biology. 2013;**14**(6):329-340

[83] Rezza A, Sennett R, Rendl M. Adult stem cell niches: Cellular and molecular components. Current Topics in Developmental Biology. 2014;**107**:333-372

[84] Schultz MB, Sinclair DA. When stem cells grow old: Phenotypes and mechanisms of stem cell aging. Development. 2016;**143**(1):3-14

[85] Sousa-Victor P, Garcia-Prat L, Serrano AL, Perdiguero E, Munoz-Canoves P. Muscle stem cell aging: Regulation and rejuvenation. Trends in Endocrinology and Metabolism. 2015;**26**(6):287-296

[86] Dumon NA, Wang YX, Rudnicki MA. Intrinsic and extrinsic mechanisms regulating satellite cell function. Development. 2015;**142**(9):1572-1581

[87] Chakkalakal JV, Jones KM, Basson MA, Brack AS. The aged niche disrupts muscle stem cell quiescence. Nature. 2012;**490**(7420):355

[88] Ratajczak MZ, Bartke A, Darzynkiewicz Z. Prolonged growth hormone/insulin/insulin-like growth factor nutrient response Signaling pathway as a silent killer of stem cells and a culprit in aging. Stem Cell Reviews. 2017;**13**(4):443-453

[89] Cavallucci V, Fidaleo M, Pani G. Neural stem cells and nutrients: Poised between quiescence and exhaustion. Trends in Endocrinology and Metabolism. 2016;**27**(11):756-769

[90] Capilla-Gonzalez V, Herranz-Perez V, Garcia-Verdugo JM. The aged brain: Genesis and fate of residual progenitor cells in the subventricular zone. Frontiers in Cellular Neuroscience. 2015;**9**:365

[91] Tang YZ, Purkayastha S, Cai DS. Hypothalamic microinflammation: A common basis of metabolic syndrome and aging. Trends in Neurosciences. 2015;**38**(1):36-44

[92] Oh J, Lee YD, Wagers AJ. Stem cell aging: Mechanisms, regulators and therapeutic opportunities. Nature Medicine. 2014;**20**(8):870-880

[93] Haller S, Kapuria S, Riley RR, O'Leary MN, Schreiber KH, Andersen JK, et al. mTORC1 activation during repeated regeneration impairs somatic stem cell maintenance. Cell Stem Cell. 2017;**21**(6):806

[94] Garcia-Prat L, Munoz-Canoves P, Martinez-Vicente M. Dysfunctional autophagy is a driver of muscle stem cell functional decline with aging. Autophagy. 2016;**12**(3):612-613

[95] Brown-Borg HM. The somatotropic axis and longevity in mice. American Journal of Physiology. Endocrinology and Metabolism. 2015;**309**(6):E503-EE10

[96] Milman S, Huffman DM, Barzilai N. The somatotropic axis in human aging: Framework for the current state of knowledge and future research. Cell Metabolism. 2016;**23**(6):980-989

[97] Sattler FR. Growth hormone in the aging male. Best Practice & Research Clinical Endocrinology & Metabolism. 2013;**27**(4):541-555

[98] Thorley M, Malatras A, Duddy W, Le Gall L, Mouly V, Butler Browne G, et al. Changes in communication between muscle stem cells and their environment with aging. Journal of Neuromuscular Diseases. 2015;**2**(3):205-217

[99] Brack AS, Conboy MJ, Roy S, Lee M, Kuo CJ, Keller C, et al. Increased Wnt signaling during aging alters muscle stem cell fate and increases fibrosis. Science. 2007;**317**(5839):807-810

[100] Kuroo M, Matsumura Y, Aizawa H, Kawaguchi H, Suga T, Utsugi T, et al. Mutation of the mouse klotho gene leads to a syndrome resembling ageing. Nature. 1997;**390**(6655):45-51

[101] Bian A, Neyra JA, Zhan M, Hu MC. Klotho, stem cells, and aging. Clinical Interventions in Aging. 2015;**10**:1233-1243

[102] Walker RG, Poggioli T, Katsimpardi L, Buchanan SM, Oh J, Wattrus S, et al. Biochemistry and biology of GDF11 and Myostatin similarities, differences, and questions for future investigation. Circulation Research. 2016;**118**(7):1125-1141

[103] Baht GS, Silkstone D, Vi L, Nadesan P, Amani Y, Whetstone H, et al. Exposure to a youthful circulaton rejuvenates bone repair through modulation of beta-catenin. Nature Communications. 2015;6:7131

[104] Villeda SA, Plambeck KE, Middeldorp J, Castellano JM, Mosher KI, Luo J, et al. Young blood reverses age-related impairments in cognitive function and synaptic plasticity in mice. Nature Medicine. 2014;20(6):659-663

[105] Sinha M, Jang YC, Oh J, Khong D, Wu EY, Manohar R, et al. Restoring systemic GDF11 levels reverses age-related dysfunction in mouse skeletal muscle. Science. 2014; 344(6184):649-652

[106] Loffredo FS, Steinhauser ML, Jay SM, Gannon J, Pancoast JR, Yalamanchi P, et al. Growth differentiation factor 11 is a circulating factor that reverses age-related cardiac hypertrophy. Cell. 2013;153(4):828-239

[107] Smith LK, White 3rd CW, Villeda SA. The systemic environment: At the interface of aging and adult neurogenesis. Cell and Tissue Research. 2018;371(1):105-113

[108] Smith LK, He YB, Park JS, Bieri G, Snethlage CE, Lin K, et al. Beta 2-microglobulin is a systemic pro-aging factor that impairs cognitive function and neurogenesis. Nature Medicine 2015;21(8):932-937

[109] Angelini F, Pagano F, Bordin A, Picchio V, De Falco E, Chimenti I. Getting old through the blood: Circulating molecules in aging and senescence of cardiovascular regenerative cells. Frontiers in Cardiovascular Medicine. 2017;4:62

[110] Chao JL, Guo YM, Li PF, Chao L. Role of Kallistatin treatment in aging and cancer by modulating miR-34a and miR-21 expression. Oxidative Medicine and Cellular Longevity. 2017;5025610

[111] Castellano JM, Mosher KI, Abbey RJ, McBride AA, James ML, Berdnik D, et al. Human umbilical cord plasma proteins revitalize hippocampal function in aged mice. Nature. 2017;544(7651):488

[112] Malaquin N, Martinez A, Rodier F. Keeping the senescence secretome under control: Molecular reins on the senescence-associated secretory phenotype. Experimental Gerontology. 2016;82:39-49

[113] Feldman N, Rotter-Maskowitz A, Okun E. DAMPs as mediators of sterile inflammation in aging-related pathologies. Ageing Research Reviews. 2015;24:29-39

[114] Gross O, Thomas CJ, Guarda G, Tschopp J. The inflammasome: An integrated view. Immunological Reviews. 2011;243(1):136-151

[115] Goldberg EL, Dixit VD. Drivers of age-related inflammation and strategies for healthspan extension. Immunological Reviews. 2015;265(1):63-74

[116] Pennisi M, Crupi R, Di Paola R, Ontario ML, Bella R, Calabrese EJ, et al. Inflammasomes, hormesis, and antioxidants in neuroinflammation: Role of NRLP3 in Alzheimer disease. Journal of Neuroscience Research. 2017;95(7):1360-1372

[117] Ratajczak MZ, Ratajczak J. Horizontal transfer of RNA and proteins between cells by extracellular microvesicles: 14 years later. Clinical and Translational Medicine. 2016;5:7

[118] Desdin-Mico G, Mittelbrunn M. Role of exosomes in the protection of cellular homeostasis. Cell Adhesion & Migration. 2017;11(2):127-134

[119] Pitt JM, Kroemer G, Zitvogel L. Extracellular vesicles: Masters of intercellular communication and potential clinical interventions. The Journal of Clinical Investigation. 2016;126(4):1139-1143

[120] Prattichizzo F, Micolucci L, Cricca M, De Carolis S, Mensa E, Ceriello A, et al. Exosome-based immunomodulation during aging: A nano-perspective on inflamm-aging. Mechanisms of Ageing and Development. 2017;168:44-53

[121] Mitsuhashi M, Taub DD, Kapogiannis D, Eitan E, Zukley L, Mattson MP, et al. Aging enhances release of exosomal cytokine mRNAs by A beta(1-42)-stimulated macrophages. FASEB Journal. 2013;27(12):5141-5150

[122] Urbanelli L, Buratta S, Sagini K, Tancini B, Emiliani C. Extracellular vesicles as new players in cellular senescence. International Journal of Molecular Sciences. 2016;17(9):1408

[123] Bouchard C, Blair SN, Katzmarzyk PT. Less sitting, more physical activity, or higher fitness? Mayo Clinic Proceedings. 2015;90(11):1533-1540

[124] Cartee GD, Hepple RT, Bamman MM, Zierath JR. Exercise promotes healthy aging of skeletal muscle. Cell Metabolism. 2016;23(6):1034-1047

[125] Marzetti E, Calvani R, Tosato M, Cesari M, Di Bari M, Cherubini A, et al. Physical activity and exercise as countermeasures to physical frailty and sarcopenia. Aging Clinical and Experimental Research. 2017;29(1):35-42

[126] Vina J, Rodriguez-Manas L, Salvador-Pascual A, Tarazona-Santabalbina FJ, Gomez-Cabrera MC. Exercise: The lifelong supplement for healthy ageing and slowing down the onset of frailty. Journal of Physiology (London). 2016;594(8):1989-1999

[127] Neufer PD, Bamman MM, Muoio DM, Bouchard C, Cooper DM, Goodpaster BH, et al. Understanding the cellular and molecular mechanisms of physical activity-induced health benefits. Cell Metabolism. 2015;22(1):4-11

[128] Chieffi S, Messina G, Villano I, Messina A, Esposito M, Monda V, et al. Exercise influence on hippocampal function: Possible involvement of Orexin-A. Frontiers in Physiology. 2017;8:85

[129] Flodin P, Jonasson LS, Riklund K, Nyberg L, Boraxbekk CJ. Does aerobic exercise influence intrinsic brain activity? An aerobic exercise intervention among healthy old adults. Frontiers in Aging Neuroscience. 2017;9:267

[130] Hernandez SSS, Sandreschi PF, da Silva FC, Arancibia BAV, da Silva R, Gutierres PJB, et al. What are the benefits of exercise for Alzheimer's disease? A systematic review of the past 10 years. Journal of Aging and Physical Activity. 2015;23(4):659-668

[131] McCay CM, Crowell MF, Maynard LA. The effect of retarded growth upon the length of life span and upon the ultimate body size. The Journal of Nutrition. 1935;**10**(1):63-79

[132] Fontana L, Partridge L. Promoting health and longevity through diet: From model organisms to humans. Cell. 2015;**161**(1):106-118

[133] Simpson SJ, Le Couteur DG, Raubenheimer D, Solon-Biet SM, Cooney GJ, Cogger VC, et al. Dietary protein, aging and nutritional geometry. Ageing Research Reviews. 2017;**39**:78-86

[134] Mattson MP, Longo VD, Harvie M. Impact of intermittent fasting on health and disease processes. Ageing Research Reviews. 2017;**39**:46-58

[135] Kennedy BK, Lamming DW. The mechanistic target of Rapamycin: The grand ConducTOR of metabolism and aging. Cell Metabolism. 2016;**23**(6):990-1003

[136] Hardie DG, Schaffer BE, Brunet A. AMPK: An energy-sensing pathway with multiple inputs and outputs. Trends in Cell Biology. 2016;**26**(3):190-201

[137] Garcia D, Shaw RJ. AMPK: Mechanisms of cellular energy sensing and restoration of metabolic balance. Molecular Cell. 2017;**66**(6):789-800

[138] Cordero MD, Williams MR, Ryffel B. AMP-activated protein kinase regulation of the NLRP3 inflammasome during aging. Trends in Endocrinology and Metabolism. 2018;**29**(1):8-17

[139] Longo VD, Antebi A, Bartke A, Barzilai N, Brown-Borg HM, Caruso C, et al. Interventions to slow aging in humans: Are we ready? Aging Cell. 2015;**14**(4):497-510

[140] Marin-Aguilar F, Pavillard LE, Giampieri F, Bullon P, Cordero MD. Adenosine monophosphate (AMP)-activated protein kinase: A new target for nutraceutical compounds. International Journal of Molecular Sciences. 2017;**18**(2):288

[141] Zhou GC, Li Y, Chen YL, Shen XL, Doebber T, Moller DE. AMP-Kinase mediates metabolic effects of metformin. Diabetes. 2001;**50**:A274

[142] Zhou GC, Myers R, Li Y, Chen YL, Shen XL, Fenyk-Melody J, et al. Role of AMP-activated protein kinase in mechanism of metformin action. The Journal of Clinical Investigation. 2001;**108**(8):1167-1174

[143] Barzilai N, Kritchevsky S, Espeland M, Crandall J. Targeting aging with metformin (tame): A study to target aging in humans. The Gerontologist. 2016;**56**:199

[144] Pryor R, Cabreiro F. Repurposing metformin: An old drug with new tricks in its binding pockets. Biochemical Journal. 2015;**471**:307-322

[145] Romero R, Erez O, Huttemann M, Huttemann M, Panaitescu B, Conde-Agudelo A, et al. Metformin, the aspirin of the 21st century: Its role in gestational diabetes mellitus, prevention of preeclampsia and cancer, and the promotion of longevity. American Journal of Obstetrics and Gynecology. 2017;**217**(3):282-302

[146] Harrison DE, Strong R, Sharp ZD, Nelson JF, Astle CM, Flurkey K, et al. Rapamycin fed late in life extends lifespan in genetically heterogeneous mice. Nature. 2009;**460**(7253): 392-U108

[147] Pinto P, Santos CN. Worldwide (poly)phenol intake: Assessment methods and identified gaps. European Journal of Nutrition. 2017;**56**(4):1393-1408

[148] Hubbard BP, Sinclair DA. Small molecule SIRT1 activators for the treatment of aging and age-related diseases. Trends in Pharmacological Sciences. 2014;**35**(3):146-154

[149] Bhullar KS, Hubbard BP. Lifespan and healthspan extension by resveratrol. Biochimica et Biophysica Acta – Molecular Basis of Disease. 2015;**1852**(6):1209-1218

[150] Novelle MG, Wahl D, Dieguez C, Bernier M, de Cabo R. Resveratrol supplementation: Where are we now and where should we go? Ageing Research Reviews 2015;**21**:1-15

[151] Kou XJ, Chen N. Resveratrol as a natural autophagy regulator for prevention and treatment of Alzheimer's disease. Nutrients. 2017;**9**(9):927

[152] Li YR, Li S, Lin CC. Effect of resveratrol and pterostilbene on aging and longevity. BioFactors. 2017;**44**:61-68

[153] Park SJ, Ahmad F, Philp A, Baar K, Williams T, Luo HB, et al. Resveratrol ameliorates aging-related metabolic phenotypes by inhibiting cAMP phosphodiesterases. Cell. 2012;**148**(3):421-433

[154] Wan D, Zhou YH, Wang K, Hou YY, Hou RH, Ye XF. Resveratrol provides neuroprotection by inhibiting phosphodiesterases and regulating the cAMP/AMPK/SIRT1 pathway after stroke in rats. Brain Research Bulletin. 2016;**121**:255-262

[155] Thiel G, Rossler OG. Resveratrol regulates gene transcription via activation of stimulus-responsive transcription factors. Pharmacological Research. 2017;**117**:166-176

[156] Morselli E, Marino G, Bennetzen MV, Eisenberg T, Megalou E, Schroeder S, et al. Spermidine and resveratrol induce autophagy by distinct pathways converging on the acetylproteome. The Journal of Cell Biology. 2011;**192**(4):615-629

[157] Madeo F, Eisenberg T, Buttner S, Ruckenstuhl C, Kroemer G. Spermidine A novel autophagy inducer and longevity elixir. Autophagy. 2010;**6**(1):160-162

[158] Eisenberg T, Knauer H, Schauer A, Buttner S, Ruckenstuhl C, Carmona-Gutierrez D, et al. Induction of autophagy by spermidine promotes longevity. Nature Cell Biology. 2009;**11**(11):1305-U102

[159] Buttner S, Broeskamp F, Sommer C, Markaki M, Habernig L, Alavian-Ghavanini A, et al. Spermidine protects against alpha-synuclein neurotoxicity. Cell Cycle. 2014;**13**(24): 3903-3908

[160] Eisenberg T, Abdellatif M, Schroeder S, Primessnig U, Stekovic S, Pendl T, et al. Cardioprotection and lifespan extension by the natural polyamine spermidine. Nature Medicine. 2016;**22**(12):1428-1438

[161] Minois N. Molecular basis of the 'anti-aging' effect of spermidine and other natural polyamines – A mini-review. Gerontology. 2014;**60**(4):319-326

[162] DiGirolamo DJ, Kiel DP, Esser KA. Bone and skeletal muscle: Neighbors with close ties. Journal of Bone and Mineral Research. 2013;**28**(7):1509-1518

[163] Girgis CM, Baldock PA, Downes M. Vitamin D, muscle and bone: Integrating effects in development, aging and injury. Molecular and Cellular Endocrinology. 2015;**410**(C):3-10

[164] Girgis CM, Cha KM, Houweling PJ, Rao R, Mokbel N, Lin M, et al. Vitamin D receptor ablation and vitamin D deficiency result in reduced grip strength, altered muscle Fibers, and increased Myostatin in mice. Calcified Tissue International. 2015;**97**(6):602-610

[165] Schlogl M, Holick MF. Vitamin D and neurocognitive function. Clinical Interventions in Aging. 2014;**9**:559-568

[166] Landel V, Annweiler C, Millet P, Morello M, Feron F. Vitamin D, Cognition and Alzheimer's disease: The therapeutic benefit is in the D-tails. Journal of Alzheimer's Disease. 2016;**53**(2):419-444

[167] Sanchis-Gomar F, Pareja-Galeano H, Santos-Lozano A, Garatachea N, Fiuza-Luces C, Venturini L, et al. A preliminary candidate approach identifies the combination of chemerin, fetuin-a, and fibroblast growth factors 19 and 21 as a potential biomarker panel of successful aging. Age. 2015;**37**(3):42

[168] Salminen A, Kaarniranta K, Kauppinen A. Integrated stress response stimulates FGF21 expression: Systemic enhancer of longevity. Cellular Signalling. 2017;**40**:10-21

[169] Iwabu M, Okada-Iwabu M, Yamauchi T, Kadowaki T. Adiponectin/adiponectin receptor in disease and aging. NPJ Aging and Mechanisms of Disease. 2015;**1**:15013

[170] Rochette L, Vergely C. "pro-youthful" factors in the "labyrinth" of cardiac rejuvenation. Experimental Gerontology. 2016;**83**:1-5

[171] Abraham CR, Mullen PC, Tucker-Zhou T, Chen CD, Zeldich E. Klotho is a Neuroprotective and cognition-enhancing protein. Vitamins and Hormones. 2016;**101**:215-238

[172] Pope CN, Brimijoin S. Cholinesterases and the fine line between poison and remedy. Biochemical Pharmacology. 2018; in press

[173] Kaushik V, Smith ST, Mikobi E, Raji MA. Acetylcholinesterase inhibitors: Beneficial effects on comorbidities in patients with Alzheimer's disease. American Journal of Alzheimer's Disease. 2018;**33**(2):73-85

[174] McHugh D, Gil J. Senescence and aging: Causes, consequences, and therapeutic avenues. The Journal of Cell Biology. 2018;**217**(1):65-77

[175] Zhu Y, Tchkonia T, Pirtskhalava T, Gower AC, Ding HS, Giorgadze N, et al. The Achilles' heel of senescent cells: From transcriptome to senolytic drugs. Aging Cell. 2015;**14**(4):644-658

[176] Kirkland JL, Tchkonia T, Zhu Y, Niedernhofer LJ, Robbins PD. The clinical potential of senolytic drugs. Journal of the American Geriatrics Society. 2017;**65**(10):2297-2301

[177] Lehmann M, Korfei M, Mutze K, Klee S, Skronska-Wasek W, Alsafadi HN, et al. Senolytic drugs target alveolar epithelial cell function and attenuate experimental lung fibrosis ex vivo. The European Respiratory Journal. 2017;**50**(2):1602367

[178] Baar MP, Brandt RMC, Putavet DA, Klein JDD, Derks KWJ, Bourgeois BRM, et al. Targeted apoptosis of senescent cells restores tissue homeostasis in response to chemo-toxicity and aging. Cell. 2017;**169**(1):132

[179] Schimke MM, Marozin S, Lepperdinger G. Patient-specific age: The other side of the coin in advanced mesenchymal stem cell therapy. Frontiers in Physiology. 2015;**6**:362

[180] Takahashi K, Yamanaka S. A decade of transcription factor-mediated reprogramming to pluripotency. Nature Reviews Molecular Cell Biology. 2016;**17**(3):183-193

[181] Soria-Valles C, Lopez-Otin C. iPSCs: On the road to reprogramming aging. Trends in Molecular Medicine. 2016;**22**(8):713-724

[182] Trounson A, DeWitt ND. Pluripotent stem cells progressing to the clinic. Nature Reviews Molecular Cell Biology. 2016;**17**(3):194-200

[183] Neves J, Sousa-Victor P, Jasper H. Rejuvenating strategies for stem cell-based therapies in aging. Cell Stem Cell. 2017;**20**(2):161-175

[184] Rebo J, Mehdipour M, Gathwala R, Causey K, Liu Y, Conboy MJ, et al. A single heterochronic blood exchange reveals rapid inhibition of multiple tissues by old blood. Nature Communications. 2016;**7**

[185] Oh J, Sinha I, Tan KY, Rosner B, Dreyfuss JM, Gjata O, et al. Age-associated NF-KB signaling in myofibers alters the satellite cell niche and re-strains muscle stem cell function. Aging-Us. 2016;**8**(11):2871-2896

[186] Rinnerthaler M, Bischof J, Streubel MK, Trost A, Richter K. Oxidative stress in aging human skin. Biomolecules. 2015;**5**(2):545-589

[187] Rinnerthaler M, Duschl J, Steinbacher P, Salzmann M, Bischof J, Schuller M, et al. Age-related changes in the composition of the cornified envelope in human skin. Experimental Dermatology. 2013;**22**(5):329-335

Permissions

All chapters in this book were first published in GERONTOLOGY, by InTech Open; hereby published with permission under the Creative Commons Attribution License or equivalent. Every chapter published in this book has been scrutinized by our experts. Their significance has been extensively debated. The topics covered herein carry significant findings which will fuel the growth of the discipline. They may even be implemented as practical applications or may be referred to as a beginning point for another development.

The contributors of this book come from diverse backgrounds, making this book a truly international effort. This book will bring forth new frontiers with its revolutionizing research information and detailed analysis of the nascent developments around the world.

We would like to thank all the contributing authors for lending their expertise to make the book truly unique. They have played a crucial role in the development of this book. Without their invaluable contributions this book wouldn't have been possible. They have made vital efforts to compile up to date information on the varied aspects of this subject to make this book a valuable addition to the collection of many professionals and students.

This book was conceptualized with the vision of imparting up-to-date information and advanced data in this field. To ensure the same, a matchless editorial board was set up. Every individual on the board went through rigorous rounds of assessment to prove their worth. After which they invested a large part of their time researching and compiling the most relevant data for our readers.

The editorial board has been involved in producing this book since its inception. They have spent rigorous hours researching and exploring the diverse topics which have resulted in the successful publishing of this book. They have passed on their knowledge of decades through this book. To expedite this challenging task, the publisher supported the team at every step. A small team of assistant editors was also appointed to further simplify the editing procedure and attain best results for the readers.

Apart from the editorial board, the designing team has also invested a significant amount of their time in understanding the subject and creating the most relevant covers. They scrutinized every image to scout for the most suitable representation of the subject and create an appropriate cover for the book.

The publishing team has been an ardent support to the editorial, designing and production team. Their endless efforts to recruit the best for this project, has resulted in the accomplishment of this book. They are a veteran in the field of academics and their pool of knowledge is as vast as their experience in printing. Their expertise and guidance has proved useful at every step. Their uncompromising quality standards have made this book an exceptional effort. Their encouragement from time to time has been an inspiration for everyone.

The publisher and the editorial board hope that this book will prove to be a valuable piece of knowledge for researchers, students, practitioners and scholars across the globe.

List of Contributors

Nora Silvana Vigliecca
National Scientific and Technical Research Council (CONICET), Institute of Humanities (IDH-CONICET), Service of Neurology and Neurosurgery of Cordoba Hospital, National University of Cordoba (UNC), Cordoba, Argentina

Radka Ivanova Massaldjieva
Health Care Management Department, Centre for Translational Neuroscience, Medical University, Plovdiv, Bulgaria

Luís Midão and Elísio Costa
UCIBIO, REQUIMTE and Faculty of Pharmacy, University of Porto, Porto, Portugal

Anna Giardini
Psychology Unit, Instituti Clinici Scientifici Maugeri Spa – Società Benefit, Care and Research Institute, IRCCS Montescano, Italy

Enrica Menditto
School of Pharmacy, CIRFF/Center of Pharmacoeconomics, University of Naples Federico II, Naples, Italy

Przemyslaw Kardas
Department of Family Medicine, Medical University of Lodz, Lodz, Poland

Lisa Pau Le Low
School of Health Sciences, Caritas Institute of Higher Education, Tseung Kwan O, N.T., Hong Kong

Neyda Ma Mendoza-Ruvalcaba and Melina Rodríguez-Díaz
University of Guadalajara CUTONALA, Tonalá, Jalisco, Mexico

Elva Dolores Arias-Merino, María Elena Flores-Villavicencio and Irma Fabiola Díaz-García
University of Guadalajara CUCS, Mexico

Alexander Morales Erazo
Internal Medicine and Geriatrics, Caldas University, Manizales, Caldas, Colombia

CES University, Medellín, Antioquia, Colombia
Cooperative University of Colombia, Pasto, Colombia
Nariño Departmental Hospital, Pasto, Nariño, Colombia
COMETA Foundation, Pasto, Nariño, Colombia

Shilpa Amarya, Kalyani Singh and Manisha Sabharwal
Lady Irwin College, University of Delhi, New Delhi, India

Jamilah Abusarah
Department of Microbiology and Immunology, McGill University, Montreal, Canada

Fatemeh Khodayarian and Yun Cui
Department of Pharmacology and Physiology, Université de Montréal, Montreal, Canada

Abed El-Hakim El-Kadiry
Department of Pharmacology and Physiology, Université de Montréal, Montreal, Canada
Department of Biochemistry, the Lebanese University, Beirut, Lebanon

Moutih Rafei
Department of Microbiology and Immunology, McGill University, Montreal, Canada
Department of Pharmacology and Physiology, Université de Montréal, Montreal, Canada
Department of Microbiology, Infectious Diseases and Immunology, Université de Montréal, Montreal, Canada

Maria Boboshko, Ekaterina Zhilinskaya and Natalia Maltseva
Laboratory of Hearing and Speech of Academician I.P. Pavlov First St. Petersburg State Medical University, St. Petersburg, Russia

Mark Rinnerthaler and Klaus Richter
Department of Biosciences, University of Salzburg, Salzburg, Austria

Index

Printed in the USA
CPSIA information can be obtained
at www.ICGtesting.com
JSHW051433221024
72173JS00006B/1456

9 781639 270095